D0830136

Advanced Practice Nursing

Michaelene P. Jansen, PhD, RN-C, GNP-BC, NP-C, is a clinical professor of nursing in the School of Nursing at the University of Wisconsin–Madison. She also works as a family and gerontological nurse practitioner in pulmonary medicine at UW Health in Madison, Wisconsin. Her professional career includes advanced practice nursing in primary care, chronic pain, and pulmonary medicine, particularly the care of adult cystic fibrosis patients. Her professional nursing career includes critical care, neurosciences, and trauma. She was co-editor of the previous three editions of this text and editor of *Managing Pain in the Older Adult*, also published by Springer Publishing.

Mary Zwygart-Stauffacher, PhD, RN, GNP/GCNS-BC, FAAN, is interim dean and professor in the College of Nursing and Health Sciences at the University of Wisconsin–Eau Claire. She also practices as a gerontological nurse practitioner and gerontological clinical nurse specialist for the Red Cedar Clinic/Mayo Health System–Nursing Home Services. She is a National Institutes of Health (NIH)-funded co-principal investigator examining multilevel interventions to promote quality improvement in the nursing home setting. She has extensive experience in gerontological advanced practice nursing, nursing education and quality improvement in long-term care. She is the co-editor of the previous edition of this text, in addition to being the author of numerous national presentations, publications, and books.

Advanced Practice Nursing

Core Concepts for Professional Role Development

FOURTH EDITION

MICHAELENE P. JANSEN, PhD, RN-C,
GNP-BC, NP-C
MARY ZWYGART-STAUFFACHER, PhD,
RN, GNP/GCNS-BC, FAAN

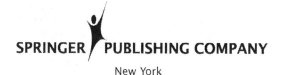

SPRINGER PUBLISHING COMPANY

New York

Springer Publishing Company, LLC
11 West 42nd Street
New York, NY 10036
www.springerpub.com

Acquisitions Editor: Allan Graubard
Project Manager: Kelly Applegate
Cover Design: David Levy
Composition: Publication Services, Inc.

ISBN: 978-0-8261-0515-8
Ebook ISBN: 978-0-8261-0516-5

14 15 16   8 7 6

Library of Congress Cataloging-in-Publication Data

Advanced practice nursing : core concepts for professional role development / [edited by] Michaelene P. Jansen, Mary Zwygart-Stauffacher. — 4th ed.
     p. ; cm.
  Includes bibliographical references and index.
  ISBN 978-0-8261-0515-8 (pbk. : alk. paper)
  1. Nurse practitioners.   2. Primary care (Medicine).   I. Mirr Jansen, Michaelene P. II. Zwygart-Stauffacher, Mary, 1955–
  [DNLM: 1. Nurse Clinicians.   2. Nurse Practitioners. 3. Nurse Anesthetists. 4. Nurse Midwives.   5. Nurse's Role. WY 128 A2437 2010]
  RT82.8.A49 2010
  610.7306'92—dc22   2009038700

Printed in the United States of America by Gasch Printing.

Contents

v

Contributors

Melissa Avery, PhD, CNM, FACNM, FAAN
Associate Professor and Chair
Child and Family Health Cooperative
Coordinator, Nurse-Midwifery
Specialty
School of Nursing
University of Minnesota
Minneapolis, MN

Kathryn A. Blair, PhD, FNP-BC, FAANP
Professor
Beth El College of Nursing and
Health Sciences
University of Colorado–Colorado
Springs
Colorado Springs, CO

Kathleen Fagerlund, PhD, RN, CRNA
Clinical Associate Professor
Coordinator, Nurse Anesthesia Area
of Study
School of Nursing
University of Minnesota
Minneapolis, MN

Karen Feldt, PhD, RN, GNP-BC
Associate Professor
Seattle University
College of Nursing
Gerontological Nurse Practitioner
Northwest Geriatrics
Mercer Island, WA

Janet Wessel Krejci, PhD, RN
Associate Professor
Coordinator, MSN Health Care
Systems Leadership
Marquette University
Milwaukee, WI

Linda Lindeke, PhD, RN, CNP
Associate Professor
Director of Graduate Studies
School of Nursing
University of Minnesota
Minneapolis, MN

Shelly Malin, PhD, RN, NEA-BC
Director, Advanced Practice
Nursing and Research
Associate Director, Children's
Research Institute
Children's Hospital of
Wisconsin
Clinical Faculty
Marquette University
College of Nursing
Milwaukee, WI

Jane Peace, PhD, RN
Clinical Assistant Professor
Informatics
School of Nursing
University of Wisconsin–
Madison
Madison, WI

Jennifer Peters, PhD, RN, GCNS-BC
Kearney, MO

Linda Reivitz, MAB
Faculty Associate
School of Nursing
University of Wisconsin–Madison
Madison, WI

Pamela F. Scheibel, MS, RN
Clinical Professor
School of Nursing
University of Wisconsin–Madison
Madison, WI

Sheila K. Smith, PhD, RN, ANP-BC
Assistant Dean and Professor
College of Nursing and Health
Sciences
University of Wisconsin–Eau Claire
Eau Claire, WI

CeCelia R. Zorn, PhD, RN
Professor
College of Nursing and Health
Sciences
University of Wisconsin–Eau Claire
Eau Claire, WI

Preface

It is hard to believe that we are publishing the fourth edition of *Advanced Practice Nursing*. Since the first edition was published in 1995, advanced practice nursing has seen incredible growth and change. Dr. Mariah Snyder, one of the first editors, envisioned a textbook to guide advanced practice nurses through the opportunities and challenges they face within a strong nursing framework. At the time of the first edition, there was only one other advanced practice text on the market. Today, there are many texts available, providing educators and students with a wide variety of choices to meet their educational needs.

This fourth edition is written for graduate students enrolled in master's or practice doctorate advanced practice nursing programs. The content will be helpful for both the beginning student in a graduate nursing program and also for those nearing completion of their program as they explore future employment as an advanced practice nurse. Major role development concepts and topics that graduate nursing students should address during their studies are highlighted. The content is not setting or role specific but addresses advanced nursing practice standards and competencies identified by professional nursing organizations, including the American Nurses Association (ANA) Standards of Practice, American Association of Colleges of Nursing (AACN), the National Organization of Nurse Practitioner Faculties (NONPF), the National Association of Clinical Nurse Specialists (NACNS), the American Association of Nurse Anesthetists (AANA), and the American College of Nurse Midwives (ACNM). The development of a new regulatory model for advanced practice registered nurses along with the development of the doctor of nursing practice as the entry level for advanced practice nursing by 2015 is reflected in the content offered here.

A brief overview of each of the four advanced practice registered nurse (APRN) roles and the historical context within which they developed provides the reader with an understanding of the richness of advanced practice nursing. Contributors to this text bring perspectives from a wide variety of practice backgrounds and settings. For example, the chapter on health policy, written by a former secretary of health and human services for the state of Wisconsin, provides unique insights into policy development.

This edition of *Advanced Practice Nursing* reflects the movement of advanced practice nursing toward the practice doctorate. The reader will find some new and revised areas of the text consistent with developing changes in advanced practice. As the doctor of nursing practice (DNP) develops, emphasis will not only focus on care and management of patients, but also how the advanced practice nurse interacts and functions within the health care arena. The chapter on leadership has been revised significantly to emphasize leadership development in practice doctorate programs. Three chapters—informatics, health care organization, and health care policy—have been added to this edition to reflect essential content identified by the AACN for DNP programs. The chapter on research has been revised to emphasize translation of research into practice and evidence-based practice. The reimbursement chapter has undergone major revision and will assist advanced practice nurses in navigating the reimbursement process. Other revisions include expansion of content on regulation, certification, and credentialing, as well as inclusion of practice agreements for advanced practice nurses. It is noted that the APRN Regulatory Model proposed by the APRN Consensus and Joint Dialogue Group uses the term *advanced practice registered nurse* (APRN) to include all four APN roles: nurse practitioner, clinical nurse specialists, certified nurse-midwives, and certified registered nurse anesthetists. As the APRN Regulatory Model is implemented, it is anticipated that APRN will be used consistently to designate all advanced practice nurses. We have used the term APN and APRN interchangeably in this edition.

As with past editions, our goal is to provide a text for students and entry-level advanced practice nurses that is easy to read, a quick reference, and a guide. With multiple APN texts available, we believe that this guide for advanced practice will assist advanced practice nurses in launching their careers, with pertinent, practical, useful, and insightful information.

Michaelene P. Jansen
Mary Zwygart-Stauffacher

Foundations of Advanced Practice Nursing

Overview of Advanced Practice Nursing

1

LINDA LINDEKE
KATHLEEN FAGERLUND
MELISSA AVERY
MARY ZWYGART-STAUFFACHER

Advanced practice nurses (APNs) are taking their place in the forefront of the rapidly changing health care system, developing a myriad of roles in organizations that aim to provide cost-effective, quality care. APNs can be found working internationally in community health, in government positions, hospitals, nursing homes, and clinics. They serve the most economically disadvantaged as well as the elite. APNs function as deans and educators, as consultants and researchers, as policy experts, and, of course, as outstanding clinicians.

Advanced practice nursing is an exciting career choice with many opportunities and challenges. Some of the challenges are related to prospective payment systems, decreased hospital stays, and spiraling costs. Evolving technology is producing amazing diagnostic and treatment results; genetic research is unraveling complex pathophysiology; and sophisticated information technology is changing the way that information is gathered, stored, and shared. Home health care programs and complimentary care clinics are now commonplace. These and other trends have resulted in a rapidly changing health care system, ready for the influence of APNs.

Graduate education prepares APNs to be key players in these complex systems, and nursing theories provide APNs with a strong conceptual base for practice. Nursing research uncovers scientific evidence for best practice, and research utilization skills enable APNs to bring fresh ideas and proven interventions to health care consumers. Complex, evolving reimbursement mechanisms require that APN education also encompass content in financial management and health policy issues. Although APNs were traditionally educated to provide advanced nursing care in a specific system or setting such as a hospital unit or clinic, it is now fairly common for APNs to work across system boundaries to follow their patients in a multifaceted care delivery arena. For example, they may see their patients in outpatient clinics, visit them during hospitalizations to assist in care coordination, and perhaps do home visits or communicate with long-term care organizations following a patient's discharge (Marten, 2000). Working in multiple systems requires APNs to be credentialed in multiple sites in order to legally provide care.

Advanced specialization of nurses beyond their formal entry-level education has a long history in nursing. Nurse anesthetists and nurse-midwives were the first to develop programs, professional organizations, and certification, beginning nearly a century ago (Hanson & Hamric, 2003). However, only recently has the preparation, certification, and licensing of these advanced nurses become more standardized (American Nurses Association [ANA], 2004a). The term "advanced practice nurse" (APN), sometimes also called "advanced practice registered nurse" (APRN), denotes nurses with formal post-baccalaureate preparation in one of four roles: nurse-midwives, nurse anesthetists, nurse practitioners, and clinical nurse specialists (ANA, 2004a).

A number of factors led nursing leaders to delineate these four roles in advanced practice nursing. A critical factor was the legal status that enabled APNs to obtain direct reimbursement for their nursing services, a gradual process first achieved by nurse-midwives 25 years ago and expanded to the other three roles over time. Reimbursement law and regulations require that nursing be able to specify the preparation of these reimbursable APNs and led to increased standardization of titling and education. The term APN became the common "umbrella" term used to designate these four roles.

Public protection was another factor that led to the APN delineation. State boards of nursing are mandated by state legislatures to safeguard the public from unsafe practice, and over time all states have implemented laws and regulations to ensure that nurses who have APN preparation have certain expertise and skills. In some states, this is done by a second-level licensure process; in other states, it is done through laws such as title protection and specific designation of scope of practice (National Council of State Boards of Nursing, 2002).

solely initiated by nurses. The early NP curricula were viewed as being based on the medical model rather than a nursing framework, although that was not the focus of Dr. Ford's original NP curriculum that emphasized child development and health promotion (Ford, 1979).

There were over 140,000 NPs in the United States as of March 2004, as reported in the *National Sample Survey of Registered Nurses March 2004: Preliminary Findings* (Health Resources Services and Administration, 2005). This report stated that 65.5% of NPs graduated from master's programs; in addition, 10.5% were prepared in post-master's certificate programs. In 2004, 87.7% of NPs were employed in nursing; of those, 65.7% held positions with the title of "nurse practitioner." The reason for this smaller percentage is that many nurse practitioners assume positions as educators, administrators, and policy makers, or choose other employment.

NPs are prepared in a multitude of specialties, including acute care, adult health, family health, gerontology, pediatrics, psychiatry, neonatology, and women's health. Specific competencies have been developed for many NP specialty areas (i.e., acute care, psychiatric mental health, etc.). After completing graduate education, NPs are eligible to sit for national certification examinations in their specialty areas. Certification is a mechanism for the nursing profession to attest to the entry-to-practice knowledge of NPs. The certification requirement has been adopted by third-party payers such as the Center for Medicare and Medicaid Services (CMS) and by most state boards of nursing as a standard that assists in protecting the public from unsafe providers (Pearson, 2009). Certification examinations are offered by a variety of bodies: the American Nurses Credentialing Center (ANCC), the American Academy of Nurse Practitioners (AANP), the Pediatric Nursing Certification Board (PNCB), the American Association of Critical Care Nurses, and the National Certification Corporation (NCC) for the obstetric, gynecologic, and neonatal specialties. Certification for nurse practitioners is discussed further in Chapter 8.

Changes in reimbursement laws, regulations, and policies that allow for direct reimbursement of NPs, the rapid increase in managed care as a mechanism to control health care costs, and the growing recognition of the significant contributions of NPs to positive patient outcomes have resulted in a rapid increase in the number of NP programs, particularly DNP programs. AACN's survey of enrollments in baccalaureate and graduate programs in nursing during the 2007–2008 academic year found that the overall number of nursing students in doctoral programs increased 20.9% between 2007 and 2008, with enrollment growth seen in DNP programs rather than research-focused doctoral programs (AACN, 2009). APNs who are savvy about ascertaining the gaps in health care and designing roles for themselves that are not merely physician-replacement roles are likely to be very successful in obtaining satisfactory employment (Hamric, Spross, & Hanson, 2009).

Scope of practice is regulated by state laws and describes the legal boundaries of health professional practice. Changes in scope of practice reflect the dynamic evolution of NP abilities to deliver quality, comprehensive care in a safe and effective manner (ANA, 2008). NPs practicing outside the designated scope of practice risk legal sanctions and potential liability (Klein, 2005). However, great variability exists regarding the regulation of acute and primary care NPs by individual states. A survey of state regulations regarding acute care nurse practitioner (ACNP) laws and regulations (Percy & Sperhac, 2007) revealed that 31 states recognized acute care certification examinations; many states were silent on differentiating between primary care and acute care certification. Many factors have influenced the growth in acute care nurse practitioner programs (Cajulis & Fitzpatrick, 2007; Chan & Garbez, 2006; Kleinpell & Hravnak, 2005; McLaughlin, 2007; Rosenfeld et al, 2003). Among these are the increasing complexity of inpatient care and technology and the regulations that limit the number of hours that physician residents are allowed to work. ACNPs have established themselves in specialty and critical care practice sites and are active in quality improvement and system redesign in those facilities. For further discussion or regulation and scope of practice, please refer to Chapters 8 and 9.

Relative to CNMs and CRNAs, NPs have a relatively short history in the health care delivery system. However, in this short period of time they have gained the respect of many health professionals and of their patients (Scherer, Bruce, & Runkawatt, 2007). Recently, television and lay publications have featured NPs and the significant contributions that they are making to improve health. New areas of practice and settings for nurse practitioners continue to arise. In many instances, NPs have succeeded in caring for persons in rural areas, in the inner city, and for other vulnerable groups. NPs have established themselves as an integral part of the health care system.

Nurse-Midwives

Nurse-midwives are unique among APNs because they are educated in two different professions. Midwifery is a profession in its own right;

nursing is not a prerequisite to midwifery in many countries around the world. The American College of Nurse-Midwives (ACNM) defines certified nurse-midwives (CNMs) as individuals educated in the two disciplines of nursing and midwifery and who possess evidence of certification according to the requirements of the ACNM (ACNM, 2004a). According to the ACNM, midwifery practice

> is the independent management of women's health care, focusing particularly on common primary care issues, family planning and gynecologic needs of women, pregnancy, childbirth, the postpartum period and the care of the newborn. The certified nurse-midwife and certified midwife practice within a health care system that provides for consultation, collaborative management or referral as indicated by the health status of the client. Certified nurse-midwives and certified midwives practice in accord with the Standards for the Practice of Midwifery, as defined by the American College of Nurse-Midwives (ACNM, 2004b, p. 1).

Although the focus of midwifery care has historically been prenatal care and managing labor and births, nurse-midwives are also primary care providers for essentially healthy women. Nurse-midwives strongly believe in supporting natural life processes and not utilizing medical interventions unless there is a clear need. This belief and others are reflected in the 2004 ACNM philosophy statement, which states that every person has a right to:

- Equitable, ethical, accessible, quality health care that promotes healing and health
- Health care that respects human dignity, individuality, and diversity among groups
- Complete and accurate information to make informed health care decisions
- Self-determination and active participation in health care decisions
- Involvement of a woman's designated family members, to the extent desired, in all health care experiences (ACNM, 2004b)

Midwives also believe in:

- Watchful waiting and non-intervention in normal processes
- Appropriate use of interventions and technology for current or potential health problems

- Consultation, collaboration, and referral with other members of the health care team as needed to provide optimal health care (ACNM, 2004b)

Midwifery is a very old profession, mentioned in the Bible. The practice of midwifery declined in the 18th and 19th centuries, and obstetrics developed as a medical specialty. In 1925, Mary Breckenridge established the Frontier Nursing Service (FNS) in Kentucky and was the first nurse to practice as a nurse-midwife in the United States. She received her midwifery education in England and returned to the United States with other British nurse-midwives to set up a system of care similar to that which she had observed in Scotland. The FNS was begun to care for individuals who were without adequate health care. The nurse-midwives of the FNS provided maternal and infant care and effectively demonstrated quality care and significantly improved outcomes.

The first U.S. nurse-midwifery education program was started at the Maternity Center Association, Lobenstein Clinic, in New York City in 1932. The American College of Nurse-Midwives was incorporated in 1955. Nurse-midwifery practice grew slowly until the late 1960s and early 1970s when nurse-midwifery experienced increased acceptance as a profession and an increase in consumer demand for nurse-midwives and the kind of care they provided (Varney, 2003). There are over 7,000 CNMs/CMs in the United States, and in 2006 they attended over 317,000 births, or 7.4% of all births and 11.3% of vaginal births in the United States (Martin, Hamilton, Sutton, Ventura, Menacker, et al., 2009). Nurse-midwives have direct third-party reimbursement and prescriptive authority in all 50 states.

In the 1970s, national accreditation of nurse-midwifery education programs and national certification of nurse-midwives was begun by ACNM. The accreditation process is recognized by the U.S. Department of Education, and the certification process now conducted by the American Midwifery Certification Council (AMCB) is recognized by the National Commission of Health Certifying Agencies.

The ACNM document, *Core Competencies for Basic Midwifery Practice* (ACNM, 2007), describes the skills and knowledge that are fundamental to the practice of a new graduate of an Accreditation Commission for Midwifery Education (ACNM) accredited education program. These competencies guide curricular development in midwifery programs and are utilized in the nationally recognized accreditation process. Categories of competencies described in the document include professional responsibilities; the midwifery management process; primary health care of women, including health promotion and disease prevention, preconception care, family planning and gynecologic care, perimenopausal and postmenopausal care, and management of common health problems; the childbearing family, including prenatal, intrapartum, and postpartum care of the childbearing woman, as well as care of the newborn. Hallmarks of midwifery practice are also delineated.

Nurse-midwifery education began with certificate programs and has progressed to graduate education. There are presently 38 ACME-accredited programs in the United States. Most midwifery programs are in schools of nursing, but two are in health-related professions schools. A direct entry (non-nursing) route to midwifery education, utilizing the same nationally recognized accreditation and certification standards, began in 1997 at the State University of New York (downstate campus). Certified midwife (CM) students are required to complete certain prerequisite health sciences courses, such as chemistry, biology, nutrition, and psychology, prior to beginning midwifery education. In addition, certain knowledge and skills common in nursing practice are required before beginning the midwifery clinical courses in the program (ACME, 2005). CMs are currently licensed to practice under the title of certified midwife in three states. Certified Professional Midwives (CPMs), another type of direct entry midwives who attend out-of-hospital births, are increasingly recognized by some states and are often confused with the ACME-educated midwives.

Nurse-midwives in the United States have consistently demonstrated that their care results in excellent outcomes and client satisfaction among the large proportion of underserved, uninsured, low-income, minority, and otherwise vulnerable women for whom CNMs provide care. Researchers have demonstrated lower caesarean section rates and outcomes comparable to a private obstetrics practice in a nurse-midwifery practice caring for underserved women (Blanchette, 1995) and fewer medical interventions, a lower caesarean section rate for nurse-midwifery clients compared with similar low-risk women cared for by family physicians and obstetricians (Rosenblatt et al., 1997). A study at the National Center for Health Statistics demonstrated significantly lower risks of neonatal mortality, low birth weight, infant mortality, and a significantly higher mean birth weight in births attended by nurse-midwives compared with those attended by physicians. These comparisons controlled for medical and sociodemographic risks (MacDorman & Singh, 1998). Births attended by CNMs and CMs occur primarily in hospitals; 99%

of births in the U.S. occurred in hospitals in 2006 (Martin, Hamilton, Sutton, Ventura, Menacker, et al., 2009).

Over the 80-plus-year history of nurse-midwifery and midwifery in the United States, a strong base of support documented by research has been developed. The number of educational programs and practitioners has grown substantially. As health care dollars continue to be carefully allocated and specific outcomes are measured more closely, certified nurse-midwives and certified midwives should play an increasing role in providing quality primary health care to women.

Clinical Nurse Specialists

The American Nurses Association has defined clinical nurse specialists (CNSs) as follows:

> The clinical nurse specialist is a clinical expert who provides direct patient care services including health assessment, diagnosis, health promotion and preventive interventions and management of health problems in a specialized area of nursing practice. The clinical nurse specialist promotes the improvement of nursing care through education, consultation, research, and in the role of change agent in the health care system (ANA, 1996, p. 3).

CNSs are registered professional nurses with graduate preparation earned at the master's or doctoral level. They may also be educated in a postmaster's program that prepares graduates to practice in specific specialty areas (Lyon & Minarik, 2001; Lyon, 2004). In 2000, 183 schools offered CNS master's programs, an increase from 147 programs in 1997 (Dayhoff & Lyon, 2001). In addition to the curriculum proposed for graduate clinical education by the American Association of Colleges of Nursing (AACN, 1996), the National Association of Clinical Nurse Specialists has developed curriculum recommendations for CNS education (NACNS, 2004). NACNS is currently developing competencies to reflect the *Essentials of Doctoral Education for Advanced Nursing Practice* (AACN, 2006). CNSs have traditionally worked in hospitals, but they now practice in many settings, including nursing homes, schools, home care, and hospice.

The CNS is one of four categories of APNs, each with distinctively different practice characteristics (NACNS, 2004). The CNS has had a long history in the United States. The Clinical Nurse Specialist role was developed following World War II. Prior to that time, specialization for nurses was in the functional areas of administration and education. Recognizing the need to have highly qualified nurses directly involved in patient care, the concept of clinical nurse specialists emerged. Reiter first used the term "nurse clinician" in 1943 to designate a specialist in nursing practice (Reiter, 1966). The first master's program in a clinical nursing specialty was developed in 1954 by Hildegarde Peplau at Rutgers University to prepare psychiatric clinical nurse specialists. That program launched the CNS role that has been an important player in the nursing profession and health care arena ever since, although the role has not been without controversy. Health care restructuring and cost-cutting initiatives in the 1980s and 1990s resulted in a loss of CNS positions in the United States. However, after increasingly frequent reports of adverse events in hospital settings in the 1990s (Institute of Medicine, 1999, 2001), it became apparent that CNSs were critical to obtaining quality patient outcomes (Clark, 2001; Heitkemper & Bond, 2004), with the result that CNSs are again seen as valuable professionals in many U.S. health care systems.

As with the NP movement, the availability of federal funds for graduate nursing education programs and the Professional Traineeship Program through HRSA that provides stipends for students has played a role in the development of many graduate CNS programs.

The development and use of complex health care technology in the management of patients in hospitals and intricate surgical procedures has resulted in increasing acuity and complexity of patient care delivery. Thus, there is a need for nurses with advanced knowledge and expertise to be integrally involved in working with staff to assess, plan, implement, and evaluate care for these patients. Many hospitals have used CNSs as care coordinators and case managers in which they coordinate the care of patients with acute or chronic illnesses during their hospital stays and prepare them for discharge to their homes or other care facilities (Wells, Erickson, & Spinella, 1996). CNSs have also been used as discharge planners working with staff to plan post-hospital care for patients who have complex health problems (Naylor et al., 1994; Neidlinger, Scroggins, & Kennedy, 1987). Their importance in care coordination over the care continuum is only now being lauded, exemplified in the work of Naylor and colleagues who reported that use of gerontological CNSs as discharge planners resulted in fewer readmissions of elderly cardiac patients.

Since its inception, the CNS role has suffered from role ambiguity (Rasch & Frauman, 1996; Redekopp, 1997). Although the initial vision was for CNSs to be integrally involved in patient care for a specific patient population, they have assumed many other roles, such as staff and patient educator, consultant, supervisor, project director, and more recently, case manager. Redekopp noted that it is difficult for CNSs to precisely describe their role to others because their roles are continually changing to meet the health needs of a changing patient population in an ever-changing health care system. Role ambiguity has made it difficult to measure the impact that CNSs have on patient outcomes. Thus, when budgetary crises have occurred in hospitals, CNSs have frequently had to advocate strongly to maintain their positions because outcome data to support the positive impact of their practice has either not been readily available or simply did not exist.

There are numerous CNS specialties and subspecialties: psychiatric/ mental health nursing, adult health, gerontology, oncology, pediatrics, cardiovascular, neuroscience, rehabilitation, pulmonary, renal, diabetes, and palliative care, to name a few. Numerous organizations offer certification examinations for CNSs. However, some organizations do not specify that master's degrees are required for certification in the specialty, causing confusion regarding the regulation and title of clinical nurse specialist. In the past, many CNSs have not sought third-party reimbursement so they have not taken specialty CNS certification examinations. With changes in state nursing practice acts and the increase in third-party payment and prescriptive privileges for advanced practice nurses, the number of certified CNSs is now increasing. Controversy regarding CNS certification continues, however, because the examinations are not available in the many specialties that CNSs perform. Exemptions from state laws and regulations for CNSs have been provided by some states because of this lack of certification. To address this need, a core CNS certification exam is under development by the American Nurses Credentialing Center.

In the late 1980s and early 1990s, many discussions and debates took place around the merging of the CNS and NP roles (Page & Arena, 1994). Several studies were conducted comparing the knowledge and skills of these two advanced practice roles (Elder & Bullough, 1990; Fenton & Brykczynski, 1993; Forbes, Rafson, Spross, & Kozlowski, 1990; Lindeke, Canedy, & Kay, 1996; Lindeke, 2004; Lindeke & Jukkala, 2005). Research indicated that there were many similarities in the educational preparation of these two groups of APNs. Many CNSs viewed the proposed merger as the demise of the CNS role. NPs were concerned that they would need to abandon the title of NP, a term that had become familiar to many patients and health professionals. A new organization, the National Association of Clinical Nurse Specialists, was formed to assist CNSs and to provide a vehicle to publicize the many contributions that CNSs have made and continue to make in providing quality patient care. The CNS role today is a dynamic and needed advanced practice nursing role, and many in the nursing profession anticipate that it will continue to exist for years to come.

Certified Registered Nurse Anesthetists

Modern nurse anesthesia traces its roots to the last two decades of the 1800s when records indicate that nurses were often asked to administer anesthesia. In fact, the practice was so common that in her 1893 textbook, *Nursing: Its Principles and Practices for Hospital and Private Use,* Isabel Adams Hampton Robb included a chapter on the administration of anesthesia. By 1912 a formal course in anesthesia had been developed in Springfield, Illinois, by Mother Magdalene Weidlocher of the Third Order of the Hospital Sisters of St. Francis. The Sisters of St. Francis went on to establish St. Mary's Hospital in Rochester, Minnesota, where nurse anesthetists became well known for their expertise in the administration of anesthesia (Bankert, 1989). Alice McGaw, one of the early nurse anesthetists for the Drs. Mayo at St. Mary's Hospital, published several papers in the early 1900s reporting on the thousands of anesthetics administered with ether and/or chloroform—all "without a death attributable to the anesthesia" (Bankert, 1989, p. 31).

A certified registered nurse anesthetist (CRNA) is a registered nurse who is educationally prepared to provide anesthesia and anesthesia-related services in collaboration with other health care professionals, such as surgeons, dentists, podiatrists, and anesthesiologists. The practice of nurse anesthesia is a specialty within the profession of nursing, and CRNAs are recognized by state licensing or regulatory agencies, primarily boards of nursing, in all 50 states (AANA, 2008a).

The CRNA scope of practice includes comprehensive patient care

1. Performing and documenting a pre-anesthetic assessment and evaluation of the patient, including requesting consultations and diagnostic studies; selecting, obtaining, ordering, and administering pre-anesthetic medications and fluids; and obtaining informed consent for anesthesia
2. Developing and implementing an anesthetic plan
3. Initiating the anesthetic technique, which may include general, regional, local, and sedation

4. Selecting, applying, and inserting appropriate noninvasive and invasive monitoring modalities for continuous evaluation of the patient's physical status
5. Selecting, obtaining, and administering the anesthetics, adjuvant and accessory drugs, and fluids necessary to manage the anesthetic
6. Managing a patient's airway and pulmonary status using current practice modalities
7. Facilitating emergence and recovery from anesthesia by selecting, obtaining, ordering, and administering medications, fluids, and ventilatory support
8. Discharging the patient from a post-anesthesia care area and providing post-anesthesia follow-up evaluation and care
9. Implementing acute and chronic pain management modalities
10. Responding to emergency situations by providing airway management, administration of emergency fluids and drugs, and using basic or advanced cardiac life support techniques (AANA, 2007a)

The CRNA scope of practice may also include responsibilities such as administration and management, quality assessment, education, research, committee appointments, interdepartmental liaison, and clinical and administrative oversight of non-anesthesia departments (e.g., respiratory therapy or the post-anesthesia care unit) (AANA, 2007a).

Nurse anesthesia educational programs are a minimum of 24 months in length and are conducted in a master's degree framework. In 2008, approximately 55% of nurse anesthesia educational programs were housed within or affiliated with university schools of nursing. The other nurse anesthesia programs offer a variety of master's degrees, including majors such as nurse anesthesiology (not housed in a school of nursing), biology, health science, or anesthesiology education. The Council on Accreditation of Nurse Anesthesia Educational Programs (COA, 2003 & 2008) accredits all nurse anesthesia educational programs. In turn, the COA is recognized by the U.S. Department of Education and the Commission on Recognition of Postsecondary Accreditation. This formal accreditation process was begun in 1952.

Although many exceed the requirements, all nurse anesthesia programs, regardless of the master's degree offered, provide a minimum curriculum, including pharmacology of anesthetic agents and adjuvant drugs including concepts in chemistry and biochemistry (105 hours);

anatomy, physiology, and pathophysiology (135 hours); professional aspects of nurse anesthesia practice (45 hours); basic and advanced principles of anesthesia practice, including physics, equipment, technology, and pain management (105 hours); research (30 hours); and clinical correlation conferences (45 hours). In addition to completing the classroom hours during the educational program, nurse anesthesia students are required to administer a minimum of 550 anesthetics, using a variety of anesthetic techniques for a wide range of procedures on healthy patients and those with comorbidities (COA, 2004).

Like all APNs in advanced practice nursing roles, CRNAs have grappled with the American Association of Colleges of Nursing (AACN) recommendation that all advanced practice nursing programs be conducted within a doctor of nursing practice (DNP) framework by 2015 (AACN, 2006). Because 45% of nurse anesthesia programs are housed within nonnursing academic units, granting a DNP degree is not possible for many programs. To address the impact of the AACN recommendation on the nurse anesthesia profession, the American Association of Nurse Anesthetists appointed a Task Force on Doctoral Preparation of Nurse Anesthetists (DTF) in 2005 (AANA, 2006). In September 2007, the AANA announced its support of the recommendation of the DTF, namely that the doctorate be required for entry into nurse anesthesia practice by 2025 (AANA, 2007b). For programs not housed within schools of nursing, the doctorate of nurse anesthesia practice (DNAP) may become the degree offered. To become a certified registered nurse anesthetist (CRNA), a nurse anesthesia graduate must successfully complete the National Certification Examination administered by the Council on Certification of Nurse Anesthetists (CCNA). Because CRNAs must graduate from a COA-accredited educational program and pass a certification examination to practice, the public can be assured that a CRNA has "met objective, predetermined qualifications for providing nurse anesthesia services" (CCNA, 2008, p. 3).

With the passage of the Omnibus Budget Reconciliation Act of 1986, CRNAs became the first advanced practice nursing professionals to be granted direct reimbursement for their services to Medicare recipients, giving them new practice options. In the 2007–2008 AANA Professional Practice Survey, the most common primary employment arrangement for CRNAs was reported as "employee of a group" (37%), followed by "employee of hospital" (35%), and "independent contractor" (15%). "Employee in other setting," "owner/partner," and "military/government/Department of Veterans Affairs" make up the remaining 13% (AANA, 2008b).

CRNAs function as sole anesthesia providers in rural hospitals, enabling these hospitals to stay open by providing surgical, obstetric, and trauma stabilization services (AANA, 2008c). Although no state statute requires anesthesiologist supervision of CRNAs, the Centers for Medicare and Medicaid (CMS) do state in their rules for participation that CRNAs must be supervised by a physician. In 2001, CMS amended this requirement by providing an opt-out or exemption ruling. Fourteen state governors have requested and received exemption from the CMS rule requiring physician supervision of CRNAs (AANA, 2008d).

International

Although the content in this chapter has focused on APNs in the United States, it is encouraging to see the continuing development of these roles in other countries. Midwifery, a profession often distinct from nursing, has a longer history internationally than in the United States. The International Confederation of Midwives, so named in 1954, has more than 90 midwifery organization members representing 80 countries (see www.internationalmidwives.org). Clinical specialization in nursing has existed in many countries for a very long time. For example, in the United Kingdom the NP role developed dramatically during the 1990s once the National Health Services recognized its legitimacy (Reverly, Walsh, & Crumbie, 2001). However, in other countries APNs are only beginning to develop programs and practices (Wang, Yen, & Snyder, 1995).

As part of the International Council of Nurses, the International Nurse Practitioner/Advanced Practice Nursing Network promotes the role of the APN globally (www.icn-apnetwork.org). Every two years, international conferences are held; there, APNs from around the world share their experiences, provide support to each other in the cause of advancing the status of nursing worldwide, and keeping alive the nursing ideal of providing quality care for all persons.

CONCLUSION

Advanced practice nurses have made significant contributions to quality health care, particularly for vulnerable populations. If all Americans are to receive quality, cost-effective health care, it is critical that greater use be made of APNs (Hooker & Berlin, 2002). A bright future awaits nursing and APNs in this new century. The APNs' advanced knowledge and skills, both in nursing and related fields, give them the capabilities to make valuable contributions to the current and future health care system, especially as our country takes on the task of meaningful health care reform. As the United States becomes more diverse, APNs can play key roles in ensuring that culturally competent care is delivered. They are poised to assume leadership in developing new practice sites and innovative systems of care to enhance health care outcomes.

REFERENCES

Accreditation Commission for Midwifery Education (ACME). (2005). *The knowledge, skills, and behaviors prerequisite to midwifery clinical coursework.* Washington DC: Author.

Advanced Practice Registered Nurses (APRN) Consensus Workgroup, & APRN Joint Dialogue Group (2008). *Consensus model for APRN regulation: Licensure, accreditation, certification, and education.* Retrieved March 29, 2009, from www.aacn.nche.edu/Education/pdf/APRNReport.pdf

American Association of Colleges of Nursing (AACN). (1996). *The essentials of master's education for advanced practice nursing.* Washington DC: Author.

American Association of Colleges of Nursing (AACN). (2003). *Faculty shortages in baccalaureate and graduate nursing programs: Scope of the problem and strategies for expanding the supply.* Retrieved August 12, 2004, from http://w2w.aacn.nche.edu/Publications/WhitePapers/FacultyShortages.htm

American Association of Colleges of Nursing (AACN). 2006. Retrieved November 13, 2008, from www.aacn.nche.edu/DNP/pdf/DNProadmapreport.pdf/

American Association of Colleges of Nursing (AACN). (2006). *The essentials of doctoral education for advanced practice nurses.* Washington DC: Author. Retrieved April 4, 2009, from www.aacn.nche.edu/DNP/pdf/Essentials.pdf

American Association of Nursing (AACN). (2009). *2008–2009 Enrollment in baccalaureate and graduate nursing programs in nursing.* Washington, DC: Author.

American Association of Colleges of Nursing (AACN). (2009). *Doctor of nursing practice programs.* Retrieved April 4, 2009, from www.aacn.nche.edu/dnp/DNPProgramList.htm

American Association of Colleges of Nursing (AACN) and National Organization of Nurse Practitioner Faculties (NONPF). (2003). *National forum on the practice doctorate.* Retrieved August 12, 2004, from www.nonpf.com/ExecSummary120803.pdf

American Association of Nurse Anesthetists (AANA). (2002). Scope and Standards for Nurse Anesthesia Practice. In *Professional practice manual for the certified registered nurse anesthetist.* Park Ridge, IL: Author.

American Association of Nurse Anesthetists (AANA). (2004). *The cost effectiveness of nurse anesthetist practice.* Retrieved June 2004, from www.aana.com/crna/ataglance.asp

American Association of Nurse Anesthetists (AANA). 2006. Retrieved November 21, 2008, from www.aana.com/professionaldevelopment.aspx?ucNavMenu_TSMenuTargetID=131&ucNavMenu_TSMenuTargetType=4&ucNavMenu_TSMenuID=6&id=1742

American Association of Nurse Anesthetists (AANA). (2007a). Retrieved November 13, 2008, from www.aana.com/uploadedFiles/Resources/Practice_Documents/scope _stds_nap07_2007.pdf

American Association of Nurse Anesthetists (AANA). (2007b). Retrieved November 16, 2008, from www.aana.com/news.aspx?ucNavMenu_TSMenuTargetID=171&ucNav Menu_TSMenuTargetType=4&ucNavMenu_TSMenuID=6&id=9678&terms=DTF

American Association of Nurse Anesthetists (AANA). (2008a). Retrieved November 16, 2008, from www.aana.com/Resources.aspx?ucNavMenu_TSMenuTargetID=52&uc NavMenu_TSMenuTargetType=4&ucNavMenu_TSMenuID=6&id=798

American Association of Nurse Anesthetists (AANA). (2008b). American Association of Nurse Anesthetists. *2007–2008 AANA annual reports*. Park Ridge, IL: Author.

American Association of Nurse Anesthetists (AANA). (2008c). Retrieved November 17, 2008, from www.aana.com/Advocacy.aspx?ucNavMenu_TSMenuTargetID=4 9&ucNavMenu_TSMenuTargetType=4&ucNavMenu_TSMenuID=6&id=1790& terms=opt+out

American Association of Nurse Anesthetists (AANA). (2008d). Retrieved November 17, 2008, from www.aana.com/aboutaana.aspx?ucNavMenu_TSMenuTargetID=179&uc NavMenu_TSMenuTargetType=4&ucNavMenu_TSMenuID=6&id=265

American College of Nurse-Midwives (ACNM). (2004a). *Definition of midwifery practice*. Washington DC: Author.

American College of Nurse-Midwives. (ACNM). (2004b). *Philosophy of the American College of Nurse-Midwives*. Washington DC. Author.

American College of Nurse-Midwives (ACNM). (2007). *Core competencies for basic midwifery practice*. Washington DC: Author.

American Nurses Association (ANA). (2003). *Scope and standards of pediatric nurse practice*. Washington DC: Author.

American Nurses Association (ANA). (2004a). *Nursing's social policy statement*. Washington DC: Author.

American Nurses Association (ANA). (2004b). *Nursing: Scope and standards of practice*. Washington DC: Author.

American Nurses Association (2008). *Pediatric nursing: Scope and standards of practice*. Silver Springs, MD: Nursebook.org.

American Nurses Association, National Association of Pediatric Nurses, & Society of Pediatric Nurses. (2008). *Pediatric nursing: Scope and standards*. Washington DC: American Nurses Association American Medical Association. (2004). Rep 24, A-06.

Bankert, M. (1989). *Watchful care, a history of America's nurse anesthetists*. New York: Continuum.

Bednash, P. (2009). *The state of the schools: Creating a professional workforce for the future*. Retrieved April 4, 2009, from www.aacp.org/meetingsandevents/Documents/ Interim2008/Feb4/ProfessionalNursingWorkforce-Bednash.pdf

Bartter, K. (2001). *Ethical issues in advanced nursing practice*. Oxford: Butterworth Heinemann.

Benner, P. (1984). *From novice to expert: Excellence and power in clinical nursing practice*. Menlo Park, CA: Addison-Wesley.

Berlin, L., & Bednash, P. (2000). *Enrollment and graduations in baccalaureate and graduate programs in nursing*. Washington DC: AACN.

Berlin, L., Stennett, J., & Bednash, G. (2003). *2002–2003 enrollment and graduations in baccalaureate and graduate programs in nursing*. Washington DC: AACN.

Blanchette, H. (1995). Comparison of obstetric outcome of a primary-care access clinic staffed by certified nurse-midwives and a private practice group of obstetricians in the same community. *American Journal of Obstetrics & Gynecology, 172*(6), 1868–1871.

Brown, S., & Grimes, D. (1995). A meta-analysis of nurse practitioners and nurse midwives in primary care. *Nursing Research, 44*, 332–339.

Brykczynski, K. (1989). An interpretive study describing the clinical judgment of nurse practitioners. *Scholarly Inquiry for Nursing Practice: An Interpretive Journal, 3*,113–120.

Cajulis, C. B., & Fitzpatrick, J. J. (2007). Levels of autonomy of nurse practitioners in acute care setting. *Journal of the American Academy of Nurse Practitioners, 19*, 500–507.

Chan, G. K., & Garbez, R. O. (2006). Education of advanced practice nurses for emergency care settings; emphasized shared competencies and domains. *Advanced Emergency Nursing Journal, 28*(3), 216–225.

Clark, A. (2001). What will it take to reduce errors in health care settings? *Clinical Nurse Specialist, 15*(4), 182–183.

Chornick, N. (2008). Advanced practice registered nurse educational programs and regulation: A need for increased communication. *JONA'S Healthcare, Law, Ethics, and Regulation, 10*(1), 9–11.

Council on Accreditation of Nurse Anesthesia Educational Programs (COA). (2004). *Standards for accreditation of nurse anesthesia educational programs.* Park Ridge, IL: Author.

Council on Certification of Nurse Anesthetists (CCNA). (2008). *2008 candidate handbook.* Park Ridge, IL: Author.

Council on Certification of Nurse Anesthetists (CCNA). (2003). *2003 candidate handbook.* Park Ridge, IL: Author.

Dayhoff, N., & Lyon, B. (2001). Assessing outcomes of clinical nurse specialist practice. In R. Kleinpell (Ed.). *Outcome assessment in advanced nursing,* pp. 103–129. New York: Springer Publishing.

Dracup, K. (2004). Peterson's nursing programs. Retrieved August 12, 2004, from www .petersons.com/nursing/articles/masters.asp?sponsor=1.

Edwardson, S. (2004). Matching standards and needs in doctoral education in nursing. *Journal of Professional Nursing, 20,* 40–46.

Elder, R., & Bullough, B. (1990). Nurse practitioners and clinical nurse specialists: Are the roles merging? *Clinical Nurse Specialist, 4,* 78–84.

Fenton, M. (1985). Identifying competencies of clinical nurse specialists. *Journal of Nursing Administration, 15,* 31–37.

Fenton, M., & Brykczynski, K. (1993). Qualitative distinctions and similarities in the practice of clinical nurse specialists and nurse practitioners. *Journal of Professional Nursing, 9,* 313–326.

Forbes, K., Rafson, J., Spross, J., & Kozlowski, D. (1990). Clinical nurse specialist and nurse practitioner core curricula survey results. *Nurse Practitioners, 15,* 45–48.

Ford, L. (1979). A nurse for all settings: The nurse practitioner. *Nursing Outlook, 27,* 516–521.

Ford, L. (2005). Opinions, ideas and convictions for NPs' founding mother, Dr. Loretta Ford. *The American Journal for Nurse Practitioners, 9*(3), 31–33.

Gallo, A., Angst, D., & Knafl, K. (2009). Disclosure of genetic information within families. *American Journal of Nursing, 109,* 65–60.

Hamric, A., Spross, J., & Hanson, C. (2009). *Advanced practice nursing: An integrative approach.* Philadelphia: Elsevier.

Hanson, C., & Hamric, A. (2003). Reflections on the continuing evolution of advanced practice nursing. *Nursing Outlook, 51*, 203–211.

Health Resources Services Administration (HRSA). (2001). National sample survey of registered nurses. Retrieved August 1, 2004, from http://bhpr.hrsa.gov/healthworkforce/reports/rnsurvey/

Health Resources Services Administration (HRSA). (2002). *Nurse practitioner primary care competencies in specialty areas: Adult, family, gerontological, pediatric and women's health.* Washington DC: Author.

Health Resources Services and Administration (HRSA). (2005). *National sample survey of registered nurses March 2004: Preliminary findings.* Retrieved April 4, 2009, from ftp://ftp.hrsa.gov/bhpr/nursing/rnpopulation/theregisterednursepopulation.pdf

Heitkemper, M., & Bond, E. (2004). Clinical nurse specialists: State of the profession and challenges ahead. *Clinical Nurse Specialist, 18*(3), 135–140.

Hooker, R., & Berlin, L. (2002). Trends in the supply of physician assistants and nurse practitioners in the United States. *Health Affairs, 21*, 174–181.

Horrocks, S., Anderson, E., & Salisbury, C. (2002). Systematic review of whether nurse practitioners working in primary care can provide equivalent care to doctors. *British Medical Journal, 324*(7341), 819–823.

Institute of Medicine. (1999). *To err is human: Building a safer health system.* Washington DC: National Academy Press.

Institute of Medicine Committee on the Quality of Health Care in America. (2001). *Crossing the quality chasm: A new health system for the 21st century.* Washington DC: National Academy Press.

International Council of Nurses. *International nurse practitioner/advanced practice nursing network.* Retrieved April 8, 2009, from www.icn-apnetwork.org

Jordan, L. (1994). Qualifications and capabilities of the certified registered nurse anesthetist. In S. Foster & L. Jordan (Eds.), *Professional aspects of nurse anesthesia practice.* Philadelphia: F. A. Davis Co.

Klein, T. (2005). Scope of practice and the nurse practitioner: Regulation, competency, expansion, and evolution. *Topic in Advanced Practice Nursing eJournal, 7*(3), 1–10.

Kleinpell, R. M., & Hravnak, M. M. (2005). Strategies for success in the acute care nurse practitioner role. *Critical Care Nurse Clinician in North America, 17*, 177–181.

Kleinpell, R. M., Ely, E. W., & Grabenkort, R. (2008). Nurse practitioners and physician assistants in the intensive care unit: An evidence-based review, *Critical Care Medicine, 36*(10), 2888–2897.

Lindeke, L, Canedy, B., & Kay, M. (1996). A comparison of practice domains of clinical nurse specialists and nurse practitioners. *Journal of Professional Nursing, 13*, 281–287.

Lindeke, L. (2004). Creating your dream job in your chosen community. *The American Journal of Nurse Practitioners, 8*, 67–68.

Lindeke, L., & Jukkala, A. (2005). Rural nurse practitioner barriers and strategies for success: One state's story. *The American Journal for Nurse Practitioners, 9*(2), 11–18.

Lyon, B. (2004). What to look for when analyzing clinical nurse specialist statutes and regulations. *Clinical Nurse Specialist, 16*(1) 33–34.

Lyon, B., & Minarik, P. (2001). Statutory and regulatory issues for clinical nurse specialist (CNS) practice: Ensuring the public's access to CNS services. *Clinical Nurse Specialist, 15*(3), 108–114.

Martin, K. (2000). Nurse practitioners: A comparison of rural-urban practice patterns and willingness to serve in underserved areas. *Journal of the American Academy of Nurse Practitioners, 12*, 491–496.

Martin, J. A., Hamilton, B. E., Sutton, P. D., Ventura, S., Menacker, F., Kirmeyer, S., & Mathews, T. J. (2009). U.S. Health & Human Services, Rockville, MD, Division of Vital Statistics.

McLaughlin, R. (2007). Preparation for negotiating scope of practice for acute care nurse practitioners. *Journal of the American Academy of Nurse Practitioners, 19*, 627–634.

Mundinger, M., Kane, R., Lenz, E., Totten, A., Tsai, W., Cleary, P., et al. (2000). Primary care outcomes in patients treated by nurse practitioners or physicians: A randomized trial. *Journal of the American Medical Association, 283*, 59–68.

National Association of Clinical Nurse Specialists (NACNS). (2004). *Statement on clinical nurse specialist practice and education.* Harrisburg, PA: Author.

National Center for Health Statistics. (2006). *Births: Final data for 2006.* Report available from National Center for Vital Statistics (Report No. 57-7). Hyattsville, MD: National Center for Health Statistics.

National Council of State Boards of Nursing (NCSBN). (2002). *Regulation of advanced practice nursing.* Retrieved August 12, 2004, from www.ncsbn.org

National Organization of Nurse Practitioner Faculties (NONPF). (1995). *Advanced nursing practice: Curriculum guidelines and program standards for nurse practitioner education.* Washington DC: Author.

National Organization of Nurse Practitioner Faculties (NONPF). (2004). *Acute care nurse practitioner competencies.* Retrieved April 4, 2009, from www.nonpf.com/ACNPCompsfinal20041.pdf

National Organization of Nurse Practitioner Faculties (2006a). *2006 domains and core competencies of nurse practitioner practice.* Washington DC: Author. Retrieved April 4, 2009, from www.nonpf.org/NONPF2005/CoreCompsFINAL06.pdf

National Organization of Nurse Practitioner Faculties (2006b). *Practice doctorate nurse practitioner entry-level competencies.* Washington DC: Author.

Naylor, M., Brooten, D., Jones, R., Lavizzo-Mourey, R., Mezey, M., & Pauly, M. (1994). Comprehensive discharge planning for the hospitalized elderly: A randomized clinical trial. *Annals of Internal Medicine, 120*, 999–106.

Newhouse, R., Stanik-Hutt, J., White, K., Johntgen, M., Zangoro, G., Heindel, L., et al. (In press). *An assessment of the safety, quality and effectiveness of care provided by advanced practice nurses.* np.

Neidlinger, S., Scroggins, K., & Kennedy, L. (1987). Cost evaluation of discharge planning for hospitalized elderly. *Nursing Economics, 5*, 225–230.

Page, N., & Arena, D. (1994). Rethinking the merger of the clinical nurse specialist and the nurse practitioner roles. *Image: The Journal of Nursing Scholarship, 26*, 315–318.

Pearson, L. (2009). The Pearson report. *The American Journal of Nurse Practitioners, 13*, 8–71. Also retrieved April 4, 2009, from www.webnp.net/downloads/pearson_report09/ajnp_pearson09.pdf

Percy, M. S., & Sperhac, A. M. (2007). State regulations for the pediatric nurse practitioner in acute care. *Journal of Pediatric Health Care, 21*(1), 29–43.

Rasch, R., & Frauman, A. (1996). Advanced practice in nursing: Conceptual issues. *Journal of Professional Nursing, 12*, 141–146.

Redekopp, J. (1997). Clinical nurse specialist role confusion: The need for identity. *Clinical Nurse Specialist, 11*, 87–91.

Reiter, F. (1966). The nurse clinician. *American Journal of Nursing, 66*, 274–280.

Reverly, S., Walsh, M., & Crumbie, A. (2001). *Nurse practitioners: Developing the role in hospital settings*. Oxford: Butterworth Heinemann.

Rosenblatt, R., Dobie, S., Hart, L., Schneeweiss, R., Gould,D., Raine, T. R., et al. (1997). Interspecialty differences in the obstetric care of low-risk women. *American Journal of Public Health, 87*, 344–351.

Rosenfeld, P., McEvoy, M., & Glassman, K. (2003). Measuring practice patterns among acute care nurse practitioners. *Journal of Nursing Administration, 33*, 159–165.

Safriet, B. (1998). Still spending dollars, still searching for sense: Advanced practice nursing in an era of regulatory and economic turmoil. *Advanced Practice Nursing Quarterly, 4*, 24–33.

Scherer, Y. K., Bruce, S. A., & Runkawatt, V. (2007). A comparison of clinical simulation and case study presentation on nurse practitioner students' knowledge and confidence in managing a cardiac event. *International Journal of Nursing Education, 4*(1), 1–14.

Varney, H. (2003). *Varney's midwifery*. Boston: Jones & Bartlett.

Wang, J., Yen, M., & Snyder, M. (1995). Constraints and perspectives of advanced practice nursing in Taiwan, Republic of China. *Clinical Nurse Specialist, 9*, 252–255.

Wells, N., Erickson, S., & Spinella, J. (1996). Role transition: From clinical nurse specialist to clinical nurse specialist/case manager. *Journal of Nursing Administration, 26*, 23–28.

Wyatt, J. (2001). Continuing the discussion of advanced practice in acute care: Past and future. *Pediatric Nursing, 27*, 419–421.

2

Advanced Practice Within a Nursing Paradigm

MICHAELENE P. JANSEN

The most important word in the title of Advanced Practice Nursing (APN) is the last one: nursing. Advanced education enables nurses to expand their knowledge base and expertise in nursing so that their practices differ not only from those of nurses with an associate's or bachelor's degree but also from that of other health professionals, particularly physicians or physician assistants. Nurses often underestimate the profound positive effect that their care can have on improving patient outcomes. Florence Nightingale, in *Notes on Nursing* (1859, reprinted 1992), noted that people in her day often thought of nursing as signifying "little more than the administration of medicines and the application of poultices" (p. 6). Efforts are still necessary to convey the full scope of nursing practice to other professionals and to the public so that nurses' contributions to positive health outcomes are understood, valued, and reimbursed. So often the media has focused on the physical assessment skills and prescriptive privileges of APNs rather than on the distinctive skills and expertise that characterize APN practice.

As advanced practice nursing moves toward the practice doctorate for entry into practice, an excellent opportunity exists to reconceptualize how advanced practice nursing is taught in APN programs. Burman, Hart, Conley, Brown, Sherard, and Clarke (2009) challenge educators to focus on health promotion and disease management incorporating theories from a variety of disciplines to improve health behavior and change as Doctor of Nursing Practice (DNP) programs develop.

WHAT IS NURSING?

Definitions of Nursing

For many years the nursing profession has sought to define nursing and to identify its scope of practice. It is critical that APNs and those aspiring to this role have a clear understanding of what nursing is in order for them to provide a clear understanding of nursing's unique contributions to health care outcomes in their interprofessional and other interactions. Therefore, we will examine several of the many definitions of nursing that have been put forth over the years.

Florence Nightingale (1859, reprinted 1992) formulated one of the earliest definitions of nursing as "having charge of the personal health of a person." The aim of nursing care, according to Nightingale, is to put the patient in the best possible condition so that nature can act upon the person. Nightingale's *Notes on Nursing*, although it was written 150 years ago, speaks to the substantive basis of nursing. Not only does Nightingale elaborate on interventions nurses can employ, she also underscores the necessity of thorough assessments before planning nursing care. Reading *Notes on Nursing* should therefore be a part of every APN curriculum.

In Virginia Henderson's (1966) definition of nursing, emphasis is placed on the nurse collaborating with the patient to enhance the patient's health status. Henderson defined nursing as

> Assisting the individual, sick or well, in the performance of those activities contributing to health or its recovery (or to a peaceful death) that he would perform unaided if he had the necessary strength, will, or knowledge. And to do this in such a way as to help him gain independence as soon as possible. (p. 15)

Henderson's definition contains many elements that constitute the substantive nature of nursing. Health promotion is a key component of her definition. In addition, the caring aspects of nursing are emphasized. Not all patients will recover from their diseases or injuries. It is the nurse's role to assist patients to achieve the goals the patient has established. Myss (1996, 2003, 2004) noted in her well-known works on healing that in curing modalities the patient is passive, but she argues that the patient must take an active role to be healed. APNs can play a key role in assisting patients in their healing process because they are able to bring additional expertise to these interactions and to perform holistic health assessments. Henderson stresses helping the patient gain independence. Independence is truly a Western belief and may not be a value in all cultures. Thus, it is important for the nurse to ascertain the personal values of each patient and realize that independence may not be one of their preferences.

Nojima (1989), a Japanese nursing theorist, defined nursing practice as "a human activity carried out by nurses to help individuals organize their health conditions so that they are able to live optimally and realize their potential" (p. 6–7). In her definition, the focus is on a person's quality of life. The partnership between the nurse and the patient is evident in Nojima's definition of nursing. With the advent of globalization, it is important to review the characteristics of nursing outside of Western medicine (Nojima, Tomikana, Makabe, & Snyder, 2003).

The American Nurses Association (ANA) has defined nursing as follows:

> Nursing is the protection, promotion, and optimization of health and abilities, prevention of illness and injury, alleviation of suffering through the diagnosis and treatment of human response, and advocacy in the care of individuals, families, communities, and populations. (2003)

Previously, the definition of nursing focused on persons and their responses to health problems, rather than specific illnesses. This definition of nursing developed in 2003, which emphasizes health promotion and optimal health, remains unchanged in current discussions of the American Nurses Association's (ANA) *Social Policy Statement* (ANA, 2008). The focus on health differentiates nursing from the practice of medicine.

Despite the frequent reference to the ANA definition of nursing, many APNs have encountered difficulty working from a nursing model. They have been forced to launch their practice within the medical model in part due to medical diagnoses used for billing and coding. Although it is important to know the cause of a person's pain or stress, much of nursing care remains the same despite the etiology. It has been encouraging to see the Agency for Healthcare Research and Quality (AHRQ) consider problems or responses, rather than disease entities, as the focus of practice guidelines. The AHRQ website (www.ahrq.gov) is an excellent resource for evidence-based practice and current clinical practices.

Advanced practice nursing builds upon the competence of the professional nurse and is characterized by the integration and application of a broad range of theoretical and evidenced-based knowledge (ANA, 2008). APNs are prepared in one of the four roles described in Chapter 1: certified nurse-midwife, clinical nurse specialist, nurse practitioner, or certified registered nurse anesthetist. Licensure, accreditation, certification, and education (LACE) should be consistent with role population (APRN Consensus Group, 2008). Specialization within advanced practice focuses beyond the six populations and provides depth within a population. One of the most important aspects of specialization in nursing is that specialization is a part of the whole field of professional nursing (ANA, 2008).

Ongoing discussions related to the revision of the ANA's *A Social Policy Statement* (2003) emphasizes the characteristics of nursing practice to include human responses, theory application, evidence-based nursing actions, and outcomes. These characteristics build the foundation for the proposed Model of Professional Nursing (ANA, 2008). Within this model, nursing's professional scope of practice, code of ethics, specialization, and certification lay the base for professional nursing. Building upon this base in a pyramid model are individual state's nurse practice acts, rules, and regulations. From this level, institutional policies and procedures guide nursing practice with self-determination as the top level of the pyramid model. This model lays the foundation not only for professional nursing, but all its expanded roles and specializations.

Scope of Practice

Gaining more knowledge about the substantive basis of nursing is an essential component of APN education. Scope of practice can be viewed in several ways. In fact, findings from the numerous studies undertaken to identify, describe, and classify the phenomena of concern to nurses have helped to clarify our understanding of scope of practice. One way to determine scope of practice from a regulatory framework is to focus on population, with each APN working within their practice population and their work determined by education and regulation. Other initiatives delineate the substantive basis of nursing. Two of these initiatives—nursing diagnoses and human responses—will be discussed further.

Nursing Diagnoses

Nursing diagnoses are one strategy nurses have used to describe phenomena for which nurses provide care. Since the First Nursing Diagnosis Conference in 1973, nurses within the North American Nursing Diagnosis Association (NANDA) have worked to identify, describe, and validate patient problems and concerns that fall within the domain of nursing. Currently there are 201 approved nursing diagnoses with a projection of over 300 diagnoses to come (NANDA, 2009). Continued efforts are necessary to identify and validate new diagnoses and to revise existing diagnoses. APNs have provided and can continue to provide leadership in the nursing diagnosis movement.

NANDA diagnoses are grouped under nine functional patterns: exchanging, communicating, relating, valuing, choosing, moving, perceiving, knowing, and feeling. According to Newman (1984), it is important for nurses to determine changes in a patient's patterns. In approaching assessment in this manner, the focus is the whole person rather than specific diagnoses.

Nursing diagnoses have been widely accepted not only in the United States but also internationally (NANDA, 2009). As the first effort to develop a common language for nursing phenomena, and despite numerous criticisms, using such diagnoses assists nurses in focusing on those aspects of care for which nursing interventions can be identified and nurse-sensitive outcomes can be determined. APNs therefore need to be familiar with both nursing and medical diagnoses.

In the United States, a number of projects to identify and classify nursing interventions have been initiated. The National Intervention Classification (NIC) has identified and classified over 430 interventions (Bulechek, Butcher, & McCloskey Docherman, 2008). A project identifying nursing outcomes links nursing diagnoses, nursing outcomes, and interventions (Johnson, Bulechek, McCloskey Dochterman, Maas, Moorhead, et al., 2005).

Human Responses

The American Nurses Association has delineated phenomena of concern to nursing (ANA, 2003). The identified phenomena were not meant to be exhaustive but rather exemplars of the types of concerns that fall within the purview of nursing. Human experiences and responses proposed by the ANA (2008) include promotion of health and wellness;

promotion of safety and quality of care; care and self-care processes; physical, emotional and spiritual comfort, discomfort, and pain; adaptation to physiologic and pathophysiologic processes; emotions related to the experience of birth, growth and development, health, illness, disease, and death; meanings ascribed to health and illness; linguistic and cultural sensitivity; health literacy; decision making and the ability to make choices; relationships, role performance, and change processes within relationships; social policies and their effects on health; health care systems and their relationships to access, cost, and quality of health care; and the environment and the prevention of disease and injury (p. 7).

As with nursing diagnoses, these identified human responses assist APNs in focusing on the health concerns for which nursing care is of primary importance in producing positive patient outcomes. Therapeutics for managing the responses or assisting the person to manage transcends medical entities. For example, despite various etiologies for sleep problems, nursing interventions, such as massage and music therapy, can be used to manage these problems. Viewing nursing from the perspective of human responses helps nurses to organize content from the nurse's point of view.

THE ART AND SCIENCE OF NURSING

The Art of Nursing

The art of nursing is integrally tied to the caring aspect of nursing. For many years, nursing was defined as an art and a science. As nursing began to give more attention to establishing a scientific basis for practice and thereby gained greater acceptance in the scientific community, the art or caring aspect of nursing received less attention. In practice settings, for example, nurses paid more attention to the high technology used in caring for patients with complex health problems. Nonetheless, the public has sustained its attachment to caring interventions, such as massage, touch, and aromatherapy, to name a few. A number of reasons for which people seek complementary therapies have been proposed: (1) they wish to be treated as a whole person by health professionals; (2) they wish to be active participants in their care; (3) they desire that the treatment not be worse than the disease; and (4) they feel that Western health care does not meet all of their needs. Therefore, it is important that APNs consider how they can integrate the art of nursing, which includes traditional and nontraditional nursing interventions, into their practice.

Caring is a critical element of nursing practice. Leininger (1990), Watson (1988), and Gadow (1980) have each put forth definitions of caring. Watson defined the art of caring as

> A human activity consisting of the following: a nurse consciously, by means of certain signs, passes on to others feelings he or she has lived through, realized or learned; others are united to these feelings and also experience them. (p. 68)

Newman, Sime, and Corcoran-Perry (1991) noted that the focus of nursing is "caring in the human health experience" (p. 3). The National Organization of Nurse Practitioner Faculties (NONPF) has identified caring as a characteristic of APNs that continues as a theme throughout their seven competency domains (NONPF, 2006).

Caring requires that a nurse be competent in assessing and intervening. Benner (1998) noted that a caring attitude was not sufficient to make an action a caring practice. The practice must be implemented in an excellent manner in order to be viewed as caring. Caring and the art of nursing convey very similar meanings, but caring nurses also seek the scientific basis for their practice and continue to update their expertise and knowledge. APNs possess the knowledge and ability to critique research about specific therapies and determine their applicability to specific patient populations.

The Science of Nursing

Significant progress has been made in developing the knowledge base that underlies nursing practice, revealing that nursing is characterized by both art and science (ANA, 2004). Although nursing is guided by standards of practice based on clinical evidence and research, additional research is needed before APNs will have a sound scientific basis from which to choose specific interventions for a patient or population (ANA, 2008). The clinical guidelines developed by professional and governmental agencies—available through the National Guideline Clearinghouse—exemplify the work that has been done, and continues to be done, in identifying "best practices" based on research findings. APNs have a key role in helping nurses review research and develop clinical guidelines that incorporate the existing knowledge base.

THEORETICAL AND CONCEPTUAL MODELS

During the past 50 years, the nursing profession has given considerable attention to theoretical and conceptual models. This attention has served to differentiate nursing from other disciplines (Marrs & Lowry, 2009; Russell & Fawcett, 2005). However, nursing theories are not new in nursing. Nightingale (1859/1992) elaborated on the relationship of the environment to health and well-being. Numerous theoretical and conceptual models exist.

What relevance do nursing theories have to practice? Can't nurses merely practice nursing? Meleis (2006) noted that a theory articulates and communicates a mental image of a certain order that exists in the world. This image includes components, and these components inform a model or perspective that guides each nurse's practice. This model may be identical to one of the publicized nursing theories, or it may be based on a theoretical perspective from another discipline. In some instances, eclectic models are used in which nurses combine elements from established nursing theories or theories from other disciplines. New nursing theories continue to be developed. Of particular importance is the delineation of nursing theories that incorporate various cultural perspectives because the Western philosophical perspective to date has not pervaded many of the existing theories.

There has been much discussion about whether one grand nursing theory for nursing is needed. Would the existence of a grand or metatheory be advantageous to the progression of the profession and discipline? Riehl-Sisca (1989) stated that nursing has benefited from having a multiplicity of theories. The wide range of perspectives elaborated in these theories has helped nurses to more clearly define the nature of the discipline and profession, to evaluate various approaches that can be employed in practice, and to respect diversity as a positive element. Alligood and Marriner-Tomey (2005) identified seven theorists who have developed grand theories or conceptual frameworks for nursing. They are Johnson (1980), King (1971), Levine (1967), Neuman (1974), Orem (1980), Rogers (1970), and Roy (1984). Many other nurses have developed midrange theories or conceptual frameworks that have served as a basis for research and practice.

More recently, nurses have turned their attention to midrange theories. Midrange theories, which focus on a limited number of variables, are more amenable to empirical testing than are grand theories by definition (Olson & Hanchett, 1997). Examples of midrange theories include: empathy

(Olson & Hanchett, 1997), uncertainty in illness (Mishel, 1990), resilience (Polk, 1997), mastery (Younger, 1991), self-transcendence (Reed, 1991), caring (Swanson, 1991), and illness trajectory (Wiener & Dodd, 1993). Many nurses give little thought to the tenets that guide their practice; however, these philosophical underpinnings have profound impact on the nature and scope of their work. Often an APN practices clinical decision making within a nursing framework but is not consciously aware of doing so. Nurses have an ethical responsibility to practice nursing with a consciously defined approach to care. The theoretical or conceptual model used by a nurse provides the basis for making the complex decisions that are crucial in the delivery of good nursing care. In this regard, Smith (1995) stated

> The core of advanced practice nursing lies within nursing's disciplinary perspective on human-environment and caring interrelationships that facilitate health and healing. This core is delineated specifically in the philosophic and theoretic foundations of nursing. (p. 3)

Thus, nursing theory is an important component of APN education. Nursing is a practice discipline, and theories achieve importance in relation to their impact on nursing care. Recently attempts have been made to relate nursing theories to practice and to begin testing these theories. However, only minimal testing of these theories in practice settings has occurred. The number of theoretical nursing studies, particularly studies examining the efficacy of nursing interventions, is an indication of the apparent separation of theories and practice that has characterized much of nursing practice. As DNP programs develop, it is anticipated that the application gap between theories and practice will narrow.

The theoretical or conceptual framework that an APN selects and uses has a major impact on the patient assessments that are made and the nature of the interventions that are chosen to achieve patient outcomes. Gordon (2007) and Johnson (1989) have noted the profound impact a nurse's theoretical perspective can have on a nursing practice. Gordon (1987) stated

> One's conceptual perspective on clients and on nursing's goals strongly determines what kinds of things one assesses. Everyone has a perspective, whether in conscious awareness or not. Problems can arise if the perspective "in the head" is inconsistent with the actions taken during assessment. Information collection has to be logically related to one's view of nursing. (p. 69)

A conceptual model provides the practitioner with a general perspective or a mindset of what is important to observe, which in turn provides the basis for making nursing diagnoses and selecting nursing interventions.

INCORPORATING NURSING INTO ADVANCED PRACTICE NURSING

Because APNs provide health care to many populations and in many settings, they have many opportunities to make major contributions to advancing the substantive basis of nursing. By focusing on the nursing elements of health care, APNs have the opportunity to demonstrate to the public and to policy makers the unique and significant contributions that nursing has on health outcomes. In using the nursing rather than the medical model as the focus of practice, APNs give the public a distinct and adjunctive model of care rather than a substitutive model (i.e., replacing physicians). APNs may carry out activities that have traditionally been a part of medicine, but the performance of these activities by APNs need to be translated into the realm of nursing.

Guaranteeing that APNs view the provision of health care from a nursing perspective has implications for graduate curricula. The American Association of Colleges of Nursing (AACN) (2006) includes nursing theory as a component of their document *Essentials of Doctoral Education for Advanced Nursing Practice*. Students also need assistance in utilizing this theoretical content in their practice. Faculty and preceptors who model this approach for APN students are critical for helping them integrate theory into practice.

REFERENCES

Alligood, M. R., & Marriner-Tomey, A. (2005). *Nursing theory: Utilization and application.* St. Louis, MO: Mosby.

American Association of Colleges of Nursing (AACN). (2006). *Essentials of doctoral education for advanced practice nursing.* Washington DC: Author.

American Nurses Association (ANA). (2003). *Nursing: A social policy statement (2nd ed.).* Washington DC: Author.

American Nurses Association (ANA). (2004). *Nursing: Scope and standards of practice.* Washington DC: Author.

American Nurses Association (ANA). (2008). Draft. *Nursing's Social Policy Statement: The essence of the profession.* Washington DC: Author. Available from www.nursingworld.org/DocumentVault/CNPE/Draft-Nursings-Social-Policy-Statement-.aspx.

APRN Consensus Workgroup and APRN Joint Dialogue Group. (2008). *Consensus model for APRN regulation: Licensure, accreditation, certification & education*. Retrieved March 29, 2009, from www.aacn.nche.edu/Education/pdf/APRNReport.pdf.

Benner, P. (1998). *Nursing as a caring profession*. Paper presented at the meeting of the American Academy of Nursing, Kansas City, MO.

Bulechek, G. M., Butcher, H., & McCloskey Dochterman, J. (Eds.). (2008). *Nursing interventions classification (NIC)* (5th ed.). St. Louis, MO: Mosby.

Burman, M. E., Hart, A. M., Conley, V., Brown, J., Sherard, P., & Clarke, P. N. (2009). Reconceptualizing the core of nurse practitioner education and practice. *Journal of the American Academy of Nurse Practitioners, 21*, 11–17.

Gadow, S. (1980). Body and self: A dialectic. *The Journal of Medicine and Philosophy, 5*, 172–184.

Gordon, M. (2007). *Nursing diagnoses* (11th ed.). Sudbury, MA: Jones & Bartlett.

Henderson, V. (1966). *Nature of nursing*. New York: Macmillan.

Johnson, D. E. (1980). The behavioral system model for nursing. In J.P. Riehl & C. Roy (Eds.), *Conceptual models for nursing practice* (2nd ed., pp. 207–216). New York: Appleton-Century-Crofts.

Johnson, M., Bulechek, G. M., McCloskey Dochterman, J., Maas, M. L., Moorhead, S., et al. (2005). *NANDA, NOC and NIC Linkages* (2nd ed). St. Louis, MO: Mosby.

King, I. M. (1971). *Toward a theory of nursing*. New York: Wiley.

Lang, N. M., & Marek, K. D. (1992). Outcomes that reflect clinical practice. In *Patient outcomes research: Examining the effectiveness of nursing practice* (NIH Publishing No. 93–3411, pp. 27–38). Washington DC: U.S. Department of Health and Human Services.

Leininger, M. (1990). Historic and epistemologic dimensions of care and caring with future directions. In J. Stevenson & T. Tripp-Reimer (Eds.), *Knowledge about care and caring* (pp. 19–31). Kansas City, MO: American Academy of Nursing.

Levine, M. (1967). The four conservation principles of nursing. *Nursing Forum, 6*(1), 45–59.

Marrs, J. A. & Lowry, L. W. (2009). Nursing theory and practice: Connecting the dots. In P. G. Reed & N. C. Shearer (Eds.), *Perspectives on Nursing Theory* (5th ed, pp. 3–12). Philadelphia: Lippincott, Williams & Wilkins.

Meleis, A. I. (2006). *Theoretical nursing: Development and progress* (4th ed.). Philadelphia: Lippincott, Williams & Wilkin.

Mishel, M. H. (1990). Reconceptualization of the uncertainty in illness theory. *Image: Journal of Nursing Scholarship, 22*, 256–262.

Myss, C. (1996). *Anatomy of the spirit*. New York: Three Rivers Press.

Myss, C. (1998). *Why people don't heal and how they can*. NewYork: Three Rivers Press.

Myss, C. (2004). *Channeling grace in your every day life*. New York: Free Press.

National Organization of Nurse Practitioner Faculties (NONPF). (2006). *Domains and competencies of nurse practitioner practice*. Washington DC: Author.

Neuman, B. (1974). The Betty Neuman health-care system model: A total person approach to patient problems. In J. P. Riehl & C. Roy (Eds.), *Conceptual approach to patient problems* (pp. 99–114). New York: Appleton-Century-Crofts.

Newman, M. A. (1984). Looking at the whole. *American Journal of Nursing, 84*, 1496–1499.

Newman, M. A., Sime, A. M., & Corcoran-Perry, S. A. (1991). The focus of the discipline of nursing. *Advances in Nursing Science, 14*(1), 1–6.

Nightingale, F. (1992). *Notes on nursing.* Philadelphia: Lippincott. (Originally published 1859).

Nojima, Y. (1989, May). *The structural formula of nursing practice: A bridge to new nursing.* Paper presented at the 19th Quadrennial Congress of the International Congress of Nurses, Seoul, Korea.

Nojima, Y, Tomikana, T, Makabe, S., & Snyder, M. (2003). Defining characteristics of expertise in Japanese clinical nursing using the Delphi technique. *Nursing Health Science, 5*(1), 3–11.

North American Nursing Diagnosis Association (NANDA). (2009). *Nursing diagnoses: Definitions and classification 2009–2011.* Ames, IA: Wiley-Blackwell.

Olson, J., & Hanchett, E. (1997). Nurse-expressed empathy, patient outcomes, and development of a middle-range theory. *Image—The Journal of Nursing Scholarship, 29,* 71–76.

Orem, D. E. (1980). *Nursing: Concepts of practice.* New York: McGraw-Hill.

Polk, L. V. (1997). Toward a middle-range theory of resilience. *Advances in Nursing Science, 19*(3), 1–13.

Reed, P. G. (1991). Toward a nursing theory of self-transcendence: Deductive reformulation using developmental theories. *Advances in Nursing Science, 13*(4), 64–71.

Riehl-Sisca, J. (1989). *Conceptual models for nursing practice.* Norwalk, CT: Appleton & Lange.

Rogers, M. (1970). *An introduction to the theoretical basis of nursing.* Philadelphia: Davis.

Roy, C. (1984). *Introduction to nursing: An adaptation model.* Englewood Cliffs, NJ: Prentice-Hall.

Russell, G. E., & Fawcett, J. (2005). The conceptual model for nursing and health policy revisited. *Policy, Politics and Nursing Practice, 6*(4), 319–326.

Smith, M. C. (1995). The core of advanced practice nursing. *Nursing Science Quarterly, 8*(1), 2–3.

Swanson, K. M. (1991). Empirical development of a middle-range theory of caring. *Nursing Research, 40,* 161–166.

Watson, J. (1988). *Nursing: Human science and human care: A theory of nursing.* New York: National League for Nursing.

Wiener, C. L., & Dodd, M. J. (1993). Coping amid uncertainty: An illness trajectory. *Scholarly Inquiry in Nursing Practice, 7*(1), 17–30.

Younger, J. B. (1991). A theory of mastery. *Advances in Nursing Science, 14*(1), 76–89.

3

Multifaceted Roles of the APN

MARY ZWYGART-STAUFFACHER

INTRODUCTION

Many see the role of the advanced practice nurse (APN) as a nurse who is directly involved in patient care. Although this may be the primary role for many APNs, it is definitely not the only one. The APN incorporates a variety of roles, including collaborator, case manager, educator, researcher, and advocate, just to name a few. How the APN puts each of these roles into operation depends on the APN and the employing agency. Certainly, direct patient care is an expected part of APN practice, particularly for the novice. In fact, it should remain a constant, ensuring a strong foundation for the development of patient care and APN expertise.

Over time, however, the issues and circumstances presented in one-to-one patient care become more predictable as the systems of care delivery become more complex. To address these issues, APNs must be equipped to utilize other APN roles to more dramatically influence these broader issues and enhance their practice. These roles may be initiated within the context of current practice or evolve to become a dominant part of the APN position. Traditionally, the roles of the APN included care provider, educator, researcher, consultant, and manager. The National Association of Clinical Nurse Specialists (NACNS) has conceptualized these various roles into spheres of practice. These spheres include the

Exhibit 3.1

ROLE OF CLINICAL NURSE SPECIALIST

Traditional	Contemporary
Direct-care Provider	Patient/Client Sphere
Educator	Nursing and Nursing Practice Sphere
Researcher	Organization/System Sphere (National Association of Consultant Clinical Nurse Specialists [NACNS], 2004)
Consultant	
Manager	

patient–client sphere, the nurses and nursing practice sphere, and the organization–system sphere (NACNS, 2004). Exhibit 3.1 compares traditional and contemporary practice roles.

As the APN assumes a more active leadership role within the health care system, the roles of patient advocate, educator, change agent, case manager, and consultant become more essential to the APN's development and the evolution of nursing, and they contribute greatly to the management of complex health care issues and systems. Although some administrators may argue that there is a loss of revenue when the APN functions outside of the direct care role, the APN must continue to market the cost-effective nature and improved outcomes or changes in care delivery that can be generated when APNs embrace the full spectrum of the their roles and functions.

Nursing management must also expand its knowledge and competence to better utilize APN expertise and to more accurately represent and advocate for the APN. For example, during the 1990s, many CNS positions were eliminated due to downsizing of hospitals and their inability to directly reimburse these nursing specialists for their activities. Recently hospitals have added many CNS positions, validating their value to the organization.

APN ROLES

Basic nursing education has provided a strong foundation to guide the APN in practice in the systematic approach of the nursing process. Graduate nursing education builds on that foundation, although each educational program has varied preparation and emphasis on the various roles performed by the APN. The APN must respect the wealth of knowledge that can be gained in each of these roles and become well grounded in that knowledge to ensure successful role development. This chapter will examine the various spheres or roles, focusing on incorporating them into the whole and consummate professional.

Advocacy in APN Practice

Advocacy for patients must remain fundamental to the practice of nursing. It is the underpinning of the nurse–patient relationship. Advocacy is defined as a way of being in a relationship that sees the patient as a whole human being in their experience with health and promotes the uniqueness of the client (Nelson, 1998). Nelson (1999) notes that advocacy has progressed to being a guardian of the patient's rights and freedoms of choice. Although several other elements may be included in advocacy, a nurse's advocacy is guided by respect for the individual.

Advocacy can be viewed from a variety of perspectives. Nelson (1998) maintains that advocacy includes legal advocacy, moral–ethical advocacy, substitutive advocacy, political advocacy, spiritual advocacy, advocacy for nursing, and advocacy for community health (Exhibit 3.2).

In legal advocacy, the nurse supports the patient's legal rights, such as informed consent or the right to refuse treatment. This may include ensuring that all patients have a copy of the institution's bill of rights. Moral–ethical advocacy requires that the nurse respect the patient's values and support decisions that are consistent with those values, such as

Exhibit 3.2

TYPES OF ADVOCACY

Legal advocacy
Moral–ethical advocacy
Substitutive advocacy
Political advocacy
Spiritual advocacy
Advocacy for nursing
Advocacy for community health

decisions regarding abortion. In substitutive advocacy, if the patient is unable to express an opinion, the nurse should continue to respect the rights of the client or surrogate and support any wishes that the patient may have previously expressed. Political advocacy includes work to change laws and policies to ensure equities for all patients, groups, and society. APNs also participate on committees and boards to help determine policy that benefits patients. In spiritual advocacy, the APN ensures that the patient has access to spiritual support such as clergy and that the plan of care includes the spiritual aspects of care. Advocacy for nursing directs the nurse to support other nurses in their professional growth and to contribute to the evolution of the nursing profession. Nelson suggests that this is an opportunity for APNs to facilitate and empower other nurses through leadership, education, and modeling standards for practice. To advocate for a community's health, nurses must advocate for the assessment of health needs in a community, consider priorities for care and resources, and determine health and environmental trends that may influence a community.

Advocacy must occur for all clients. APNs should advocate for all clients to complete living wills and advanced directives to make sure that health care issues are well documented and patient wishes are respected. On occasion, issues of competency may arise in areas such as substitutive advocacy and moral–ethical advocacy. When competency is a concern, the APN must be familiar with laws governing competence, including criteria for the assessment of competence. At the same time, the APN should be instrumental in establishing policies for direct action when a patient is judged incompetent. In such a case, the APN must communicate the patient's expectations, if they are known, to the surrogate and/or the patient's family to support any requests and decisions to be made based on the patient's past recommendations. Because there can be confusion and conflict among family, friends, surrogates, and even health care professionals during these times, the APN should have no reservation about convening family–client conferences and implementing ethics committee evaluations if questions or controversies arise.

Because advocacy carries with it a significant ethical dimension, principles of ethics can help to evaluate a nurse's effectiveness (Nelson, 1998). Pinch (1996) points out that some ethical principles may conflict. For example, the principle of autonomy (self-determination) could conflict with distributive justice (fair, equitable distribution of goods or services) if the patient's decisions were to impact the community's greater need or safety. If a patient requested no treatment and is discharged with a dangerous communicable disease that may infect the community, or if a patient demanded resources that jeopardized the financial or medical resources of a community, the patient's autonomy may be at risk of being overshadowed by what is best for the majority. In maintaining advocacy, the APN would need to be sure that there was indeed a conflict in distributive justice and no prejudices existed toward an individual or group.

Concerns exist regarding the ability of a nurse to be an advocate given our current health care systems and associated cost containment measures (Donagrandi & Eddy, 2000; Nelson, 1998; Watson, 1989). Is the APN in a position to maintain advocacy despite the demands of the system? Nelson (1998) contends that the APN can rise above these constraints. It is believed that the APN is in a unique position of influence through interaction with other team members, ensuring advocacy through policy formulation that directs patient care and through legislative involvement. It is also critical that the APN be well versed in the areas of evidence-based practice, standards of care, ethics policies, accreditation criteria, nursing licensure regulations, and professional association standards that can help to support an APN's advocacy position.

Educator

Grounded in the reality of patient care, the APN is in a unique position to assume the role of educator with patients, their families, students, and staff. In this environment the APN has a workshop of experiences for developing standards for practice, strategies for use of equipment and procedures, assessment of patient issues and concerns, and evaluations of nursing staff capabilities and limitations. Advanced practice nursing education makes the APN a resource for current knowledge in content areas, supportive resources, research findings, and the implementation of evidence-based practice. When providing education to students and staff, the APN can provide sound clinical examples that enhance the application of content. APNs may find it helpful to seek assistance from their colleagues in academic settings when they are initially developing educational content. It takes considerable knowledge and skill to develop a sound teaching–learning plan.

Whether the APN is teaching students, colleagues, or patients, an assessment of the person's current knowledge base is essential. A thorough assessment should include the APN's capabilities (e.g., able to use the computer), limitations (unable to read), disabilities (difficulty hearing), and availability of resources, to name a few. A patient's readiness to learn is also a factor. To plan for the best teaching strategies, the APN needs to know the learner. Knowles and Associates (1984) developed a list of assumptions about adult learners that will assist the APN in educational planning.

1. The learner is self-directed, needing a sense of involvement and control.
2. Experience is a rich resource for learning.
3. Readiness to learn occurs with a perceived need to know or do something.
4. Orientation to learning is problem-centered or task-centered.
5. Internal motivation is more potent than external motivators.

Although isolated teaching events can be provided, a planned content series is most effective in ensuring learner outcomes and competencies. When planning for the patient, student, or staff, an assessment first needs to be completed to determine what knowledge is needed so the APN can focus the content. This may be guided through planned curriculum, observed problems in patient care, standards or protocols for practice, or common client questions, to name a few. The assessment identifies what type of learner outcomes (competencies) are to be achieved.

When the assessment is complete, the APN needs to develop content objectives to achieve these outcomes. Guidelines for the development of objectives were established by Bloom (1956) who divided objectives into three domains of learning: cognitive, affective, and psychomotor. Objectives are developed with action verbs like "identify" or "demonstrate" with these action verbs dictating a certain level of complexity. For instance, the expectations of the learner would be very different if they were required to "identify" the steps to doing cardiopulmonary resuscitation (CPR) as opposed to actually "demonstrating" CPR. The action verb also guides the educator in selecting teaching strategies. To have the learner "identify," lecturing may be adequate. However, to have the learner "demonstrate" requires some guided lab activity. Demonstrating outcomes or competencies also is consistent in evaluating whether learning has occurred. Identification could be done with a written test and a demonstration that would require a lab so the learner could show a particular skill. Support content such as handouts or videotape may also need to be developed. These, too, should reflect the level of learning being addressed. With staff, the APN has the unique opportunity of continuing to work beside a staff member. In this way, a staff member can continue to pursue clarification and assistance, and the APN can evaluate the staff member for their grasp of the information.

Sparks (1999) offers these principles when teaching:

1. Proceed from the simple to the complex
2. Build on what is known to learn the unknown
3. Use terminology that is familiar to the learner
4. Set short-term and long-term goals
5. Plan a sequence of incremental learning activities
6. Application of content enhances learning
7. Learner objectives direct content and learning experiences
8. Use positive reinforcement
9. Evaluate outcomes of the learning process

Patients and students alike are using the Internet as a primary source of information. Some sources have information that is directed to health care professionals and is more likely to be reliable. The information that individuals gather is generated from a wide variety of Internet sources such as chat rooms and/or blogs. Information also comes from advertisements, brochures, newspapers, television, health kiosks, nontraditional care providers, or family and friends. This information can be skewed, inaccurate, or incomplete. The APN should take the time to access and review these sources to appraise the accuracy and reliability of the information that is being provided.

Patients may experience fears or preconceived ideas regarding care strategies and inappropriate outcomes. These apprehensions can either motivate them to become very knowledgeable or to remain very uninformed about their health concern. Just as you might ask a student for content references, the APN should ask the patient for their information sources. The APN needs to make a point of screening related health information made available by the health care organizations. Most printed educational content should be constructed at a fifth- to eighth-grade reading level. Background, color, and print format are all considerations. Many patients are overwhelmed simply by their diagnosis, much less their medication, treatment course, or plan of care. Printed information can be given to a patient to reinforce verbal information.

For students, the opportunity to learn from an APN can complement their education by providing a strong emphasis in nursing practice. Murphy (2000) described a collaboration in which a nurse educator, a researcher, and a practitioner were brought together. The practitioner in this study was an RN, but the use of an APN in both undergraduate and graduate curriculums could certainly give the student the same clinical opportunities. This collaboration would also benefit the development of the APN by providing opportunities to share with nursing educators and researchers in academia. Driver and Campbell (2000) also described the role of having a lecturer–practitioner in a 50–50 clinical and academic position. Although there was no significant difference in learning outcomes, the students appreciated the opportunities of working with a practitioner and subjectively described a sense of better preparation for practice.

Case Manager

Case management has become a more common dimension of the APN role, coinciding with the expansion of managed care programs. Coffman (2001) describes case management as a collaborative process promoting quality care and cost-effective outcomes to specific patients and groups. Umberell (2006) outlines the value of an advanced practice trauma case manager in orchestrating a comprehensive plan to reduce fragmentation of care and better utilization of resources. The key features of the case manager as outlined by Benoit (1996) include (1) standardized resources for a length of stay for selected patient care, caregiver, and system outcomes; (2) collaborative team practice among disciplines; (3) coordinated care over the course of an illness; (4) job enrichment for the caregiver; (5) patient and physician satisfaction with the care; and (6) minimized costs to the institution.

Taylor (1999) initially described the two primary types of case management as (1) the patient-focused model, which supports the patient throughout the continuum of care and helps them access health care, and (2) the system-focused model, which involves the service environment and is structured for cost containment of a specific group of patients and use of critical pathways for cost-effective outcomes. However, Taylor advanced her model of comprehensive case management that incorporates elements of cultural competency, consumer empowerment, clinical framework, and multidisciplinary practice in addition to other activities of assessment, service, planning, plan implementation, coordination and monitoring, advocacy, and termination. The focus in health care is on patient empowerment and quality service based on process improvement, outcome measurements, and performance-based expectations. In the past, case management was associated with the utilization of clinical pathways to drive the plan of care—therefore focusing on process—but the focus since the early 2000s has been on outcome measures. Taylor asserts that this new model is optimal because it incorporates components of both patient and system models to ensure that the patient receives needed services.

Ethical concerns have persisted as to how APNs who are active in nursing and case management can remain advocates for patients in a managed care environment (Donagrandi & Eddy, 2000). However, nursing is bound by ethics, and now with capitation legislation and Joint Commission on the Accreditation of Healthcare Organizations (JCAHO) emphasis on outcomes management and patient empowerment, the focus is changing. Taylor (1999) notes that managed care's success now rests in ensuring that access and utilization are appropriate, with managed care working to control high costs and ineffective treatment modalities. Taylor contends that the case manager is the person who makes managed care work well.

The utilization of APNs as case managers has been advocated by multiple authors (Donagrandi & Eddy, 2000; Taylor, 1999). APNs have enhanced capabilities in interdisciplinary coordination, advanced clinical decision making, autonomy, synthesis, and critical thinking. Taylor (1999) believes that the primary case manager should be an APN, with an RN doing case management in specialty areas under an APN's guidance. In this time of economic constraints, it may be a concern to have an APN managing day-to-day coordination of patient services. It would seem practical to utilize the APN in supervision of patient care providers with a focus on direct involvement on more complex patient cases. The APN expertise would also be valuable in the development of outcome standards, communication and coordination between disciplines, and analysis of patient care trends. In addition, a focus on complex patient populations requiring extended lengths of stay or long-term care resources are very ably managed by the APN (Abdallah et al., 2005). APN case management is believed to be best focused on health and disease prevention (Taylor, 1999).

Change Agent

Particularly in the unpredictable health care market, organizations will need to identify needs and make changes in order to survive. A change agent is an individual who identifies, plans, and implements that change.

According to Freed (1998), the change agent is distinguished by an ability to move from analysis to synthesis and show results.

Barker (1990) asserts that a change agent must have resilience, flexibility, creativity, and responsiveness. Recognizing the need for change is critical. For the best change, Price Waterhouse (1995) suggests that the change be (1) integral to and focused on the strategy of the organization; (2) leading to high-performance, significantly improved results with measurable differences; (3) helped by the energy and creative ideas of people in the organization; (4) supported by empowered and motivated employees; (5) driven by specific customer needs; (6) guided by a limited number of balanced performance measures; (7) able to build revenue; and (8) institutionalized in a culture that values continuous improvement.

Three models of organizational change are described by Kaluzny and Hernandez (1988). They are (1) the rational model, which focuses on the internal needs of the organization; (2) the resource dependency model, which is focused on the relationship and interdependence between the organization and the environment; and (3) organizational ecology model, which emphasizes the concept of an evolutional natural process. Wheatly (1992) describes a fourth model, the chaos model, in which the organization is in a necessary disequilibrium, making change continuous. Change occurs due to internal or external elements that motivate change. Hansen (1999) believes that the ecology and chaos models may be more useful in understanding the health care organization today.

Anderson and Ackerman Anderson (2001) now indicate that the organization has three types of change: (1) developmental change, which primarily deals with improvement in elements such as skill, methods, or performance standards, and is the simplest of changes; (2) transitional change, which does more than improve on what is, instead replacing the current situation with something new; and (3) transformational change, which is the most complex type of change, moving from one state of being to another, changing culture, behavior, and mindset. Developmental change is usually accomplished through sharing of information and process improvement. The threat in this change is low. Transitional change is needed when a problem exists, an opportunity for a worthwhile objective is not being pursued, or something needs to change or be created to serve current or future demands. This change requires a dismantling of the old ways of being and pursuit of a new state; it also requires a comprehensive plan, which includes building the case for change and involving employees in its design and implementation.

Transformational change is required when leadership is aware of two things: (1) the current process must be changed to reach the objectives, and (2) the scope of this change is so significant that it requires a fundamental shift in people's culture, mindset, and behavior in order to be successful. In transformational change, leadership must first be transformed for the change to occur.

Hansen (1999) describes both internal and environmental forces for change. Internal pressures come from behavioral and process sources such as a need for increased efficiency, improved staff competence, or analysis and reassessment of the work process. Environmental forces are elements outside of the organization that require the organization to change, such as new technology, client dissatisfaction, or legislation. Anderson and Ackerman Anderson (2001) define the drivers of change as being the environment, the marketplace, a business imperative, organizational imperatives, cultural imperatives, leader and employee behavior, and leader and employee mindset. Such change is viewed as a progression with the initial event (environment) triggering the next event and progressing through each stage until it finally reaches leader and employee mindset.

A discussion of change would not be grounded in the literature if the work of Lewin (1951) were not included. Lewin describes the change process as consisting of three phases: (1) unfreezing (realizing the need for change), (2) moving (forces for change are identified and altered), and (3) refreezing (establishing a new equilibrium). Hansen (1999) recommends these principles for effecting change: (1) selecting and focusing on the change opportunity or benefit; (2) building and maintaining relationships that will help in the change effort; (3) planning and guiding the change; and (4) continuously monitoring the situation, getting and receiving feedback, and making adjustments.

Price Waterhouse (1995) has now developed a change readiness assessment to evaluate the chance for success, scoring each factor on a scale of 1 to 5. If the assessment score is between 15 and 34, the change agent should "watch out." If the score is between 35 and 55, the situation needs to be closely watched, and if the score is between 56 and 75, change is likely to succeed. The use of this assessment may help the change agent identify areas of weakness and areas of strength to improve the change plan or realize its worth or necessity. Failed change can leave people less inclined to embrace another change.

In order to achieve a positive change, the change agent must be prepared to work through or avoid some specific issues. One situation in which there is potential for failure is if there is no sense of dissatisfaction with a current situation (Oates, 1997). If a change is introduced in this environment, resistance will occur. McPhail (1997) notes that people will be reluctant to leave what they perceive as a secure situation. Also, employees may not share the same vision of the change. It is critical that participants be aware of the plan and participate in its construction.

Early in the planning, the change agent should identify the people who will be actively involved in the change and determine which people will be supportive and which people will resist the change and the rationale for it. Many times resistance can be as simple as feeling left out or uninformed. Price Waterhouse (1995) suggests that those who are planning for a change must consider all the areas that may be affected, and each of these areas should be addressed to ensure that the plan will be effective in addressing each issue, whether to it is to redesign jobs or to modify procedures. Likewise, the change agent should avoid pitting people against each other, which can be very disruptive and can waste energy. Price Waterhouse identified 11 issues that may create problems for the change project.

1. Failure to deliver early, tangible results. If change is ongoing for longer than 6 months, anticipate that your support will decrease by half and your barriers will double.
2. Talk about breakthroughs but don't drown in the detail. Focus on the outcomes, not the process.
3. Pick the most important priorities, always refining your priorities as the project progresses.
4. Use performance measures appropriate to the plan. Avoid the old long-established measures. However, do be sure to measure because what gets measured gets done.
5. Assure that competing projects support each other and are not divisive or competitive. Show how all the changes are connected.
6. Listen to and involve your consumer.
7. Involve your employees in the project. This can build commitment.
8. Ensure that management is well informed, has a stake in the plan, and endorses the plan.
9. Explain how the change will improve the situation, making it tangible for employees.
10. Ensure that the change is based on that organization's facts and is tailored to that organization's need. Avoid just inserting something that has worked elsewhere.

11. Engage another set of employees, not just those who have always been involved. This can lead to new ideas that promote the change rather than maintain the status quo.

The APN as change agent should utilize strategies that will help to ensure a positive change and a positive experience in that change. Freed (1998) provides several suggestions. One recommendation is that change agents should not wait for organizational readiness because it is unlikely that readiness will ever happen. Instead they should plan to avoid the consequences of not changing and adapting soon enough. Also, the right change agent must be selected. A person internal to the organization, even if the person is well known, is not always viewed as being the most credible. Outside consultants are more likely to be effective promoters of change.

Another strategy operates on the idea that even small successful changes can build credibility and that a successful long-term change has many short-term milestones. Freed notes that any meaningful change will disenfranchise someone. When change occurs, the change agent must plan and be prepared to step in with the new order or risk the return of the status quo. Freed indicates that it is not reasonable for the change agent to expect infinite inclusion, consensus, and popularity. For some changes, it is simply necessary to help people realize the lack of good alternatives. Although it may be comfortable for people to remain as they are, the reality is that they will eventually have to change. Freed also believes that some people just have to be "kidnapped" and moved to the new change so that they don't have to contemplate the change for too long. The people who created the current system are unlikely to help change it. Change will not be orderly, but Freed indicates that this disorder helps to signal the advent of a change and the need to refine a new model. Finally, having too many options can paralyze change. Sometimes it is best to proceed with what you have available.

Price Waterhouse (1995) lists the following principles for implementing change.

1. Confront reality
2. Focus on strategic contexts
3. Summon strong mandates (i.e., top management)
4. Set a reasonable amount of change
5. Build a case for the change and work for consensus
6. Get the consumer involved in making the change

7. Know who the powerful individuals or groups are, who can help with the change
8. Communicate
9. Reshape your performance measures
10. Use anything that will help to effect the change (rewards, technology, etc.)
11. Encourage and generate big and creative ideas
12. Encourage the use of diverse populations of staff who may be able to see the issues differently
13. Build skills
14. Make sure that the plan addresses all the major issues
15. Balance creative initiatives with focused strategies

The APN has the knowledge, competence, and motivation to plan complete change (Oates, 1997), and is also in a position to notice opportunities to improve a structure, process, or outcome (Hansen, 1999). APNs are often in positions that Hansen refers to as "boundary spanning" and are able to communicate to a variety of people. Change that is best suited for the APN will occur at the case level and will have an effect on patient outcomes, cost, and quality of care. Therefore, APNs should be encouraged to position themselves to make changes in delivery of care to the chronically ill and to underserved and vulnerable populations.

APNs must perfect the skills of organizational politics, interpersonal influence, group leadership and decision making, collaboration and conflict management, systems thinking, quality improvement, and program planning and management. To ensure that APNs have the knowledge and skill sets necessary to influence change, graduate nursing curriculums must address the topics that will prepare the APN as a change agent in areas such as systems analysis, budget, and business management.

Consultation

The consulting activities of the APN are well documented in the literature (Noll, 1987; Broom, Shirk, Pehrson, & Peterson, 2008). The APN's consultation role is often referred to in the Magnetism Force 8 (Consultation and Resources), which addresses the influence of clinical experts on patient outcomes (ANCC, 2008; Broom et al., 2008). An APN may be an internal (inside the organization) or external (outside the organization) consultant. Generally an internal consultant has been hired to manage ongoing issues (i.e., specific client populations) that have a high prevalence or require long-term management. Edlund et al. (1987) describe several advantages and disadvantages to both types of consulting.

The advantages of the internal consultant are that they are less likely to be viewed by staff as an agent of administration; they know the system's issues better than an external consultant would; and they function better in a client consultation because of availability and follow-up. In contrast to this position, Lippitt and Lippitt (1978) believe that an internal consultant is viewed by staff as being subordinate to administration and is therefore viewed as an agent of administration. Edlund et al. (1987) do note that the internal consultant is more likely to be perceived as having less ability, credibility, and power (i.e., they are not viewed as expert in their own backyard). In practice, this author has found that the day-to-day presence of an internal consultant can reinforce certain practices, ensure the consultant's availability to manage changes, and provide immediate alternatives. If an internal consultant is perceived as being limited in authority and ability, it may be more an issue of the person than the position.

An external consultant is often perceived as having greater administrative sanction, more knowledge, easier access to information sources, and fewer preconceived ideas about a situation. They can often provide the impetus for change and, because they have no long-term investment, they can be the "scapegoat" of staff anxieties about the change, which shields the permanent administration from the rancor (Harris, 1995). Limitations are that the external consultant must gain the trust of staff, spend substantial time acquiring knowledge about the system, and may still have diminished long-term effects, especially in a client or consultee consultation (Edlund et al., 1987). It is also difficult involving an external consultant in direct client care in that there is not the staff interface or day-to-day follow-up. If an APN provides external consultation on client care (for example, at a workshop), it may be practical and wise to contract for an assessment opportunity to review the clinical setting and a post-education practicum with staff to model care expectations.

As possibly the best of all alternatives, Ulschak and SnowAntel (1990) suggest that the internal and external consultants work together. To utilize this approach, the external consultant should give the internal consultant plenty of opportunities to participate in the planning, implementation, and education process. The external consultant should work to enhance the organization's perception of the internal consultant's expertise and authority. This approach definitely increases the probability of long-term impact.

Certainly consultation could be considered a primary vehicle for the dissemination of an APN's expertise. Caplan (1970) notes that consultation can be described by the type of client served, the type of activities requested in the consultation, the method of consultation (formal or informal) provided, and the relationship of the consultant to the organization (internal or external). Consultation is categorized in four ways: (1) client-centered case consultation; (2) consultee-centered case consultation; (3) program-centered administrative consultation; and (4) consultee-centered administrative consultation.

Consultation requires much planning prior to the actual consultation meeting. Lippitt and Lippitt (1978) provide a six-phase guide that has been utilized in a variety of consultation situations: (1) contact and entry; (2) formulating a contract and establishing a helping relationship; (3) problem identification and diagnostic analysis; (4) goal-setting and planning; (5) taking action and cycling feedback; and (6) contract completion, continuity, support, and termination.

In APN practice, Caplan's client-centered consultation often uses an informal approach in Phases 1 and 2 because of the casual nature and frequency of this type of consult in nurse-to-APN interaction. Although this informal approach can be educational and save time, Manian and Janssen (1996) warn that the consultant and client's care can be vulnerable to incomplete information and examination, especially if the consult is of a complex nature. It is always important to establish areas of responsibility for the consultant and consultee. The APN who elects to function as a consultant must respect the confines of a consultant's practice and the authority that role assigns to others.

Consultation is a function into which the individual APN must evolve. It is based on the APN's knowledge, experience, and confidence. The beginning APN will generally first serve in the area of direct practice and client-centered consultations. Holt (1984) describes an evolution of development with many of the areas of consultation occurring much later in the professional development of the APN. Certainly, the beginning APN will need time in the application of newly acquired skills to be recognized as competent by others and to develop the personal confidence to provide expert consultation.

How the APN consultant evolves will depend on the definition and parameters of the client group, the framework of the consultant's practice, and the inherent rewards for maintaining consultation as part of the APN practice. Over time, consultation should demonstrate growth, diversity, and mentorship as the practice is refined.

In the early years of practice, an APN may choose to remain in a consultation area in which the parameters are those of a defined client group with specific known problems. The APN should always retain this client-oriented consultation because it is a way to gain and explore new knowledge and a mechanism for implementing evidence-based practice. However, as the consultant's practice evolves, the definition of "client" should change to represent groups of patients, staff, or organizations. This evolution is both economical and growth-producing. The consultant should ask these questions:

1. What is needed?
2. Why is it needed? (What has happened or changed that created the need?)
3. What has been tried?
4. What outcome is desired?
5. What outcome is reasonable?
6. What is the time frame?
7. What are the obstacles to and resources for achieving the outcome?
8. What areas and options of change are comfortable or uncomfortable?
9. Who is important to the process?
10. What are the limits or boundaries of the consultation?

The APN should take the following steps in preparing for a consultation.

1. *Become familiar with the client, organization, and environment.* This can be accomplished by reading the philosophy statements, procedures, and models of care of the organization, and by getting descriptions of the locale and other demographics. In client care, the consultant might explore a client's finances, environment, etc., to ensure a realistic plan of care that the client is likely to accomplish (Larson, Risor, & Putnam, 1997).
2. *Identify a primary contact in the organization.* Then ensure that the contact has the ability to access needed information and has the authority to carry out the recommendations. If there are other parties involved, these persons should be identified. There

are no greater obstacles to a plan than persons who have been left out of the process.

3. *Be honest about the consultant role and the expectations about what is to be accomplished.* Know whether recommendations are to be treated as suggestions or mandates. State your limitations as a consultant whether these are due to expertise, conflicts of interest, or administrative restrictions. Stay within the confines of what has been requested. If other issues are identified, these can be noted if they affect the area of the consult, but they should not be acted on unless they are acceptable to the consultee.

4. *Allow adequate time to accomplish the work required for the consultation.* In client-based consultation, allow at least 1 to 2 hours for the initial visit. Subsequent follow-up can be shortened to 5 to 15 minutes. Consultation to an organization will vary in time, depending on the size and complexity of the organization and its issues. Time should be allotted for preparation and evaluation as well as the actual visit.

5. *Know why the consult was requested and whether it is related to a need for change.* Continue to keep the client focused on a defined area.

6. *Respect the client and consultee.* Their knowledge of the problem and their ideas for practical solutions are essential for accomplishing the recommendations.

7. *Know when to leave.* There are two reasons for leaving: (1) completion of the consult and (2) disregard for the recommendations. If your recommendations are not followed and if a comfortable compromise is not reached, the consultant can be of no value and should terminate the contract. On the other hand, in many cases the clients embrace the recommendations and function well with them. The best consultation outcomes occur when consultants hear their own recommendations being verbalized by the client who is expressing a sense of ownership. This is the best of all changes that can be made by a consultant and is evidence of completion.

Depending on the type of consultation, the consultant can behave in a variety of ways. Lippitt and Lippitt (1978) describe a continuum of consultant behaviors that require the consultant to be more directive or more nondirective. The consultant assumes a greater leadership role when a more directive behavior is needed. Lippitt and Lippitt's eight consultant behaviors are (1) objective observer/reflector; (2) process counselor; (3) fact finder; (4) alternative identifier; (5) linker, joint problem solver; (6) trainer education; (7) information expert; and (8) advocator. The consultant's directive behavior increases as the latter behaviors are used more frequently.

The use of the intervention model developed by McEvoy and Egan (1979) is a very effective framework for developing the consultant's practice. This model helps the consultant identify commonalities of a population and test interventions to promote reliable outcomes. In doing this, a consultant can move from the client/consultee-specific practice to the more group-related model of practice that we see in program development and administration-centered consultation. The intervention model provides a systematic way for the consultant to collect and analyze information while looking for characteristics and trends about the population.

Meyer et al. (1996) reviewed the use of consultation expertise when it was applied to a computerized program that would ask the nurse questions regarding a clinical issue. In this system (the urological nursing information system, or UNIS), the program was placed in a nursing facility and compared with the actual consultant practitioner. On initial evaluation, the UNIS asked more questions and had more recommendations than the actual practitioner. However, on retrospective analysis, there were clear limitations with the UNIS. Therefore, an analyst followed an APN during consultation in an effort to understand the consultation process and eventually modify the program. It was discovered that the problem was that UNIS had to ask many more questions and nurses were its only data source. This differed from the APN consultant who used multiple sources. Also, the use of rule-changing for interfacing and the inability to interface with the patient record limited the UNIS. It was believed that eventually these issues could be corrected. However, it is questionable whether information procured through multiple levels of nursing staff and without direct examination of the patient can accurately replace the assessment, diagnosis, and intervention planning of the APN consultant. The APN needs to be vigilant about the development of these types of systems. Questions of accountability and the impact on nursing practice without a licensed practitioner should be explored to ensure integrity of the nursing profession, reliable content, and patient safety.

Because of the APN's unique role, knowledge, and position of influence, the APN has many issues of ethical boundaries and power about which it must be responsible and cognizant. Lippitt and Lippitt (1978) provide a code of ethics for the professional consultant that requires that the consultant have objectivity and integrity, competence to do the work, adherence to moral and legal standards, avoidance of misrepresentation, confidentiality, primary concern for the client's welfare, adherence to professional rather than economic standards, integrity in interpersonal relationships, fair remuneration, respect for the rights and reputation of the organization, and accurate promotional activities.

The issue of the power available to the consultant is also a concern. Van Bree Sneed (1991) states that the consultant's power is legitimate (power of the position held), referent (based on personality), and expert (based on the possession of special knowledge and skills). With this power comes responsibility, and the APN should consider the following issues carefully.

1. Respecting the fact that power places the consultant–client in an unequal relationship
2. Understanding that the consultant's knowledge has a limited scope
3. Resisting the practice of withholding information with the intention of creating dependency
4. Being honest in the presentation of your abilities and limitations
5. Expecting the aura of influence generated by consultants and avoiding its misuse
6. Working to ensure a balance with regard to the client's perception of that power by providing positive reinforcement to the client

The consultant must remain vigilant in other areas as well. When they are in a consulting role, consultants should not push their personal opinions, beliefs, values, or biases upon a client. Also, when working in an organization, the consultant should be careful not to stress ideas that may conflict with the mission or capabilities of that organization. The boundaries of professional and personal conduct should be guarded. If there are potential differences between client and consultant, resolution or clarification should be sought before proceeding. The APN must let go of the information that has been shared in the consultation. There can be a tendency to want to cling to certain turf. Always clarify the reasons for retaining certain professional responsibilities and removing or limiting others.

STRATEGIES FOR IMPLEMENTATION OF APN ROLES

It is critical that APNs be familiar with any organization with which they interact. Ulschak and SnowAntel (1990) describe a CPR+F model representing the organization's purpose, roles, feedback in communication, and commitment with the organization's environment (trends, regulatory bodies, licensing groups, vendors, and professional groups), which encompass the entire model. Using this model, the APN can look at the culture of the organization and better understand its elements. The APN should be familiar with policy, procedure, resources, affiliations, and the structure of the organization's framework in order to market an advanced practice.

The APN also should prepare a written statement of APN capabilities along with fiscal and patient outcome potentials that could be realized through these advanced roles. This can help the administrative team realize the expanded potential of the APN. Because administrators may not be familiar with these capacities, the APN should continue to provide regular updates that extend beyond direct patient care. The APN should outline these capabilities when interviewing for a position and mention the roles that have taken on in regular updates to immediate supervisors. Maintenance of patient outcome statistics will help management advocate and support the APN position. APNs must become more visible on community boards, organizational committees, and in legislative activities to promote the ideas of disease prevention and health care through APN practice. Opportunities for collaboration with academic institutions can also promote an expanded role.

SUMMARY

For the APN to fully participate in these roles, administration needs to be educated about the many aspects of their position and the benefits that accrue to patient care and the institution in supporting expanded APN practice. The APN should initially market these capabilities to many groups of people from management to legislators. Although providing direct patient care is valuable and rewarding, the APN can continue to evolve and actually have greater impact in patient care, community and social health, and the development of nursing as a profession by pursuing advanced APN roles. Whether she works as part of a practice or in a separate position, the opportunity to function in these advanced roles will give the APN personal satisfaction, enhance the care of patients, and contribute to the profession of nursing.

Acknowledgment

The author acknowledges the contributions of Deborah Moniken who contributed to this chapter in a previous edition.

REFERENCES

Abdellah, L, Fawcett, J., Kane, R., Dick, K., & Chen, J. (2005). The development and psychometric testing of the Evercare Nurse Practitioner Role and Activity Scale (ENPRAS). *Journal of the American Academy of Nurse Practitioners, 17*(1), 21–26.

American Nurses Credentialing Center (ANCC). (2008). Magnet recognition program application. Silver Springs, MD: ANA.

Anderson, D., & Ackerman Anderson, L. (2001). *Beyond change management. Advanced strategies for today's transformational leaders.* San Francisco: Jossey-Bass/Pfeiffer.

Barker, A. M. (1990). *Transformational nursing leadership: A vision for the future.* Baltimore: Williams and Wilkins.

Benoit, B. C. (1996). Case management and the advanced practice nurse. In J. Hickey, R.Ouimette, & S. Venegoni (Eds.). *Advanced practice nursing. Changing roles and clinical application* (pp. 107–125). Philadelphia: Lippincott.

Bloom, B. S. (Ed.). (1956). *Taxonomy of educational objectives.* New York: David McKay.

Broom, C., Shirk, M. J., Pehrson, K. M., & Peterson, K. (2008). Perspectives on psychiatric consultation liaison nursing. *Perspectives in Psychiatric Care, 44*(2), 131–134.

Caplan, G. (1970). *The theory and practice of mental health consultation.* New York: Basic Books.

Coffman, S. (2001). Examining advocacy and care management in managed care. *Pediatric Nursing, 23*(3), 287–289, 304.

Donagrandi, M. A., & Eddy, M. (2000). Ethics of case management: Implications for advanced practice nursing. *Clinical Nurse Specialist, 14*(5). 241–246.

Driver, J., & Campbell, J. (2000). An evaluation of the impact of lecture practitioners on learning. *British Journal of Nursing, 9*(5), 293–300.

Edlund, B., Hodges, L., & Poteet, G. (1987). Consultation: Doing it and doing it well. *Clinical Nurse Specialist, 1*(2), 86–90.

Freed, D. (1998). Please don't shoot me: I'm only the change agent. *Health Care Supervisor, 17*(1), 56–61.

Hansen, H. (1999). The advanced practice nurse as change agent. In M. Snyder & M. Mirr (Eds.). *Advanced practice nursing: A guide to professional development* (2nd ed., pp. 187–205). New York: Springer Publishing Company.

Harris, M. (1995).Consultants. An administrator's report. *Journal of Nursing Administration, 25*(7/8), 12–14.

Holt, F. (1984). A theoretical model for clinical specialist practice. *Nursing and Health Care, 5,* 445–449.

Kaluzny, A. D., & Hernandez, S. R. (1988). Organizational change and innovation. In S. M. Shortell & A.D. Kaluzny (Eds.). *Health care management: A text in organizational theory and behavior* (2nd ed., pp. 374–417). Albany, NY: Delmar.

Knowles, M. S., & Associates (1984). *Androgogy in action.* San Francisco: Jossey-Bass.

Larson, J., Risor, O., & Putnam, S. (1997). P-R-A-C-T-I-C-A-L: a step-by-step model for conducting the consultation in general practice. *Family Practice, 14,* 295–301.

Lewin, K. (1951). *Field theory in social science.* New York: Harper and Row.

Lippitt, G., & Lippitt, R. (1978). *The consulting process in action.* LaJolla, CA: University Associates.

Manian, F., & Janssen, D. (1996). Curbside consultation. A closer look at a common practice. *Journal of the American Medical Association, 275* (2), 145–147.

McEvoy, M., & Egan, E. (1979). The process of developing a nursing intervention model. *Journal of Nursing Education, 18*(4), 19–25.

McPhail, G. (1997). Management of change: An essential skill in nursing in the 1990s. *Journal of Nursing Management, 5,* 199–205.

Meyer, K., Sather-Levine, B., Lauvent-Bopp, D., Gruenewold, D., Nichol, P., & Kimmerle, M. (1996). The impact of clinical information systems research of advanced practice nursing. *Advanced Practice Nursing Quarterly, 2*(3), 58–64.

Murphy, F. (2000). Collaborating with the practitioners in teaching and research: A model for developing the role of the nurse lecturer in a practice area. *Journal of Advanced Nursing, 31*(3), 704–714.

National Organization of Clinical Nurse Specialists. (2004). *Statement on clinical nurse specialist practice and education.* Harrisburg, PA: Author.

Nelson, M. (1998). Advocacy. In M. Snyder & R. Lundquist (Eds.), *Complimentary/alternative therapies in nursing* (3rd ed., pp. 337–352). New York: Springer Publishing.

Nelson, M. (1999).Client Advocacy. In M. Snyder and M. Mirr (Eds.), *Advanced practice nursing: A guide to professional development* (2nd ed., pp. 235–253). New York: Springer Publishing.

Newman, M. (1994). *Health as expanding consciousness* (2nd ed.). New York: National League for Nursing Press.

Oates, K. (1997). Models of planned change and research utilization applied to product evaluation. *Clinical Nurse Specialist, 11*(6), 270–273.

Pinch, W. J. (1996). Ethical issues in case management. In D.L. Flarey & S.S. Blancett (Eds.), *Handbook of nursing case management: Health care delivery in world of managed care* (pp. 443–460). Gaithersburg, MD: Aspen Publishers.

Price Waterhouse Change Integration Team. (1995). *Better change. Best practices for transforming your organization.* Chicago: Irwin Professional Publishing.

Sparks, R. K (1999).The APN as educator. In M. Snyder & M Mirr (Eds.), *Advanced practice nursing: A guide to professional development* (2nd ed., pp. 119–134). New York: Springer Publishing.

Taylor, P. (1999). Comprehensive nursing case management. An advanced practice model. *Nursing Case Management, 4*(1), 2–9.

Umberell, C. E. (2006). Trauma case management: A role for the advanced practice nurse. *Journal of Trauma Nursing, 13*(2), 70–73.

Upshaw, R., & Snow-Ante, S. (1990). *Consultation skills for health care professionals.* San Francisco: Jossey-Bass.

Van Bree Sneed, N. (1991). Power: Its use and potential for misuse by nurse consultants. *Clinical Nurse Specialist, 5*(1), 58–62.

Watson, J. (1989). Transformative thinking and a caring curriculum. In E. O. Bevis & J. Watson, (Eds.), *Toward a caring curriculum: A new pedagogy for nursing.* New York: National League for Nursing.

Wheatley, M. J. (1992). *Leadership and the new science: Learning about organization from an orderly universe.* San Francisco: Barrett-Kohler.

The Role of Organizations in Advanced Practice Nursing

MARY ZWYGART-STAUFFACHER

INTRODUCTION

The U.S. health care system has undergone innumerable changes during the last few decades. These changes have required the advanced practice nurse (APN) not only to be clinically competent, but also to have an understanding of the organizations in which care is presently being delivered. The APN must also have knowledge and ability to create the systems of care that will ensure the high-quality and cost-effective care needed in the future.

The economics of health care have become increasingly complex. In an attempt to achieve cost efficiencies, merging health care organizations have given birth to giant health care corporations. However, the goal of demonstrated cost savings has not necessarily been consistently and nationally achieved. This is evidenced by ever-increasing health care costs and the percentage of the national budget being spent on health care today, with less than ideal outcomes for all citizens (Levit et al., 2003; National Center for Health Statistics, 2006).

THE U.S. HEALTH CARE SYSTEM

Health care delivery systems in the United States are unlike those of any other country in the world. Although most other developed countries have national health insurance programs run by governments and financed through general taxes, so that almost all citizens are entitled to receive health care, the United States does not. The U.S. health care delivery system is not in fact a system in the true sense, even though it is commonly referred to in that way. Its central feature perhaps is that it is unnecessarily fragmented (Shortell et al., 1996).

In truth, the U.S. health care system is comprised of multiple types of organizations, complicated by innumerable governmental and private funding and payment sources. These payment sources, such as third-party reimbursement (for example: insurance and Medicaid) can vary from state to state and region to region of the country. For instance, the federal government does specify overall coverage requirements for the Medicaid program, although individual states have substantial autonomy in the depth and breadth of services for several diagnoses, such as treatments for infertility or family planning.

There also are no national requirements for private health insurance. Again, insurance coverage varies greatly from plan to plan, state to state, and region to region. A major insurance provider may include a certain type or degree of coverage in one enrollee's existing plan, but that does not mean such coverage will be included in the plan offered to another employee in the same company in another state or in a plan offered by another employer. Not only does this affect the APN's personal coverage, it is an extraordinarily complex maze to address.

There is convincing evidence that health insurance coverage improves access and quality of health and medical care, contributing to the overall health of individuals and their families. According to 2005 data from the National Ambulatory Medical Care Survey and the National Hospital Ambulatory Care Survey (Centers for Disease Control, 2009), it has been found that

- In emergency departments, the visit rate for patients with no insurance was about twice that of those with private insurance.
- Conversely, the number patient visits to physician's offices was higher for individuals with private health insurance compared to those with no insurance.

More and more U.S. citizens are uninsured or underinsured, presenting even greater challenges in ensuring that health care is available to all. In 2006, 43.6 million Americans, or 14.8% of the U.S. population, were underinsured or uninsured, including working-age adults (those aged 18–64); in 2006, 19.8% of Americans did not have health insurance, which was an increase in the percentage of uninsured from 18.9% the year before. Approximately 9.3% of children under the age of 18 did not have health insurance in 2006 (CDC, 2009; Barnes & Schiller, 2007).

Even more striking is the inequity of coverage based on race and ethnicity, with higher rates of uninsured and underinsured for Hispanics and African-Americans than for non-Hispanic whites. Uninsured persons are defined as persons without private health insurance, Medicare, Medicaid, State Children's Health Insurance Program (SCHIP) coverage, a state-sponsored or other government-sponsored health plan, or a military plan. Also included among the underinsured and uninsured are persons who have only Indian Health Service coverage or a private plan that pays for only one type of service, such as accidents or dental care. (CDC, 2009).

The complexities of the various systems of care—which include nonprofit and proprietary organizations; large and small corporations; local, regional, and worldwide conglomerates; small and multisystem plans; multistate health care systems and payment mechanisms; and regulatory requirements—can be overwhelming to the new APN. Few nurses have a strong background or experience in the organizational influences of health care. Content on the complexity of health care coverage has historically been minimal in nursing undergraduate education. This knowledge deficit is compounded by the fact that most nurses have limited experience with the organizational dimensions of health care coverage while they are employed as staff nurses (Ladden et al., 2006).

Organizational Influences

How does an understanding of these organizational influences affect the APN's roles and functions? Many factors are involved, and these influences can clearly change during the tenure of the APN's career. A beginning APN needs to understand these organizations when selecting future employment and providing care to clients. As APNs become more confident in their role as care providers, they can expand their role as change agents and influence their organizations. To do so requires enhanced knowledge and skills in organizational design, systems, function, and complexity. Therefore, advanced knowledge in such fields as organizational behavior, cost analysis, risk management, patient satisfaction, safety, and quality are necessary to fully implement the role of the APN. To ensure that the APN is on the forefront of new and innovative care delivery practices, an understanding of the health care systems and organizations that are and should be in place where the APN practices is a needed prerequisite.

Even though these rapidly changing health care systems settings are ripe for innovation, the APN may find it a daunting task to understand and negotiate them. Traditionally educated to provide advanced nursing more closely aligned to a specific system or setting of care, the APN is now faced with the challenge of a multisystem arena for care delivery. Understanding system issues has been identified as a necessary component of graduate education for nurse administrators and APNs for many years, but the recommendation has not been fully embraced. As early as 1988, Lynn, Layman, and Englebardt (1998) identified the importance of incorporating such topics as leadership, financial management polices, health policy, and organizational culture and structure into course content in advanced practice educations programs.

The American Association of College Nurses (ACCN) *Essentials of Master's Education for Advanced Practice Nursing* (AACN, 2009) identifies policy, organization, and financing of health care as core curricular content. In this environment of ongoing changes in the organization and financing of health care, this document asserts that it is imperative that all graduates of master's degree nursing programs have a keen understanding of health care policy, organization, and financing of health care. The purpose of this content is to prepare a graduate to provide quality cost-effective care, to participate in the design and implementation of care in a variety of health care systems, and to assume a leadership role in managing human, fiscal, and physical health care resources. The recently developed AACN *Essentials for the Doctor of Nursing Practice* identifies the need to expand these content areas even more fully in doctor of nursing practice (DNP) programs.

Analysis of Organizations

For the new APN, understanding health care organizations is vital in determining the most appropriate place or setting for employment. The ability to understand an organization is based on several factors. APNs should ask such questions as

- What is the organizational structure of the organization?
- What is the philosophical underpinning of the organization?
- What are the directions and goals of the organization?
- What are the culture and climate of the organization?

Organizational structure is one dimension that is important to understand. Historically, health care organizations have been structured in the more traditional hierarchical and bureaucratic organizational models. Many experts in organizational functioning believe that these traditional models will no longer work in the emerging health care arena. They have proposed that the new models needs to be flat, innovative, nimble, and responsive to change. The health care organizations that will survive in the frenetic pace of today's world will promote greater flexibility and have the ability to deal with ambiguity and uncertainty (Porter-O'Grady & Malloch, 2007).

The APN should evaluate the structure of the organization and how it will influence their ability to provide care and perform the various aspects of the APN role. For instance, organizational structure clearly affects communication in a health care system and influences how and by whom decisions are made. The APN should identify how many layers of the organization lie between the APN and the person or persons who are responsible for making decisions that will affect the APN's clinical decisions, the latitude of the APN's daily practice, and the costs of care related to patient care. The APN should understand the "official" organizational structure and recognize the "informal" lines of communication and decision-making networks.

Every organization has different philosophical underpinnings that frame the organization's direction for the future and give the APN insight into how decisions will be made. An organization's mission, vision, values, philosophy, and organizational objectives are important. The mission of the organization describes the purpose for which that organization exists. The mission statement provides valuable information about the organization's direction and goals for the future. Mission statements allow the reader to understand what is meaningful to the organization, how that meaning may be measured, and clearly define the organization's reason for existing. They can also lead to an enhanced understanding of the ethics, principles, and standards for which the employees will be held accountable (Danna, 2009).

Mission statements should provide vision for the organization. The vision should be an image of the future, while value statements should bond people and set behavioral standards in the organization. The philosophy of the organization outlines values, concepts, and beliefs that establish the organization's care practices. Mission and vision statements can help a prospective employee understand the value placed on the clients and workers in an organization. Having a clear understanding of these foundational aspects of an organization can help inform the APN about an agency's present and future goals and expected outcomes. For instance, an APN who has a strong belief in providing care to all people regardless of their ability to pay, or a strong belief in a certain ethical orientation, is wise to identify that the organization they are considering has values that are consistent with that person's belief system. Simply hoping that an organization promotes the same level of quality care that the individual APN aspires to give or believing that all organizations are the same is naïve and will affect whether the APN will survive or strive in the practice setting.

A common method of analyzing health care organizations is to utilize a systems theory approach. The health care organization is considered an open system; it has permeable boundaries that are affected by the society in which it operates. Change in society forces internal change in the operation of an organization. The rapidity with which these changes have occurred recently is responsible for the chaotic situations in which many health care practitioners and administrators operate today (Yoder-Wise, 2006). Due to the extraordinary complexity of these health care systems, an emerging field of science has been suggested as an alternative approach to understanding them (Plsek, 1999). This emerging field, termed complexity science, offers alternative leadership and management strategies for the chaotic, complex health care environment.

One method to evaluate an organization is to examine an organization's outcomes or its "organizational effectiveness." Danna (2009) provides a helpful listing of indicators to monitor organizational effectiveness. Those indicators include patient satisfaction with care; family satisfaction with care; staff satisfaction with work; staff satisfaction with rewards, intrinsic and extrinsic; staff satisfaction with professional development; staff satisfaction with organization; management's satisfaction with staff, community relationships; and organizational health. A malfunctioning organization would be reflected by such elements as focusing on the wrong elements of the operation, having too many meetings attended by too many people accomplishing little work, and having too many levels of administration, to name a few.

Healthy environments support meaningful work and provide an environment in which the APN can excel and feel an important part of the team. The American Organization of Nurse Executives (AONE, 2009) has identified six critical factors to improve workplace initiatives, extracted from a study of workplace implementation and innovation. These factors are leadership development; empowered collaborative decision making; work design and service delivery innovation; a values-focused organizational culture; recognition and rewards systems; and professional growth and accountability.

Organizational Climate and Culture

All health care organizations have a climate and culture. Climate is described as the emotional states, feelings, and perceptions shared by the members of the organization. Climate can be described by such terms as positive or negative, hopeful or negative, trusting or suspicious, and competitive or nurturing. The APN can influence the climate or be influenced by it. Climate can influence interactions and responses by patients and co-workers alike. It is a component of job satisfaction and enjoyment in one's work life. An organizational climate that is inconsistent with an APN's preferred orientation can cause dissatisfaction and limit the ability to excel. However, the seasoned APN can be pivotal in establishing the day-to-day climate in the practice setting.

An organization's social system, including its beliefs, norms, mission, philosophies, traditions, and values, make up an organization's culture. It represents the perspectives, values, assumptions, language, and behaviors that have been effectively used by the members of the organization. Culture influences the formal and informal methods and styles of communication. When considering employment in an organization, an APN should assess the culture and climate of an organization to assess whether it is an appropriate fit. The APN may wish to practice with a specific population or within a specialty area. However, without an appreciation of the organization's climate and culture, they may be unable to implement the changes and level of care they hope to provide. Finding an organization that is consistent with the preferences of the APN's preferred culture and climate can provide a solid and more comfortable practice arena for an individual practitioner.

The Culture of Safety and Quality

Beginning in the 1980s and continuing with increased emphasis during the past decade, there has been a nationwide agenda to address the culture of safety and quality in health care organizations. National health care quality accreditation and regulatory agencies have taken major steps to enhance quality and safety by identifying evidence-based best practices and encouraging measurement and monitoring of these practices and care outcomes. The Joint Commission on the Accreditation of Health Care Organizations (JCAHO), the Institute of Medicine (IOM), the Agency of Healthcare Research and Quality (AHRQ), the Centers of Medicare and Medicaid Services (CMS) of the U.S. Department of Health and Human Services (HHS) are just a few of the many organizations and agencies focused on enhancing health care quality and safety.

The IOM has identified safety concerns and problems with quality of care. It defines quality as "the degree to which health services for individuals and populations increase the likelihood of desired health outcomes and are consistent with current professional knowledge" (IOM, 2001).

A series of IOM reports help to illustrate how wide the quality chasm is and how important it is to close the gulf between our standards of high-quality care and the prevailing norm in practice. Two landmark reports released by the IOM, *To Err is Human: Building a Safer Health System* (1999) and *Crossing the Quality Chasm: A New Health System for the 21st Century* (2001), moved the national dialogue, asserting that reform is not accomplished by simply addressing the issues around its margins. The third phase of the IOM's *Quality Initiative* is currently in process and focuses on making the vision of a future health system described in the *Quality Chasm* report a reality.

The overall goal for the Quality and Safety Education for Nurses (QSEN) project (2009) is to meet the challenge of preparing future nurses who will have the knowledge, skills, and attitudes (KSAs) necessary to continuously improve the quality and safety of the health care systems in which they work.

Using the IOM (2003) competencies, QSEN faculty and a national advisory board have defined quality and safety competencies for nursing and proposed targets for the knowledge, skills, and attitudes to be developed in nursing prelicensure programs for each competency. These competencies serve as a guide to curricular development for formal academic programs, transition to practice, and continuing education programs (Bargagliotti & Lancaster, 2007; Cronenwett et al., 2007). QSEN is now developing standards that will assist APNs in understanding and measuring quality of care they should provide.

CMS launched their initiatives to develop quality measures of nursing homes, home care agencies, and hospitals following the Office of Budget Reconciliation Act (OBRA) 1987 nursing home reform legislation. One approach was to provide the consumer with information on the quality of agencies that are the recipients of federal monies. These measures found on the CMS website provide easy-to-read data regarding care practices, staffing, and costs. The APN should be aware of these outcome measures when considering a place of employment and use them as a mechanism to monitor the quality of services provided by their organization. There are now innumerable quality and safety initiatives nationwide, and astute APNs will understand what is occurring in their place of employment and will help to shape its practices to enhance quality.

SUMMARY

The APN of today and tomorrow will need to address organizational and system issues. Although it may seem daunting in our changing health care landscape, APNs must develop the knowledge to analyze organizational variables and the skills and abilities to enhance quality and safety. The APN must be a change agent instrumental in creating the care delivery systems that will be needed in the future.

REFERENCES

American Association of Colleges of Nursing (AACN). (2009). www.aacn.nche.edu/

American Association of Nurse Executives. (2009). www.aone.org

Bargagliotti, L, & Lancaster, J. (2007). Quality and safety education in nursing: More than new wine in old skins. *Nursing Outlook, 55* (3), 156–158.

Barnes, P., & Schiller J. (2007). Early release of selected estimates based on data from the 2006 National Health Interview Survey. Washington: National Center for Health Statistics.

Centers of Disease Control (CDC). (2009). Retrieved on April 30, 2009, from www.cdc.gov/features/uninsured/health.

Cronenwett, L., Sherwood, G., Barnsteiner, J., Disch, J., Johnson, J., Mitchell, P., et al. (2007). Quality and safety education for nurses. *Nursing Outlook, 55* (3), 122–131.

Danna, D. (2009). Organizational structure and analysis. In L. Roussel. (Ed.). *Management leadership for nurse administrators* (5th ed). Boston: Jones and Bartlett.

Institute of Medicine (IOM). (2003). *Health professions education: A bridge to quality.* Washington DC: National Academies Press.

Institute of Medicine (IOM). (1999). *To Err is human: Building a safer health system.* Washington DC: National Academy Press.

Institute of Medicine (IOM). (2001). *Crossing the quality chasm: A new health system for the 21st century.* Washington DC: National Academy Press.

Ladden, M., Bednash, G., Stevens, D., & Moore, G. (2006). Educating interprofessional learners for quality, safety, and systems improvement. *Journal of Interprofessional Care, 2,* 497–505.

Levit, K., Smith, C., Cowan, C., Lazenby, H., Sensenig, A., & Catlin, A. (2003). Trends in U.S. health care spending. *Health Affairs, 22,* 154–164.

Lynn, M., Layman, E., & Englebardt, S. (1998). Nursing administration research priorities, a national Delphi study. *Journal of Nursing Administration, 15,* 7–11.

National Health Interview Survey. (2006). www.cdc.gov/nchs/data/nhis/earlyrelease

National Center for Health Statistics. (2006). *Health, United States, 2006: With chartbook on trends in the health of Americans.* Hyattsville, MD: Department of Health and Human Services.

Plsek, P. (1999). Innovative thinking for improvement of medical systems. *Annals of Internal Medicine, 131,* 438–444.

Porter-O'Grady, T., & Malloch, K. (2007). *Quantum leadership: A textbook of new leadership.* Sudbury, MA: Jones and Bartlett.

Quality and safety education for nurses. Retrieved April 30, 2009, from www.qsen.org

Shortell, S., Gillies, R., Anderson, D., Erickson, K., & Mitchell, J. (1996). *Remaking health care in America: Building organized delivery systems.* San Francisco: Jossey-Bass.

Yoder-Wise, P. (2006). *Leading and managing in nursing.* St Louis: Mosby.

5

Leadership Competencies for APNs: Challenges and Opportunities

JANET WESSEL KREJCI
SHELLY MALIN

INTRODUCTION

Advanced practice nurses (APNs) can be the difference between chaos and quality in today's complex health care system if—and only if—they develop leadership competencies for the current environment. The revolutionary advances in technology, pharmaceutical research, and surgical innovations, coupled with organizational complexities created by competition for resources, present unprecedented challenges as well as opportunities for APNs. In the midst of these advances, however, something else is clear: The sobering unintended consequences of a complex, highly regulated, and yet fragmented system, first identified by the Institute of Medicine (IOM) almost 10 years ago (IOM, 1999, 2001, 2004), have not yet been solved. At a time when cloning of a human is possible, ensuring the basics, such as hand-washing for all providers or accurate patient identification, remains elusive. APNs have incredible opportunities, but they still face obstacles related to the hierarchy of the health care system that have plagued nurses for decades. According to O'Neil et al. (2008), if the persons instrumental in health care outcomes do not commit to a deep investment in leadership development, the future of health care is at risk.

This chapter will emphasize the importance of leadership competencies for APNs who have major responsibilities for delivery of quality care, evidence-based practice, patient safety, and innovations in nursing practice. Different leadership development models and curricula related to leadership in doctorate of nursing practice (DNP) programs will be explored. Application of leadership competencies to specific scenarios common to APNs will also be presented.

RECENT CHANGES INFLUENCING THE APN ROLE

Those practicing in APN roles are aware of major changes both in practice and in educational requirements. In 2004, the American Association of Colleges of Nursing decided that the credential necessary to perform the APN role will be the doctor of nursing practice (DNP) beginning in 2015, which will affect credentialing and educational preparation in the future (AACN, 2006). The role of the APN in the practice setting is also changing. In the last decade, the influence of the APN has been expanding exponentially as the evidence related to APNs' influence on positive patient outcomes builds (Brooten et al., 2004, 2005; Burns & Earven, 2003; Cunningham, 2004; Gawlinski et al., 2001; Kleinpell, 2007; Larkin, 2003; Lenz et al., 2004; Russell et al., 2002). More APNs are responsible for outcomes and providing care at academic health centers, acute care facilities, primary care facilities, and specialty clinics and in rural areas. At a time when over 40 million people are uninsured in the United States and clear disparities exist for minority populations, costs are skyrocketing, reimbursement is dropping, and health care providers are scrambling to protect their compensation (IOM, 2004).

What does all this mean for APNs who are working in a variety of settings with increasing responsibilities, whether as a clinical nurse specialist (CNS) or as a direct-care provider nurse practitioner (NP)? In order to be successful in today's complex and political health care system, APNs cannot rely solely on their expertise in practice or naïve optimism about collaboration and cooperation. As the American Association of Colleges of Nursing indicated, one of the reasons for the move to requiring a DNP was to prepare APNs with a blend of "clinical, organizational, economic and leadership skills" because of the complexity they face in trying to influence patient outcomes (AACN, 2006). Although great strides have been made in APN licensure, recognition, and reimbursement (Pearson, 2004), patients are still at risk for losing the best of what APNs offer unless those APNs develop skills, knowledge, and competencies, not only in clinical practice but in leadership as well.

Senge (1990; Senge et al., 1994) has articulated that the systematic structure of any organization (e.g., the incentives, interdependencies, policies, and group norms) provides the context in which all behavior, relationships, and outcomes result. We believe that understanding and mastering this context, and developing the *competencies to lead* in complex health environments is as, or more, important for APNs than any other clinical competency they might develop. Additionally, we propose that at present this competency is, at best, not effectively nurtured in either education or practice settings and, at worst, it is undermined. For these reasons, historical influences, along with leadership models, will be explored, including the DNP curriculum with a sampling of programs related to leadership, and recommendations for obtaining leadership competencies for APNs will be made.

THE INFLUENCE OF HISTORY

In order to successfully progress into the future, it is imperative to understand the historical context of nursing, which has influenced the present state of the profession as well as the role of the APN as a leader. Nursing's history has resulted in both a light and shadow side of nursing (Ashley, 1979; Roberts, 1983, 2005; Nightingale, 1946). Two powerful influences of the profession will be highlighted here. The first is the position of power (or lack thereof) that nurses held in the hierarchy of health care systems; the second is the way the profession articulated and lived its philosophy and values, specifically as they contrasted with the philosophy and values of medicine.

Historically, the predominant thinking and design in other industries has influenced the design of hospitals and health care. In the 20th century, the assembly line design was prominent. Most of these industries resembled what Mintzberg would call a "machine bureaucracy," in which roles were clearly delineated with the strategic apex (e.g., the thinkers) of the organization making the decisions and creating the standardized processes that those in the operating core (e.g., the doers) carried out. The place of nursing was clearly in the operating core whereas physicians straddled both spheres, enacting their practice in the operating core but influencing decisions in the strategic apex (Mintzberg, 1983). It is important to recognize that the historical differences in gender in these two professions, nursing being predominantly female and medicine predominantly male, also influenced the alignment within the hospital structure. As Weber poignantly pointed out, once a hierarchical system is in place, it is easier to annihilate it completely than to make any incremental changes in its structure that are long lasting, as those holding power have no incentive to relinquish it and those without power do not have the leverage to obtain it easily (Weber, 1987).

In addition, nurses have always been steadfast in grounding their values, philosophy, and vision in a framework of care (Gordon, Benner, & Noddings, 1996; Reverby, 1987, 2001). Reverby, a philosopher who studied the nursing profession, said that in contrast to medicine, nurses focused on the *duty to care* rather than the *right to care*, whereas medicine understood that in order to fulfill the *duty to care*, they needed to focus on the *right to care*, which necessitated prioritizing protection of their economic viability and their place in the hierarchy where they could influence decisions. It is important to note that the hierarchical positions were influenced, not by differences in inherent contributions to patient care, but by philosophical and political positioning.

APNs AND THE CONCEPT OF POWER

Given this history, philosophy, and values, the concept of power holds ambivalence for many nurses, even APNs. In a graduate course on systems taught by one of the authors, an imagery exercise is conducted on the concept of power (Krejci, 1997). Over the years, images of power experienced in this exercise continue to include negative militaristic, violent, and/or hierarchical images. APNs are sometimes ambivalent about the concept of power, given how they may have experienced or witnessed the use of power throughout their nursing career. The imagery exercise mentioned also includes a question: "Who wants to be powerful?" Many are tentative about raising their hands, and those who do admit that they were hesitant because the desire for power seemed to conflict with the prototype of an expert nurse committed to patient care. Although, in response to the next question, "Who wants to avoid being powerless?" everyone raises their hand. This is a dilemma; APNs resent powerlessness and yet are ambivalent about wanting to be powerful. Although many arguments could be made related to the word *power* and its meaning, it is not coincidental that this ambivalence exists, given our history and our values, contrasted with a health care system that is clearly traditional and hierarchical. In contrast, when this imagery exercise is held with a predominantly male audience, almost all participants raise their hands in response to the question "Who wants to be powerful?"

For many APNs, the focus on clinical competence and holistic care is paramount as it should be. Unfortunately, without development of leadership competencies and influence at decision-making tables, clinical competence will not be enough to affect care. Although APNs usually clearly believe in and align with Benner's transformational "power with" (2001/1984), they may be uncomfortable making a concerted effort at enhancing the traditional bases of power as articulated in the classic work by French and Raven (1950) and still used today. Nurses tend to rely heavily on their expert power base. Although expert power is crucial, APNs would benefit from developing other bases of power in order to advocate more successfully for their patients.

Nurses by nature strive toward collaboration, often using accommodation as a primary approach to negotiation. Accommodation as a hopeful conduit to collaboration is often a learned approach for women, and nurses use it, often believing it may be the only way to ensure high-quality care for patients, at least in the short term (Valentine, 2001). Unwittingly, they may be creating the very thing they are wishing to avoid, a continual experience of being at what Kritek calls the "uneven table" (2002). The systematic structure in most health care settings does not unfortunately reward the essence of nursing (Fagin, 1993) nor the unique contribution of APNs; rather the system rewards actions and outcomes that facilitate the traditional medical model. This can create a fine line between collaboration and competition, especially for APNs and physicians (Stewart-Amidei, 2003). Consequently, nurses must develop the leadership, negotiation, and system skills needed in order to influence systems that may not be designed to naturally highlight their unique contribution.

LEADERSHIP DEVELOPMENT IN NURSING EDUCATION

Leadership development in nursing became more formally recognized and integrated into education with the advent of programs that awarded the bachelor of science in nursing (BSN) degree. The inclusion of leadership content in the curriculum was indeed one of the hallmarks that distinguished a BSN education. The new *Essentials for Baccalaureate Education* (AACN, 2008), emphasizes the importance of leadership as it identifies "Basic Organizational and Systems Leadership for Quality and Patient Safety" as the second essential for baccalaureate education. Subsequently, BSN programs have all required some type of leadership and management course in the curriculum. Most of these courses are traditional leadership courses that include content on delegation, nurse practice acts, magnet hospital designation, evidence-based practice, quality improvement endeavors, and some management content on staffing, productivity, and budgeting.

All of these concepts are important, but mastery of them is insufficient for true leadership development. Nurses usually receive all of their leadership training in one senior leadership course, and soon thereafter they will be responsible for advocating for clients who may be confused about their bills, their disease, the many providers they encounter, and the technology that they may have to depend on when they are discharged.

In graduate nursing programs, graduate students, except for those on the nursing leadership or administrative tracks, may only get one course that covers health care systems and has limited leadership content. Given the importance of covering the necessities and the demands on curriculum content occasioned by the knowledge explosion, most of the curricula for students pursuing clinical degrees focus on nursing theory, pathophysiology, pharmacology, technology, research, education, professional issues, and the assessment and management of conditions. In reality, however, once in practice, APNs are expected to be exquisite agents of change, skilled negotiators, astute group leaders, incisive systems thinkers, innovators of practice, and flexible collaborators with a variety of other leaders. Adding complexity to their role (Ebright et al., 2006), APNs operate from a basis of expert power, usually in staff roles, whereas many of the administrative and physician leaders APNs negotiate with on a daily basis often hold line positions of authority within the organization.

LEADERSHIP DEVELOPMENT OUTSIDE OF NURSING

Industries outside of health care have long understood that leadership development is crucial to productivity, satisfaction, profitability, and retention (Buckingham & Coffman, 1999). There have been prestigious fellowships, such as the Kellogg Fellowship, through universities, and in-depth training of business leaders through centers such as the Center for Creative Leadership (CCL) (Center for Creative Leadership, 2008).

Interestingly enough, 65% of the leaders trained in the CCL, one of the top-ranked executive education providers worldwide, were men. Many industries have also invested in consultants in order to provide leadership development for leaders throughout the organization.

However, it is not common for nurse leaders to participate in these leadership fellowships in the same numbers as leaders from other disciplines, including leaders of health care systems. As a case in point, the American Council on Education (ACE) has a very highly regarded leadership fellowship for leaders in academic settings. This fellowship has launched many presidents and provosts in their careers, yet when we reviewed the credentials from ACE fellows in the past 40 years, fewer than 10 academic nurse leaders have participated in this fellowship (less than 0.007%).

Physician leadership development is also alive and well. An Internet search using the words *physician leadership development* revealed leadership development and leadership fellowship programs focused exclusively on physicians at Harvard, Stanford, Johns Hopkins, Duke, and others. The American Association of Medical Colleges (AAMC) created a publication that identified 31 leadership development programs available to physicians (Hall, 2005). It is clear to the AAMC and many academic health centers that it is crucial to provide in-depth leadership development for physicians in order to gain leverage in today's health care system. Crites, Ebert, and Schuster (2008) have recommended a curriculum revision to incorporate in-depth leadership competencies in every year of medical school education because they believe these skills are crucial to the future success of the profession. They also believe it is imperative to develop physicians as leaders early in their careers to make the biggest difference. They agree with Goleman (2001) that leadership competencies are easier to develop and longer lasting when professionals are at the beginning of their careers rather than mid-career development.

LEADERSHIP DEVELOPMENT IN NURSING

Although nursing leadership development programs are not as extensive or numerous as physician and traditional CEO programs, several significant and influential programs exist. These programs elucidate the competencies needed for nurses who are agents of change and leaders in the health care system today. One of the most prestigious leadership development programs in nursing is the Robert Wood Johnson Foundation's Executive Nurse Fellowship (RWJFENF) Program (Bellack & Morjikian, 2005). This program develops nurse leaders from practice and educational environments so that nurses can influence health policy and patient outcomes. The RWJFENF program identifies five main competencies needed for nurses to make a difference in today's health care environment. These competencies are self-awareness, interpersonal and communication effectiveness, risk taking and creativity, strategic visioning, and inspiring and leading change.

The University of South Carolina created a Center for Nursing Leadership in 1994. The center focuses on the competencies of organizational communication, self-awareness, resolving and negotiating conflict, the impact of globalization and complexity of organizations, the circle of influences, leading and managing complex systems, and strategic thinking. The Center has offered a fellowship program for the last 13 years, developing nurses in all roles in many different settings to become stronger leaders and to influence health care throughout the southeastern United States.

Recently O'Neil et al. (2008) canvassed the leadership development programs available to nurse leaders. They found that most of the activity related to leadership development has occurred since 2000, although leadership development in other industries had strong development in the 1970s (CCL, 2008). They surveyed nursing and non-nursing leaders to ascertain the competencies needed in nursing leaders and found that leaders—both within nursing and outside of the field—valued first and foremost building effective teams, followed by communicating vision, managing conflict, translating vision into strategy, and maintaining focus on the patient and consumer. The authors found that health care leaders had a clear preference for developing leadership competencies in nurses but that leadership development of nurses was undercapitalized compared to other industries.

Although these leadership development programs are a great resource for nurses in all roles, it is incumbent upon both nursing practice and education to ensure that APNs have sufficient leadership competencies to leverage their clinical contributions and influence health care as we move forward in a new political and economic climate (Fagin, 2000). Although the AACN highlights leadership as one of the main essentials of the DNP curriculum, many programs have yet to integrate leadership development to the degree that is seen in medical schools.

Leadership Development in DNP Curriculum

The current explosion of doctorate of nursing practice (DNP) programs provides good evidence of the belief within the nursing community that the health care system, the profession, and the public need nurses who are prepared to be practice leaders. The American Association of Colleges of Nursing developed its *Essentials for Doctoral Education for Advanced Nursing Practice* in 2006 (AACN, 2006), identifying eight main essentials for inclusion in the curriculum of any DNP program. This document specifically addresses the importance of leadership in Essential II, "Understanding Organizations and Systems Leadership for Quality Improvement and Systems Thinking," and Essential VI, "Inter-professional Collaboration for Improving Patient and Population Outcomes."

A review of the AACN website reveals over 90 schools currently offering DNP degrees, with more than 50 additional schools working on developing programs. A comparison of the core curricula of 12 programs, including the oldest in the country and a mix of public and private universities and colleges, in relationship to their requirements for effective leadership reveals variations in goals and curricula.

In order to review programs for leadership content in course titles or course descriptions available on websites, a model of leadership competencies developed by the authors (Krejci & Malin, 1997) was used as a framework for analysis (Figure 5.1). The model is based on 20 years of teaching and consulting in the area of leadership development with nurses in a variety of roles (Krejci & Malin, 1997) and encompasses leadership development for all nurses, not just those in executive or administrative roles. The foundation of the model is self-awareness, as the literature on leadership has consistently identified self-awareness as a prerequisite for successful leadership (Covey, 2004; Goleman, 2001; Guthrie & Kelly-Radford, 1998; O'Neil et al., 2008; Senge, 1990). The components in this model are congruent with the AACN's *Essentials* document (2006). Self-awareness and mission occupy the center of the model, which is surrounded by the supporting competencies of systems thinking, circle of influence (personal power), interpersonal communication, building teams, negotiating conflict, moving vision to action, coaching and developing others, and implementing change.

This analysis was an exercise to begin to identify what types of leadership competencies are included in a cross section of DNP programs for which course titles and descriptions were available on the websites

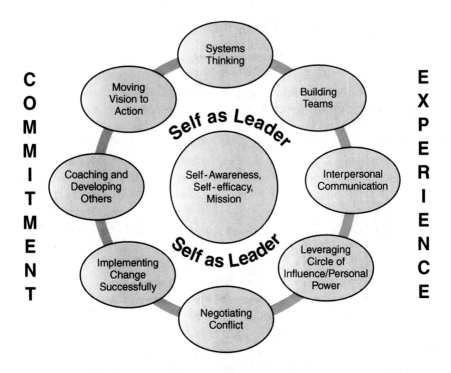

KNOWLEDGE, SKILL, COMPETENCIES

Figure 5.1 Krejci and Malin Leadership Model of Competencies.

of schools of nursing. See Table 5.1 for a summary of results. Although it is understood that programs may have integrated leadership development in ways that are not visible on their websites, it still presents an interesting starting point for a discussion on how DNP programs overtly articulate their curriculum and how they will prepare APNs to be practice leaders.

No program appeared to have courses incorporating all of the competencies. Many programs have one course on leadership in practice, but looking specifically for the identified competencies provided some interesting results. Systems thinking was evident in 7 of 12 programs; change implementation was evident in 11 of 12 programs, and although effective change requires effective teams, it was difficult to identify any program referring to this knowledge and skill. Communication, conflict, and negotiation were covered in 4 of 12 programs; aspects of leadership in practice were identified in 10 of 12 programs; and a clear focus on self-

Table 5.1

REVIEW OF WEB SITES FOR 12 DNP PROGRAMS FOR LEADERSHIP CONTENT IN EITHER COURSE TITLE OR COURSE DESCRIPTION (KREJCI & MALIN MODEL)

Colleges/Universities	1	2	3	4	5	6	7	8	9	10	11	12
Self Awareness		X				X	X		X	X		X
Systems Thinking		X	X	X	X		X	X			X	
Building Teams						X						
Interpersonal Communication						X	X	X	X		X	
Circle of Influence (Personal Power)												X
Negotiating Conflict						X		X	X		X	
Implementing Change	X	X	X	X	X	X	X	X	X	X		X
Coaching and Developing Others												

awareness was identifiable in 6 of 12 programs. All of the programs offer electives, so students might choose to augment the core curriculum and obtain leadership competencies through other courses. Although comparing competencies and course titles according to other models such as the RWJFENF or the University of South Carolina's Center for Nursing Leadership might produce some differences; many of the competencies share similarities across models.

Although there seems to be much agreement that leadership competencies are a prerequisite for successful APNs, at this point nursing education has not overtly delineated this content in their curricula as compared to the recommendations to medical school curricula or other industries. As more DNP programs are created, nursing education has a stunning opportunity to create stronger leaders and implore those seeking admittance into DNP programs to evaluate the leadership competency content in the curriculum.

In addition, we believe there is a need for leadership development that augments what is learned in formal graduate education programs. Although the numbers of non-degree leadership development programs have grown exponentially, many are created for and offered to those in formal administrative roles, with few focusing on practice leaders. Interestingly, this is not the case in medicine where practice leadership development programs flourish (Hall, 2005). A brief review of the websites of national nursing organizations relevant to advanced practice nursing revealed very little focus on leadership development. The same was true of most advanced practice nursing sites for nurse practitioners, certified nurse specialists, and nurse-midwives. It is strongly recommended that faculty teaching in DNP programs evaluate the DNP curriculum and ensure that there is material on overt, in-depth leadership development throughout the curriculum. APNs roles are strongly encouraged to seek out the leadership development and fellowship opportunities that exist locally, regionally, and nationally.

APPLICATION OF COMPETENCIES TO APN ROLE

In order to demonstrate the importance of leadership competencies, four scenarios will be presented. Common issues occurring in many practice settings provide context for examining the critical need for leadership development among APNs. Both authors have been working with APNs and other nurses over the last 20 years in leadership development sessions. One has been leading a department of advanced practice for several years. The following scenarios are typical examples of common problems that an APN is likely to encounter.

Implementing Change, Moving Vision to Action

Jeanne is a seasoned nurse practitioner who has what she believes is an exciting, excellent idea for creating a new clinic that could be staffed solely by the APNs in the practice. The clinic would allow their physician colleagues to spend more time in the operating room, and it would provide a satisfying role for the NPs. She presents a detailed proposal for the new clinic to the provider group only to have it dismissed by her physician colleagues as being cost-prohibitive. Her APN colleagues who agreed to support the proposal before the meeting didn't speak in support of the proposal during the meeting. When she asks why, they shrug and walk away. Jeanne is left confused, disappointed, angry, and unsure of what to do next. The leadership competencies of implementing change successfully and moving vision to action may have helped Jeanne to strategize by partnering with early adopters, proposing a low-cost pilot, and presenting a compelling vision aligned with physician goals. Even if her proposal was not accepted, Jeanne would then have been able to reframe the conclusion from "defeat" to "new information" that can be incorporated into her next proposal.

Systems Thinking, Building Teams, Developing and Coaching Others, and Interpersonal Communication

Bruce, an experienced APN, is approached by a staff nurse working in the practice who is fuming about the encounter she just had with an APN in the practice. She found her encounter with the APN discounting and believes this APN holds herself above others and devalues nurses as "mere staff nurses." Bruce believes everyone should be responsible for their own "stuff," and although he enjoys the nurse and values her role in the practice, he's not sure how to be helpful. He tells the nurse to shake it off and assures her the APN didn't really mean it. The staff nurse leaves feeling discounted again and begins to question whether she wants to stay. She avoids the other APN and Bruce, not seeking their consultation. The use of many leadership skills by either APN may have produced better results for the APNs, the patients they serve, and the system. Systems thinking competencies would have allowed both to see this situation from a larger perspective helping them understand that individual tensions, events, and relationships are influenced by systematic structure and inherent system patterns. Unfortunately, in this situation, accidental adversaries, a common system archetype (Senge, 1990) has now been created. Competencies in building teams, interpersonal communication, and developing and coaching others might also have kept this situation from escalating into powerlessness and frustration.

Negotiating Conflict and Circle of Influence (Personal Power)

Many APNs are hired into practices by physicians who value their contributions but do not always maximize the APNs' competencies, nor do they always include APNs in important decision making related to the practice. APNs often succumb to feeling powerless, acting more from the role of victim rather than as a powerful contributor. A cycle begins and continues as APNs find themselves caught off guard and sometimes demoralized by the changes their physician colleagues decide to make without asking for their input or involvement in the decision-making process. Leadership competencies in negotiation and acknowledgment of personal power by maximizing one's own circle of influence could create leverage for negotiating a more effective role when partnering with physicians. Imagine the potential outcomes if APNs spent time strategizing, identifying mutually beneficial reasons for their inclusion in the process, and then drafting a proposal for involvement.

Self-awareness

An effective APN is one who is self-aware and spends time learning through practice. Betty is a highly productive APN who consistently works 12 hours a day. She finds herself dreading getting up and going to work these days. Over the past 6 months, she has had a number of formal patient complaints and is mortified by this development. She is hoping that no one will mention the complaints, yet she is very concerned about what has happened because patients have always enjoyed having her work with them in the past. Many APNs practice in busy practices with little time for interacting with their colleagues, mentoring, development, or reflection. Leadership development in the area of self-awareness could have helped Betty to understand her particular strengths and challenges and manage her boundaries more effectively. Understanding the importance of self-awareness and exploring growth through strengths is likely to lead to more effective, congruent professional relationships. The habit of learning through practice is key to excellence in practice.

IMPLICATIONS

Understanding the historical context and areas of leverage for APNs is necessary but not sufficient in ensuring that humans have access to the best APNs have to offer. In order to advocate for patient care and enhance outcomes for individuals and populations, APNs need strong leadership competencies. The responsibility to promote evidence-based leadership skills in the APN lies with graduate education, professional organizations, and the individual APN. All three entities need to make the development of leadership in APNs a priority. These leadership and system skills are as crucial to the success of APNs in health care organizations as their clinical prowess.

Although the ability to operationalize leadership in a measurable way remains elusive, there is now a growing body of literature that has correlated outcomes with leadership, even when it has been measured or articulated in different ways (Bennis et al., 1969; Buckingham & Coffman, 1999; Farkas & Wetlaufer, 1996; Fisher & Ury, 1991; Heifetz, 1994; Heifetz & Linsky, 2002; Goleman, Boyatzis, & McKee, 2002; Kouzes & Posner, 1995; Kritek, 2002; Perra, 2000; Porter-O'Grady & Malloch, 2003; & Senge, et al., 1994). Buckingham and Coffman (1999), leaders in the research conducted by Gallup on managers and outcomes, have identified that strong leadership is correlated with retention, productivity, profitability, and satisfaction. The research on magnet hospitals has supported a need for strong leadership. AACN has now identified a need for stronger leadership presence in the health care system in order to enhance quality care by mandating the DNP for advanced practice after 2015 (American Association of Colleges of Nursing, 2006). The IOM (1999, 2001, 2004). reports clearly indicate that mastering and coordinating the context of care are important variables for quality. APNs not only need to use evidence-based practice in clinical phenomena but also in system phenomena, for which there is a growing body of supportive evidence (Pfeffer & Sutton, 2006). The National Association for Clinical Nurse Specialists (NACNS) clearly identifies that one dimension of the scope of practice for APNs is leadership in the organization or system (National Association for Clinical Nurse Specialists, 2004).

APNs may gain skills in a variety of ways, by reading, attending workshops and training, taking courses, and working with a mentor. How they acquire these skills is not nearly as important as a focused systematic effort to enhance their competencies. Hopefully future DNP programs will include a more intense focus on systems and leadership. Today most organizations are investing heavily in leadership development for those in administrative positions because they know the impact strong leaders can have on an organization. APNs should inquire about participating in these development opportunities.

Second, APNs need to understand the system and system politics. They should be socialized during their graduate education as well as by professional organizations to study the systems where they are or will be employed. All APNs should understand the organizational chart, both formal and informal (Mintzberg, 1983, 1987), to examine where they are placed within the hierarchy and the place and role of the person to whom they report. They should carefully review their job descriptions and ascertain how words such as *supervision* and *collaboration* are defined. In essence, how APNs are described by the organization, where they are located on the organization chart, and the decisions over which they have influence are equally as important as their clinical expertise in terms of affecting outcomes of care.

Finally, and quite simply, APNs need to *show up* at the table. APNs are often so immersed in practice that they may make the mistake of being unintentionally absent or even intentionally avoiding important system decision-making bodies (formal and informal) because they don't want to engage in "politics." APNs should network with their colleagues to make sure they provide adequate representation themselves or by other strong nursing leaders when discussions or decisions are being carried out that affect their role. APNs must take every opportunity to be present, particularly when they are invited to the table. When APNs miss these opportunities, they signal disinterest and a lack of professional involvement.

CONCLUSION

Demonstrated leadership competencies are critically important to ensuring effective, high-quality APN practice in health care systems. Being knowledgeable about the current state of their organization and understanding when and how to choose high-leverage targets for change are essential competencies for APNs if they are to achieve the appropriate level of respect in that system. When this happens, they will have universal access, receive appropriate compensation for services rendered, and sit at the appropriate decision-making tables. Other health professionals clearly understand the importance of in-depth leadership development. It is imperative that APNs be leaders and take their place at the table because patient care outcomes depend on their leadership.

REFERENCES

American Association of Colleges of Nursing (2006). *Essentials of doctorate of nursing practice education.* Washington DC: Author.

American Association of Colleges of Nursing. (2008). *Essentials of baccalaureate education for professional nursing practice.* Washington DC: Author.

Ashley, J. (1979). *Hospitals, paternalism, and the nurse.* New York: Teachers College.

Bellack, J. P., & Morjikian, R. L. (2005). The RWJ executive nurse fellows program, part 2. *Journal of Nursing Administration, 35*(12), 533–540.

Benner, P. (1984, reprinted 2001). *From novice to expert: Excellence and power in clinical nursing practice.* Upper Saddle River, NJ: Prentice Hall.

Bennis, W. G., Benne, D., & Chin, R. (Eds.). (1969). *The planning of change.* New York: Holt, Rinehart & Winston.

Brooten, D., Youngblut, J. M., Kutcher, J., & Bobo, C. (2004). Quality and the nursing workforce: APNs, patient outcomes and health care costs. *Nursing Outlook 52*(1), 45–52.

Brooten, D., Youngblut, J., Blais, K., Donahue, D., Cruz, I., & Lightbourne, M. (2005). APN-physician collaboration in caring for women with high-risk pregnancies. *Journal of Nursing Scholarship. 37*(2), 178–184.

Buckingham, M., & Coffman, M. (1999). *First, break all the rules: What the world's greatest managers do differently.* New York: Simon & Schuster.

Burns S. M., & Earven, S. (2003). Improving outcomes for mechanically ventilated medical intensive care unit patients using advanced practice nurses: A 6-year experience. *Critical Care Nursing Clinics of North America. 4*(3): 231–243.

Center for Creative Leadership (CCL). 2008. Retrieved November 8, 2008, from www.ccl.org/leadership/index.aspx.

Covey, S. (2004). *The 8th habit.* New York: Free Press.

Crites, G., Ebert, J., & Schuster, R. (2008). Beyond the dual degree: Development of a five-year program in leadership for medical undergraduates. *Academic Medicine,* *83*(1), 52–58.

Cunningham, R. S. (2004). Advanced practice nursing outcomes: A review of selected empirical literature. *Oncology Nursing Forum, 31*(2), 219–232.

Ebright, P. R., Kooken, W. S., Moodey, R. C., & Hassan, A. (2006). Mindful attention to complexity: Implications for teaching and learning patient safety in nursing. In M. Oermann and K. Heinrich (Eds.), *Annual Review of Nursing Education* (Vol. 4, pp. 339–360). New York: Springer Publishing.

Fagin, C., & Schwarz, M. R. (1993). Can APNs be independent gatekeepers? *Hospitals & Health Networks, 67*(11), 8-9.

Fagin, C. M. (2000). *Essays on nursing leadership.* New York: Springer Publishing.

Farkus, C., & Wetlaufer, S. L. (1996). The way chief executive officers lead. In H. Mintzber, J. Kotter, A. Zaleznik, J. Badatacco, D. Farkas, R. Heifetz, et al., *Harvard Business Review on Leadership* (pp. 115–146). Boston: Harvard Business School.

Fisher, R., & Ury, R. (1991). *Getting to yes: Negotiating agreement without giving in.* B. Patton (Ed.), Boston: Houghton Mifflin.

French, J. R., & Raven, B. (1959/1986). The bases of social power. In D. Cartwright (Ed.), *Studies in social power* (pp. 150–167). Ann Arbor: Institute for Social Research, University of Michigan.

Gawlinski, A., McCloy, K., & Jesurum, J. (2001) Measuring outcomes in cardiovascular APN practice. In R. Kleinpell (Ed.), *Outcome Assessment in Advanced Practice Nursing* (pp. 131–188). New York: Springer Publishing.

Goleman, D. (2001). What makes a leader? In *Harvard Business Review: On what makes a leader* (pp. 53–86). Boston: Harvard Business School Publishing.

Goleman, D., Boyatzis, R., & McKee, A. (2002). *Primal leadership: Realizing the power of emotional intelligence.* Boston: Harvard Business Review.

Gordon, S., Benner, P., & Noddings, N. (1996). *Caregiving: Readings in knowledge, practice, ethics, and politics.* Philadelphia: University of Pennsylvania.

Guthrie, V., & Kelly-Radford, L. (1998). Feedback-intensive programs. In C. McCauley, R. Moxley, & E. VanVelor (Eds.), *The center for creative leadership: Handbook of leadership development* (pp. 66–105). San Francisco: Jossey-Bass.

Hall, L. (2005). *National leadership development programs.* Washington DC: American Association of Medical Colleges.

Heifetz, R. (1994). *Leadership without easy answers.* Cambridge, MA: Belknap Press of Harvard University.

Heifetz, R., & Linsky, M. (2002). *Leadership on the line: Staying alive through the dangers of leading.* Boston: Harvard Business School.

Institute of Medicine. (1999). *To err is human: Building a safer health system.* Washington DC: National Academies of Science.

Institute of Medicine. (2001). *Crossing the quality chasm: A new health system for the 21st century.* Washington DC: National Academies of Science.

Institute of Medicine. (2004). *Insuring American's Health: Principles and recommendations.* Washington DC: National Academies of Science.

Kleinpell, R. M. (2007). APNs: Invisible champions? *Nursing Management, 38*(5), 18–22.

Kouzes, J., & Posner, B. Z. (1995). *The leadership challenge.* San Francisco: Jossey-Bass.

Krejci, J. W. (1997). Imagery: Stimulating critical thinking by unearthing mental models. *Journal of Nursing Education, 36*(10), 482–484.

Krejci, J. W., & Malin, S. (1997). Impact of leadership development on leadership competencies. *Nursing Economics, 15*(5), 235–241.

Kritek, P. (2002). *Negotiating at an uneven table: Developing moral courage in resolving our conflicts.* San Francisco: Jossey-Bass.

Larkin, H. (2003). The case for nurse practitioners. *Hospitals & Health Networks, 77*(8), 54.

Mintzberg, H. (1983). *Structure in fives: Designing effective organizations.* Englewood Cliffs, NJ: Prentice Hall.

Mintzberg, H. (1987/1979). The five basic parts of the organization. In J. M. Shafritz & J. S. Ott (Eds.), *Classics of organization theory* (2nd ed., pp. 219–233). Pacific Grove, CA: Grove.

National Association of Clinical Nurse Specialists. (2004). *Statement on clinical nurse specialist: Practice and education.* Glenview, IL: NACNS.

Nightingale, F. (1946). *Notes on nursing: What it is and what it is not.* Philadelphia: Lippincott.

O'Neil, E., Morjickian, R. L., Cherner, D., Hirschkorn, C., & West, T. (2008). Developing nursing leaders: An overview of trends and programs. *Journal of Nursing Administration, 38*(4), 178–181.

Perason. L. (2004). Sixteenth annual legislative update. *Nurse Practitioner, 29*(1), 26.

Perra, B. M. (2000). Leadership: The key to quality outcomes. *Nursing Administration Quarterly, 24*(2), 56–61.

Pfeffer, J., & Sutton, R. I. (2006). *Hard facts, dangerous half-truths and total nonsense: Profiting from evidence-based management.* Boston: Harvard Business Publishing.

Porter-O'Grady, T., & Malloch, K. (2003). *Quantum leadership.* Boston: Jones and Bartlett.

Reverby, S. (1987). *Ordered to care: The dilemma of American nursing, 1850–1945.* New York: Cambridge University Press.

Reverby, S. (2001). A caring dilemma: Womanhood and nursing in historical perspective. In E. C. Hein (Ed.), *Nursing issues in the 21st century: Perspectives from the literature* (pp. 10–25). Philadelphia: Lippincott.

Roberts, S. (1983). Oppressed group behavior: Implications for nursing. *Advances in Nursing Science, 5*(4), 21–30.

Roberts, S. (2005) Oppressed Group Behavior and Nursing. In K. Wolf & P. Nicholas, *A History of Nursing Ideas.* Jones & Bartlett Publishers.

Russell, D., VorderBruegge, M., & Burns, S.(2002). Effect of an outcomes-managed approach to care of neuroscience patients by acute care nurse practitioners. *American Journal of Critical Care. 11*(4), 353–364.

Senge, P. (1990). *The fifth discipline: The art and practice of the learning organization.* New York: Doubleday.

Senge, P.M. et al. (1994). *The fifth discipline fieldbook: Strategies and tools for building a learning organization.* New York: Currency, Doubleday.

Stewart-Amidei, C. (2003). Collaboration or competition. *Journal of Neuroscience Nursing, 35*(4), 183.

University of South Carolina College of Nursing. Center for Nursing Leadership. Retrieved November 10, 2008, from www.sc.edu/nursing/CNL/docs/Current%20Cockroft%20Desription%206-16-08.pdf

Valentine, P. B. (2001). A gender perspective on conflict management strategies for nurses. *Journal of Nursing Scholarship, 33*(1), 69–74.

Weber, M. (1987). Bureaucracy. In J. M. Shafritz & J. S. Ott (Eds.), *Classics of organization theory* (2nd ed., originally published in 1946). Pacific Grove, CA: Grove.

Implementation of the APN Role

PART II

Clinical Decision Making in Advanced Practice Nursing

SHEILA K. SMITH

Clinical decision making in advanced practice nursing occurs as a continuous, purposeful, theory- and knowledge-based process of assessment, analysis, strategic planning, and intentional follow-up. It is both a cognitive and affective problem-solving activity for defining patient problems and selecting appropriate management approaches (Buckingham & Adams, 2000). Lunney (2009) states, "The personal strengths of tolerance for ambiguity and reflective practice need to be developed because decisions are so complex in nursing and the use of clinical judgment needs to be an ongoing learning process. Each decision is relative to context of situation and specific nature of the individual, family, or community" (p. 7).

The role of the advanced practice nurse (APN) is multifaceted, and the scope of decision making is similarly complex. It incorporates health promotion, disease prevention, risk reduction, management of functional health needs, subjective concerns, program planning, biomedical diagnostics, and disease management. Large amounts of data are elicited, sorted, and organized into meaningful patterns. Conducted within the context of nurse–patient relationships, APN clinical decision making is frequently characterized by changing health circumstances and complex social variables. The nursing and biomedical decision making involved may be straightforward, of moderate complexity, or of high complexity.

The level of patient health risk may range from very low to very high. The amount and quality of evidence-based health information available may demonstrate a wide degree of variability.

From a societal perspective, recipients of health care and health policy makers are demanding ever greater transparency in the decisions made by health care professionals and greater accountability for outcomes (Thompson & Dowding, 2002). Advanced practice clinical decision making thus necessitates careful and conscientious attention to a wide range of cognitive skills, with an eye toward deliberately applying and improving the critical thinking and knowledge base required for practice.

PROCESSES, FOCUS, AND FRAMEWORKS

To understand clinical decision making at the APN level, it is necessary to examine at least three interrelated aspects of practice: decision-making processes; the focus of APN practice; and APN frameworks for practice. Each of these components contributes essential elements to the process of clinical decision making in advanced practice nursing, resulting in a unique and valuable clinical practice role.

Decision-Making Processes: Research in Clinical Reasoning

Research in clinical judgment and decision making has been an important area of study for over 50 years. Much of the decision-making and problem-solving research began in the cognitive sciences (Newell & Simon, 1972; Tversky & Kahneman, 1974), with early application to diagnostic reasoning and clinical problem solving in nursing and medicine (Elstein, 1976; Elstein, Shulman, & Sprafka, 1978; Hammond, 1964; Hammond, Kelly, & Castellan, 1966). Strong interest in this field of study has continued with distinctions more clearly discerned between clinical problem solving in nursing and medicine. Nursing problem solving frequently focuses on expert judgment about changes in a patient's overall status; anticipating and preventing potential problems; ensuring safe passage through uncertain health–illness trajectories; addressing the functional needs and capacities and quality-of-life issues for the whole person; understanding and responding to complex human responses; and protecting individuals and groups in their health–illness vulnerabilities (Benner, Hooper-Kyriakidis, & Stannard, 1999; Carnevali

& Thomas, 1993; Tanner, Benner, Chesla, & Gordon, 1993). Medical reasoning, in contrast, focuses more specifically on the management of illness, pathology and disease, biomedical hypothesis generation with probability determination, and medical treatment decisions (Elstein & Schwartz, 2000). In medicine, a very different set of problem-solving skills and knowledge bases are required: pathophysiologic causal reasoning, use and interpretation of diagnostic tests, prognostic determination, and disease-oriented therapeutic decision making (Kassirer & Kopelman, 1991). Advanced practice nursing involves a complex blending of both nursing and medical decision making. It is important to be able to synthesize decision-making skills from both fields.

Commonalities in Clinical Reasoning Across Health Disciplines

Several common or core features of clinical reasoning across health disciplines have been identified in the research (Higgs & Jones, 2000). First, clinical reasoning and clinical knowledge are now accepted as being strongly interdependent. At one time, particularly in medicine, it was hypothesized that clinical reasoning and clinical knowledge could be learned independently (Patel & Kaufman, 2000). Many educational programs attempted to deal with the rapidly escalating volume of biomedical information by emphasizing the development of problem-solving skills and devoting less time to content. Research has shown, however, that the development of expertise in clinical reasoning requires considerable depth and organization of domain-specific clinical knowledge (Boshuizen & Schmidt, 1992). Growth in clinical expertise is accompanied by increasing depth and complexity of knowledge structures (Higgs & Jones, 2000).

Another core feature of clinical reasoning across health disciplines is that an array of higher order cognitive skills and processes is necessary for effective clinical reasoning. Various theorists identify these higher-order cognitive skills differently, but some that have been emphasized in the literature are clinical appraisal (Brookfield, 2000), categorization (Hayes & Adams, 2000), and propositional knowledge (Titchen & Higgs, 2000). Clinical appraisal consists of critically evaluating the totality of presenting information for the key or most salient clinical features and accurately defining what those features represent. Categorization is both a way of learning complex content and using salient features and pattern recognition to relate novel instances to known categories. For instance, categorization would be used to judge the level of severity or acuity of patient presentation. Risk stratification is an important current application of categorization, selecting management approaches based on the level of severity or risk and statistically predicted patient care outcomes. Propositional knowledge incorporates hypothesis generation and the development of plausible and probabilistic relationships between events. For example, the APN uses propositional knowledge to hypothesize the most probable diagnosis given a certain patient presentation. When clinicians make prospective predictions about the likely course of a condition based on clinical signs and symptoms, they are engaging in a combination of categorization and probabilistic reasoning.

The third feature associated with clinical reasoning is that it is highly context dependent. The context within which clinical reasoning occurs is determined by the client's health concern(s); the specific health setting; the care provider's disciplinary background and level of experience; the client's unique personal context; the stage of case management (e.g., initial diagnosis versus long-term stabilization versus exacerbation management, etc.); and elements of the wider health care environment (Higgs & Jones, 2000). Research attending to context-specific factors (e.g., Benner, Hooper-Kyriakidis, & Stannard, 1999) demonstrates that expert clinical reasoning is complex, interpretive and personalized: "A good clinician is always interpreting the present clinical situation in terms of the immediate past condition of the patient" (p. 10). In addition, a good clinician interprets present status in light of most probable future trajectories, given analyzed risk factors, comorbidities, treatment effectiveness, and known patterns of disease progression. The expert clinician attends to the direction of change in the client's condition and interprets ambiguous and unfolding client information as it becomes available.

Clinical Reasoning in Nursing

Multiple approaches have been used to study clinical reasoning in nursing, including information processing theory (Corcoran, 1986a), analytical decision making (Corcoran, 1986b), skill acquisition or hermeneutic processes (Benner, 1984), cognitive continuum theory (Lauri & Salantera, 2002), and the use of heuristics (Cioffi & Markham, 1997). Information processing derives primarily from the cognitive sciences. It focuses on memory capacity, the "chunking" or clustering of complex information into recognizable patterns, weighing alternative options, and searching for pathways to solutions (Elstein, 1976; Newell & Simon, 1972).

Information is accessed from long-term memory and cue assessment, then transformed into units that can be cognitively manipulated in short-term memory. In nursing, information processing has been used with verbal or "thinking aloud," protocols to study cognitive processes used in clinical decision making (Corcoran, 1986a; Simmons, 2002). The tendency of information-processing models to be overly linear and mechanistic has been addressed through the addition of heuristics, contextual variables, varying degrees of task complexity, and varying levels of uncertainty (Higgs & Jones, 1995; Narayan & Corcoran-Perry, 1997; Tanner, Padrick, Westfall, & Putzier, 1987). This recent development provides a better theoretical match for the dynamic environments and ambiguity of decisions in clinical practice.

Analytical decision making relies on a more structured process of identifying options and possible outcomes, assigning values to the outcomes, and determining probability relationships between the options and anticipated outcomes. Formal (mathematically based) or informal (conceptually based) models are used to systematize decision making using grids or decision flow diagrams (Corcoran, 1986b; Narayan, Corcoran-Perry, Drew, Hoyman, & Lewis, 2003). Decision analysis has been reported as useful for evaluating medical treatment options, cost analysis, quality improvement decisions, and policy decisions (Narayan, Corcoran-Perry, Drew, Hoyman, & Lewis, 2003).

Skill acquisition theory, also referred to as the hermeneutic model, has been used by Benner and colleagues (Benner, 1984; Benner & Wrubel, 1989; Benner, Tanner, & Chesla, 2009) to study expertise in clinical nursing practice. Benner and colleagues argue that experienced nurses frequently use the nurse–patient relationship and their intimate knowledge of a patient's response patterns to make clinical judgments about patient care. From their contributions, definitions of clinical judgment, particularly at the level of expert practice, have been expanded to include both deliberate analytic thinking and nonconscious holistic discrimination of a patient's clinical status. In the hermeneutic model, expert judgment includes ethical decision making on what is good and right, a repertoire of extensive knowledge from practice, emotional engagement with patients and with one's practice, and a deep understanding of specific contexts for care (Benner, Tanner, & Chesla, 2009). Components of the hermeneutic model have been identified as pattern recognition, similarity recognition, common-sense understanding, skilled know-how, sense of salience, and deliberative rationality (Dreyfus & Dreyfus, 1986).

As language has evolved in nursing to name and examine the cognitive processes and activities of expert clinical decision making, reference is frequently made to "intuition" in expert nursing practice (Benner, 1984; Pyles & Stern, 1983; Smith, 1987; Rew, 1988). "Intuition" refers to the capacity of the expert clinician to process quickly large amounts of complex data, simultaneously discern patterns, and act on hypotheses without consciously naming all the factors involved in their decision making. The term *intuition* is invoked in an attempt to capture episodes when the complexity of expert knowledge combines with the artistry of expert practice, resulting in a "flow" of engaged practice that seems beyond the capacity of available language to describe. Using Heideggerian and other phenomenologic methodologies, the goal of such inquiries is not necessarily a reductive analysis of linear thought, but an in-depth understanding of the complex experiential knowledge embedded in practice. Intuition is the understanding of a phenomenological gestalt of nurse–client interaction, characterized by intense involvement in an evolving health scenario and the ability of the expert clinician to apply heuristics, attribute meanings, and enact effective care. Intuition is not an uninformed or irrational process. Rather, it is the highly expert application of rational processes and cue analysis, occurring at a pace too rapid for each step to be discretely named or recognized.

Cognitive continuum theory (Hamm, 1988; Lauri & Salantera, 2002) posits a range of analytical thinking approaches with varying combinations of intuitive and analytical thinking. In this theory, the task to be accomplished exhibits features that determine the degree of intuition and/or analysis used by the decision maker. Particularly salient here are these three features: the complexity of task structure (number and redundancy of cues, form of an accurate organizing principle); the ambiguity of task content (availability of organizing principles, familiarity with the task, possibility of high accuracy); and the form of task presentation (task decomposition, cue definition, and response time). In this model, greater analytical thinking is assumed to be related to fewer cues, less redundancy of cues, and more complex procedures for combining evidence to result in correct answers. The availability of organizing principles, greater task familiarity, and the possibility for high accuracy also contribute to greater use of formal reasoning.

The use of heuristics, as proposed by Tversky and Kahneman (1974), is a method for reducing the complexity of judgment tasks by cognitively estimating probabilities, typically based on prior experience via these three categories: representativeness, availability, and anchoring-adjustment.

Representativeness can be used to compare signs and symptoms in a new clinical situation to previously encountered clinical conditions. *Availability* is the ease with which particular instances or cases of a condition can be brought to mind. *Anchoring-adjustment* is used to determine a baseline set of indicators for a condition, then shifting that baseline to account for the clinical factors present in a specific situation. For their part, Cioffi and Markham (1997) examined relationships between the use of heuristics and task complexity in midwifery. In simulated clinical decision-making situations, heuristic processes were used more frequently in situations of greater clinical risk and complexity, less predictability, and when less clinical information was available. Heuristic techniques were used effectively (i.e., with a high rate of accurate diagnoses) and more frequently as task complexity increased. Cioffi (1997) has proposed that heuristic strategies are an important component of nurses' decision making in ambiguous clinical situations and in deriving intuitive judgments.

A small number of studies have focused specifically on the clinical reasoning of advanced practice nurses. Using an information-processing model to study diagnostic reasoning among nurse practitioners, White, Nativio, Kobert, and Engberg (1992) concluded that study participants made decisions reflective of hypothetic–deductive models proposed in the information-processing literature. Experienced nurse practitioners demonstrated greater expertise in making hypothesis-driven choices about what data was necessary for making accurate diagnoses. Nurse practitioners with less expertise in a clinical area used data widely rather than focusing assessments on the basis of diagnostic hypotheses. Not all participants had the content expertise needed to correctly interpret the significance of findings or to make correct management decisions. Findings from this study demonstrate that both the process of clinical decision making and the nurse practitioner's content expertise were necessary for effective client care.

In a study of 70 entry-level nurse practitioners, Sands (2001) found that 76% of the participants were able to develop differential diagnoses, acquire relevant data, refine their hypotheses, and make an accurate diagnosis with a common health concern (pregnancy). Characteristics of novice practice were demonstrated in the tendency of participants to acquire a great deal of data, "seemingly in an effort 'not to miss something'" (p. 137). Entry-level nurse practitioners with at least 5 years of RN experience demonstrated stronger scores on the test of diagnostic reasoning. Participants with less than 2 years of RN experience were at increased risk for inadequate reasoning through the clinical problem.

Ritter (2003) examined the diagnostic reasoning of 10 expert nurse practitioners using both information-processing and hermeneutic models. Specific steps of either information processing or hermeneutics accounted for 99% of participants' think-aloud responses. Within information processing, gathering information accounted for 32% of the responses. Within hermeneutics, skilled know-how accounted for 25% of the responses. Information processing was found to begin the process. Hermeneutics were then used for cue acquisition, thereby bringing structure to the clinical problem and determining what information was salient.

APN Phenomena of Concern

One factor that can be used to distinguish clinical decision making in advanced practice nursing from other autonomous health care providers is the focus of APN practice, or the phenomena of concern. Smith (1995) identified the core of advanced practice nursing as lying within nursing's disciplinary perspectives on health, healing, person–environment inter-actions, and nurse–client relationships. Huch (1995) echoes this in iden-tifying the need to use nursing theory as the basis for advanced nursing practice. Many authors argue that the inclusion of nursing theory and nursing's disciplinary perspectives is an area that needs to be strength-ened in advanced practice nursing.

Advanced practice nurses focus their clinical decision making on health promotion, health protection, disease prevention, and the man-agement of health concerns (NONPF, 2006; NACNS, 2004). As outlined by nurse practitioner and clinical nurse specialist organizations, health promotion activities include lifestyle concerns, principles of lifestyle change, and behavioral change. Health protection includes knowledge of health risks, use of epidemiologic principles, and community/popu-lation-level measures to protect health. Disease prevention includes primary and secondary prevention measures addressing major chronic illness, disability, and communicable disease. Management of health concerns focuses on assessing, diagnosing, monitoring, and coordinating the care of individuals and populations (NONPF, 2006; NACNS, 2004). Depending on the APN's role and specialty preparation, phenomena of concern include both disease- and nondisease-based etiologies that affect health, wellness, and quality of life. For nurse practitioners, the focus is generally on providing direct patient care. For clinical nurse specialists, the focus tends to be on influencing the outcomes of care more widely within an area of specialization, at individual patient, population, and health system levels. Human responses to health and illness, evidence-based nursing interventions, and expertise in the health care needs of a specialty population are frequently emphasized by the CNS.

APN Practice Frameworks

Advanced practice nursing has been consistently characterized as based in holistic perspectives, the formation of partnerships with patients or populations, the use of research and theory to guide practice, and the use of diverse approaches in health and illness management (Brown, 2000; Davies & Hughes, 2002). These characteristics are now built into nationally recommended educational guidelines for advanced practice educational programs (AACN, 2006; NONPF, 2006; NACNS, 2004). For example, the National Organization of Nurse Practitioner Faculties (NONPF) (2006) core competencies for nurse practitioner clinical decision making incorporate the following expectations for practice: "Demonstrates critical thinking and diagnostic reasoning skills in clinical decision making" (p. 1). The core competencies and associated domains of practice were developed based on studies by Benner (1984), Brykcyznski (1989), and Fenton (1983). As advanced practice education moves to the practice doctorate level, AACN (2006) has provided criteria for developing advanced clinical decision making: "Demonstrates advanced levels of clinical judgment, systems thinking, and accountability in designing, delivering and evaluating evidence-based care to improve patient outcomes" (p. 17).

An important feature of clinical decision making in advanced practice nursing is that the phenomena of concern continue to be evidenced in daily practice. This can be done, for example, by making an effort to understand the meanings that patients attribute to their health situation; by learning about the patient's lived social world, support systems, and role responsibilities; and by working with the patient to identify personal and social health obstacles or facilitators. Several additional approaches for incorporating basic nursing perspectives into APN care are listed in Exhibit 6.1.

In addition to the specialty knowledge required for health and illness management, these patient-centered, holistic dimensions of clinical decision making are necessary to maintain the quality of APN care and the ability to distinguish advanced practice nursing from other forms of autonomous health practice.

Exhibit 6.1

APPROACHES FOR INCORPORATING CORE NURSING PERSPECTIVES INTO APN CARE

- Make an effort to understand meanings that patients attribute to their health situation.
- Learn about the patient's lived social world, support systems, and role responsibilities.
- Work with the patient to identify personal and social health obstacles or facilitators.
- Determine the patient's preference for and ability to participate in health care decision making and self-health management.
- Jointly determine appropriate health care goals and priorities.
- Work with patients as they struggle through personal crises, losses, or transitions.
- Learn about the patient's spiritual point of view and how they view the relationship between their health status and spirituality.

CLINICAL DECISION MAKING AS UNDERSTOOD FROM PRACTICE

In addition to influences from nursing research, theory, and professional organizations, much has been learned about APN clinical decision making directly from clinical practice as well as research and practice experiences from other disciplines.

Skilled communication and interaction are essential components of clinical decision making at all levels, whether the APN is posing wide-field or focused inquiries, clarifying diverse perspectives, providing guidance for lifestyle health behaviors, or evaluating a client's responses to treatment. As Chase (2001) points out, clinical decision making is not a process that occurs with the APN in isolation. It occurs as dialogue and interaction between the patient and provider, with experiences of satisfaction significantly influenced by the quality of communication and engagement with the clinical situation (Benner, Stannard, & Hooper, 1996).

Most descriptions of APN clinical decision making begin with an expanded nursing process model that integrates elements of hypothetic–deductive reasoning. Carnevali and Thomas (1993) describe the diagnostic reasoning process in nursing as reviewing pre-encounter data, entry into the assessment situation, collecting the database, coalescing cues into working clusters, selecting pivotal cues or cue clusters, determining possible diagnostic explanations, further comparison of the clinical situation with diagnostic categories, and assigning the diagnosis.

White, Nativio, Kobert, and Engberg (1992) outlined a clinical decision-making framework for advanced practice nurses that adds elements from hypothetic–deductive reasoning. Hypotheses formed are used to guide the process of inquiry, (i.e., decisions about how to focus the history, exam, and diagnostic testing). The process outlined by White, Nativio, Kobert, and Engberg adds many of these elements to nursing clinical decision making: reviewing pre-encounter data, early hypothesis generation, engaging in clinical inquiry, determining working hypotheses, conducting diagnostic testing, testing the final hypothesis, specifying the diagnosis, determining client management, and evaluating the total clinical situation.

Chase (2004) configures this process specifically for nurse practitioner practice. She lists the phases of clinical judgment as: an early wide-field search for the primary concerns; early hypothesis generation on probable causes of the concerns; focused data acquisition related to supporting the active hypotheses and ruling out other serious conditions; evaluating various hypotheses by clustering and analyzing the data for the appropriate fit with diagnostic categories; naming the priority problems; determining appropriate therapeutic goals; determining an appropriate management plan; evaluating the effectiveness of the clinical process; and confirming or revising the diagnoses and plans. Table 6.1 provides a comparison of these three approaches.

In advanced practice nursing, each of these approaches might be appropriate for differing clinical scenarios or problems. The decision-making processes can be used with both disease- and nondisease-based concerns, as well as with medical or nursing diagnoses. Clinical nurse specialists might place less relative emphasis on the biomedical diagnostic content, tending more often to work collaboratively with medical care providers for these decision-making components. Nurse practitioners emphasize greater autonomy in medical diagnostic and treatment elements but place less overall emphasis on specialty nursing care and system-level thinking. With either role, however, keys to the process are clinician characteristics of perception and engagement, discipline-specific knowledge, commitment to quality practice, and knowing how to "think clinically" under differing clinical role expectations. Skilled clinical decision making occurs as an intentional

Table 6.1

COMPARISON OF NURSING AND APN CLINICAL DECISION-MAKING FRAMEWORKS

Carnevali & Thomas (1993), Diagnostic Reasoning in Nursing	White, Nativio, Kobert, & Engberg (1992), APN Clinical Decision Making	Chase (2004), Process of Clinical Judgment for Nurse Practitioners
Collecting pre-encounter data	Reviewing pre-encounter data	Wide-field data search
Entry into the assess-ment situation	Early hypothesis generation	Hypothesis generation
Collecting the database	Clinical inquiry	Data acquisition
Coalescing cues	Determining working hypotheses	Hypothesis evaluation
Selecting pivotal cues	Diagnostic testing	Naming priority problems
Determining diagnostic explanations	Final hypothesis testing	Determining therapeutic goals
Comparison with diag-nostic categories	Specifying the diagnosis	Determining management plan
Assigning the diagnosis	Determining client management	Evaluating effectiveness
	Evaluation	Confirming or revising

process of problem solving, critical thinking, and reflection in action (Benner, Stannard, & Hooper, 1996). It is guided by content expertise and deliberate decisions about how to proceed through the current clinical encounter as well as reasoning through the anticipated trajectory of the health concern.

Relationship between Critical Thinking and Clinical Decision Making

Critical thinking skills can assist with sorting out the above complexities. In a 1990 consensus statement on critical thinking, Facione defines critical thinking as a tool of inquiry characterized by "purposeful, self-regulatory judgment" resulting in "interpretation, analysis, evaluation, and inference" (Facione, 1990, p. 3). It is not "rote, mechanical, unreflective" (p. 8) or disconnected from other thought activities. Critical thinkers are able to examine and evaluate their own reasoning processes and apply critical thinking skills in a variety of contexts. The consensus components of critical thinking are provided in Table 6.2.

Table 6.2

CONSENSUS COMPONENTS OF CRITICAL THINKING

Critical Thinking Skill	Identified Components of the Skill
Interpretation	Categorizing
Evaluation	Clarifying meanings
Inference	Assessing claims and arguments
Explanation	Examining evidence
Self-regulation	Drawing conclusions
Dispositional skills	Proposing alternatives
	Stating results
	Presenting arguments
	Justifying procedures
	Self-examination
	Self-correction
	Inquisitiveness
	Eagerness for reliable information

Scheffer and Rubenfeld (2000) used a Delphi method to develop a consensus statement on critical thinking in nursing, describing both its affective and cognitive components. In addition to the components described by Facione (1990), the nursing study identified creativity and intuition as two additional affective components.

Although critical thinking is defined by educators as a broad set of cognitive skills and habits of mind, applying these skills in clinical practice requires large amounts of discipline-specific knowledge. Research-based understandings of relationships between critical thinking and clinical decision making are not yet well developed. Clearly, however, the skills of interpretation, analysis, evaluation, and inference are highly necessary in advanced clinical practice, where both nursing and medical knowledge must be distinguished and applied. Well-developed critical thinking skills and habits of mind are an important foundation for the discipline-specific processes of clinical thinking required in advanced practice nursing.

Thinking Clinically

As suggested above, the meaning of "thinking clinically" will vary widely from one advanced practice nursing clinical setting and role to another. General elements can be described, however. From these elements it becomes incumbent upon nurses in advanced practice who are pursuing future research agendas to discern the particulars for their practice areas.

Organizing Clinical Knowledge for Practice

Ultimately, cognitively organizing diagnostic and treatment concepts for clinical practice is hard work that individual practitioners must do for themselves (Carnevali & Thomas, 1993). A systematic approach is recommended, based on building a repertoire of specific diagnostic/prognostic/treatment concepts and exemplars from practice. For knowledge from nursing, such cognitive categories could be built around human response categories, broad nursing diagnostic categories, functional health patterns, or population health needs. As the depth of knowledge increases with various phenomena, increasing expertise is developed relating to manifestations, underlying mechanisms, risk factors and complications, prognostic variables and anticipated trajectories, and the efficacy of treatment options. Increasing depth of medical knowledge, on the other hand, relates to the complexity of pathophysiologic explanations and relationships, variations in disease attributes and manifestations, use and interpretation of diagnostic tests, increasingly precise probabilistic and prognostic thinking, and increasingly sophisticated risk–benefit analyses. Building interprofessional and nursing knowledge for advanced clinical practice is an ongoing process of study and practice.

Clinical Decision Making within Human Responses to Health–Illness

In the realm of advanced nursing knowledge and human responses, APN clinical decision making is characterized more by differences in the depth and complexity of skills and knowledge than by differences from professional nursing in the decision-making processes themselves. Relationships between and among human responses to health–illness concerns are more deeply understood, and purposeful engagement with the human responses becomes a larger focus of practice. Benner, Tanner, and Chesla (2009), for example, describe one focus of expert nursing practice as attending to human concerns such as easing suffering, protecting from vulnerability, and preserving dignity. At the advanced practice level, these attributes of expert practice might be the primary focus of a nurse–client interaction enacted from expert palliative care knowledge, derived through the study of nursing research and theory on suffering or vulnerability within a specific population or disease process.

One approach to modeling nondisease-based problems is to seek an understanding of the mechanisms or dynamics most fundamental to the clinical issue that needs to be addressed. For example, inadequate self-health management might be a common nursing diagnosis among individuals with poorly controlled chronic illness. Dynamics underlying such a diagnosis, however, may range from lack of knowledge to situational depression, inadequate self-monitoring, specific self-care skill deficits, or inadequate social support. Once some of the situation-specific dynamics are understood, realistic decisions about where and how to intervene can be made much more effectively.

Clinical Decision Making in Health–Illness Management

In the realm of biomedical knowledge, diagnosis and management of health–illness places greater emphasis on probabilistic thinking and inferential or inductive reasoning, with greater attention to the specificity of the data and the precision of decisions. Rational justification, confirmation and elimination strategies, and judging value are critical reasoning skills within this domain. As outlined by Kassirer and Kopelman (1991), the first step in the diagnostic process is hypothesis activation, or the identification of diagnostic possibilities. Hypothesis activation is based on preliminary information such as the patient's age, medical history, clinical appearance, and presenting concerns. The next step is information gathering and interpretation. This step is strongly influenced by probabilistic thinking and inductive reasoning. The likelihood of various diagnostic hypotheses is carefully considered, with new data used to assist with confirming, eliminating, or discriminating between diagnoses. The working diagnosis is then selected based on causal attribution (i.e., whether all physiologic features are consistent with the favored diagnosis and underlying cause).

The working diagnosis becomes the basis for therapeutic action, prognostic assessment, or further diagnostic testing. Final verification of the diagnostic hypothesis is determined through tests of adequacy and coherence. Adequacy ascertains whether the suspected disease process encompasses all of the patient's findings. Coherence determines whether all of the patient's illness manifestations are appropriate for the suspected health concern. The final diagnostic hypothesis then becomes the basis for treatment decisions, in combination with evidence-based analysis of treatment options and patient-specific cost–benefit analyses for each of the treatment options. Experience and mentoring are clearly necessary to learn biomedical decision making. Kassirer and Kopelman (1991) also advise parsimony in medical reasoning (i.e., seeking a simple, direct, and clear explanation for the patient's health–illness findings whenever possible).

Heuristics in Advanced Practice Nursing

Heuristics are specific cognitive techniques used by skilled clinicians to make reasoning more efficient by reducing complex tasks to simpler and more automatic processes (Tversky & Kahneman, 1974). Heuristics are domain specific (i.e., medical–surgical nursing, critical care nursing, mental health nursing) and are thought to operate strongly in what has been understood as the "intuitive" knowing of clinical experts.

Simmons (2002) identified 11 heuristics used by experienced nurses to reason about assessment findings: recognizing patterns, enumerating lists, forming relationships, searching for information, setting priorities, providing explanations, judging value, stating practice rules, stating propositions, drawing conclusions, and summing up.

Other heuristics used by expert nurses have been identified by Benner and colleagues. These include clinical grasp (making qualitative distinctions, clinical puzzle solving, recognizing changing clinical relevance, and developing population-specific clinical knowledge), and clinical forethought (future think, clinical forethought about specific diagnoses or conditions, anticipating crises, risks and vulnerabilities, and seeing the unexpected) (Benner, Hooper-Kyriakidis, & Stannard, 1999).

Central to clinical grasp are understanding and recognizing clinical patterns and attending very closely to the clinical situation. It is essential to get an accurate story, then observe carefully for patient responses and trends. Clinical forethought involves thinking ahead to common eventualities and using this knowledge to be prepared for or, when possible, to prevent the unfolding of detrimental scenarios. Expertise in clinical forethought requires not only expert textbook knowledge but an array of personal case experiences, providing firsthand experience from which to generate understandings of the clinical terrain, timing issues, and practical knowledge on how to read and interpret clinical cues. Chase (2004) and Dains, Baumann, and Scheibel (2007) describe multiple heuristics specific to nurse practitioner judgment and decision making.

The heuristics described are too numerous to elaborate here, but these and other clinical reasoning texts provide very valuable compendiums of practice knowledge central to nurse practitioner decision making.

Errors in Clinical Reasoning

Several types of clinical practice errors are described in the literature, broadly grouped as skill-based errors, knowledge-based errors, and errors caused by psychoemotional factors. Skill- and knowledge-based errors in this context are not the same as not possessing the necessary skills or knowledge. Rather, the assumption is made that the necessary skills and knowledge are present, but errors are made in their application. Skill-based failures include lack of attention at crucial moments, distraction or preoccupation resulting in missed crucial events, failure to carry out specific activities or intentions, and errors resulting from mixing up behaviors or activities.

Knowledge-based failures include errors due to the use of heuristics. Despite the value of heuristics, overuse has the potential to increase errors in clinical judgment. Care must be taken to maintain a reflective balance between formal reasoning and the use of knowledge from practice. Overconfidence about the correctness of one's knowledge (overconfidence bias), using personal case experience alone as the basis for a decision (hindsight bias), and neglecting the underlying base rate of a health condition when diagnosing or treating (base rate neglect) are three common types of errors in the application of practice knowledge (Thompson, 2002). Conservatism is the failure to revise diagnostic probabilities as new data are presented. Pseudodiagnosticity, or confirmation bias, is the tendency to seek information that confirms a diagnosis but failing to efficiently test competing hypotheses (Elstein & Schwartz, 2000). A psychoemotional error occurs (value-induced bias) when the clinician exaggerates the probability of a diagnosis when one possible outcome is perceived as exceedingly unfavorable compared with others (Buckingham, 2002; Kassirer & Kopelman, 1991).

Errors in the information processing components of practice are also categorized using terminology from hypothesis testing. Type I errors, claiming a significant difference when there is none (analogous to rejecting a true null hypothesis), occurs in clinical decision making through naming a clinical problem when there is none. In this situation, the disease model employed by the clinician may be too broad, perhaps causing the clinician to overestimate the allowable range of variation for findings in a given diagnosis and not recognizing that the actual findings are at odds with the favored diagnosis.

Type II errors, claiming no significant difference when there is one (analogous to accepting a false null hypothesis), occurs with failing to name a clinical problem when there is one. This may occur through missing significant clinical indicators of a health problem or failing to realize the significance of specific signs or symptoms. A correct diagnosis may have been eliminated even though the findings are consistent with the diagnosis.

Type III errors, solving the wrong problem, involve phasing a clinical problem incorrectly, setting the boundaries or scope of the problem too narrowly, or failing to think systematically (Kassirer & Kopelman, 1991). Based on this information, habits of practice that promote sound clinical reasoning can be cultivated by the advanced practice nurse. These are summarized in Table 6.3 (revised from Chase, 2004).

Tools to Support and Enhance Clinical Decision Making in Advanced Practice Nursing

A final aspect of APN decision making is the increasingly important role of a variety of tools that can be used to support and enhance clinical decision making. A listing of these tools is provided in Exhibit 6.2.

Multiple nursing standards of practice have been developed by the American Nurses Association and by specialty nursing organizations. These are organized both by specialty practice areas and by practice-related frameworks such as the nursing code of ethics and the nursing social policy statement. They continue to serve as basic frameworks for nursing practice and are especially important documents for clinical nurse specialists. The NANDA/NIC/NOC taxonomies, although not necessarily complete and not universally used, help to organize ways of naming nursing diagnoses and begin the process of building common expectancies for interventions and outcomes. Mid-level theories help to guide practice by addressing the needs or experiences of specific populations, typically relative to one or more human responses or areas of concern. Incorporating information or concepts from mid-level theories is an excellent way to begin addressing the holistic care considerations of health care populations and build depth at an advanced practice level.

Evidence-based practice has been described as basing clinical decisions and practice on the best available evidence (Higgs, Burn, & Jones, 2001). Not all elements of practice are based on empirical evidence,

Table 6.3

HABITS THAT PROMOTE SOUND CLINICAL REASONING IN ADVANCED PRACTICE NURSING

Phase of Clinical Reasoning	Habits that Promote Sound Reasoning
Data acquisition	Use a systematic and comprehensive approach. Use nursing and medical hypotheses in combination with a systems approach to focus the data collection. Integrate new findings into the emerging model. Search for and attend to both confirming and disconfirming data. Critically evaluate the significance and reliability of findings. Attend to variations in clinical attributes and manifestations.
Hypothesis generation	Formulate preliminary hypotheses early in the encounter. Develop reasonable competing hypotheses. Remain vigilant for serious or life-threatening conditions. Use the hypotheses as models against which to seek and compare findings. Adjust the hypotheses as new data emerge. Carefully compare the hypotheses to reliable information on manifestations, prevalence, and probability. Eliminate hypotheses that fail to remain tenable.
Diagnostic testing	Consider test results as further probability information. Decide if a test result could alter the probability of disease enough to alter management. Use highly sensitive tests (low rate of false negatives) to exclude serious disease. Use highly specific tests (low rate of false positives) to confirm a diagnosis.
Hypothesis evaluation	Determine the "working hypothesis." If competing hypotheses remain, determine a strategy for discriminating between them. Test the hypothesis for coherence, adequacy, and parsimony. Avoid premature closure. Continue testing the working hypothesis against test results, clinical course, and response to therapy.
Comprehensive care	Identify the most fundamental problems and concerns. Incorporate risk stratification. Include disease- and nondisease-based perspectives. Incorporate nursing theory, human responses, and personhood. Include health promotion, disease prevention, and risk reduction. Engage the patient as a partner in care.

(Continued)

Table 6.3 (Continued)

Phase of Clinical Reasoning	Habits that Promote Sound Reasoning
Establishing goals	Include the patient in establishing goals. Determine management priorities and plan care accordingly. Identify specific and realistic goals for treatment. Incorporate clinical standards in goal setting.
Determining management plans	Employ intervention modalities from both nursing and medical perspectives. Initiate effective care for emergency or life-threatening conditions. Consult with appropriate colleagues in complex care situations. Consider patient's social context, preferences, abilities, lifestyle, and individual needs. Anticipate and discuss possible conflicts in values, priorities, and beliefs. Use evidence-based therapies appropriately. Consider treatment efficacy as compared to risks, costs, and desired outcomes. Think ahead to probabilistic disease progression needs. Incorporate evidence-based approaches, accepted treatment guidelines, and current standards of care. Provide effective and appropriate management for comorbidities.

Source: Adapted from Chase (2004).

Exhibit 6.2

TOOLS TO SUPPORT AND ENHANCE CLINICAL DECISION MAKING IN ADVANCED CLINICAL PRACTICE

Nursing Standards of Practice
NANDA/NIC/NOC
Mid-level theories
Evidence-based practice
Clinical practice guidelines
Web-based information systems

however. Many areas of practice do not have adequate bodies of evidence. In addition, context-specific problems sometimes warrant decisions not addressed by the research literature. Thus, it is imperative that critical thinking, research appraisal, and clinical decision making skills be used in combination with one another. Typically, evidence-based practice is assumed to refer to external, population-based evidence derived through systematic research. Many authors caution against the application of external evidence without careful consideration of its appropriateness to a specific individual's needs and circumstances. There is a growing expectation, however, that advanced practice nurses will seek the available evidence and use this evidence to inform their decision making.

Clinical practice guidelines can be formalized by specific managed-care organizations with the expectation that the guidelines are used to direct practice, or they may simply refer to concise informational outlines and algorithms intended to assist clinicians with the massive amounts of diagnostic and management information available. In either case, they are tremendously useful, but they can also constrain and oversimplify practice by focusing more uncommon problems (Tracy, 2009). If they are overly relied upon, clinical guidelines can result in failing to attend to the individual needs and nuanced presentations of a patient's condition. Many Web-based information systems have been developed that are now viewed as part of the standard support tools for practice. These include intranet and Internet systems, as well as online journals, databases, and governmental and organizational websites. One entry-level advanced practice competency is the ability to access, search, and critically evaluate the appropriateness of clinical guidelines and electronic resources for practice.

CONCLUSIONS

Expertise in clinical decision making is vital for clinical competency. At the advanced practice level, this is a complex undertaking for both the individual provider and the profession. Keeping the core of nursing theory and perspectives central and visible while gaining competency in the knowledge base and probabilistic thinking of advanced practice requires continuous attention to practice-based cognitive skills and processes. It is recommended that advanced practice clinical decision making be approached as a continuous and deliberate process of knowledge expansion and reflective practice, maintaining the personhood and holistic needs of the patient and the importance of the nurse–patient relationship central to practice.

REFERENCES

American Association of Colleges of Nursing (AACN). (2006). *The essentials of master's education for advanced practice nursing.* Washington DC: Author.

Benner, P. (1984). *From novice to expert: Excellence and power in clinical nursing practice.* Upper Saddle River, NJ: Prentice Hall.

Benner, P., Hooper-Kyriakidis, P., & Stannard, D. (1999). *Clinical wisdom and interventions in critical care: A thinking in action approach.* Philadelphia: W. B. Saunders Company.

Benner, P., Stannard, D., & Hooper, P. L. (1996). A "thinking-in-action" approach to teaching clinical judgment: A classroom innovation for acute care advanced practice nurses. *Advanced Practice Nursing Quarterly, 1*(4), 70–77.

Benner, P., Tanner, C. A., & Chesla, C. A. (2009). *Expertise in nursing practice: Caring, clinical judgment, and ethics* (2nd ed.). New York: Springer Publishing.

Benner, P., & Wrubel, J. (1989). *The primacy of caring.* Menlo Park, CA: Addison-Wesley.

Boshuizen, H. P. A., & Schmidt, H. G. (1992). On the role of biomedical knowledge in clinical reasoning by experts, intermediates, and novices. *Cognitive Science, 16,* 153–184.

Brookfield, S. (2000). Clinical reasoning and generic thinking skills. In J. Higgs & M. Jones (Eds.), *Clinical reasoning in the health professions* (2nd ed., pp. 62–67). Oxford: Butterworth-Heinemann.

Brykczynski, K. A. (1989). An interpretive study describing the clinical judgment of nurse practitioners. *Scholarly Inquiry for Nursing Practice: An International Journal, 3*(2), 75–111.

Buckingham, C. D., and Adams, A. (2000). Classifying clinical decision making: A unifying approach. *Journal of Advanced Nursing, 32,* 981–989.

Buckingham, C. D. (2002). Psychological cue use and implications for a clinical decision support system. *Medical Informatics and the Internet in Medicine, 27*(4), 237–251.

Carnevali, D. L., & Thomas, M. D. (1993). *Diagnostic reasoning and treatment decision making in nursing.* Philadelphia: J. B. Lippincott.

Chase, S. K. (2001). The art of diagnosis and treatment. In L. M. Dunphy & J. E. Winland-Brown (Eds.), *Primary care: The art and science of advanced practice nursing* (pp. 85–103). Philadelphia: F. A. Davis.

Chase, S. K. (2004). *Clinical judgment and communication in nurse practitioner practice.* Philadelphia: F. A. Davis.

Cioffi, J. (1997). Heuristics, servants to intuition in clinical decision making. *Journal of Advanced Nursing, 26,* 203–208.

Cioffi, J., & Markham, R. (1997). Clinical decision making by midwives: Managing case complexity. *Journal of Advanced Nursing, 25,* 265–272.

Corcoran, S. A. (1986a). Task complexity and nursing expertise as factors in decision making. *Nursing Research, 35*(2), 107–112.

Corcoran, S. A. (1986b). Planning by expert and novice nurses in cases of varying complexity. *Research in Nursing & Health, 9,* 155–162.

Dains, J. E., Baumann, L. C., & Scheibel, P. (2007). *Advanced health assessment and clinical diagnosis in primary care* (3rd ed.). St. Louis: Mosby.

Davies, B., & Hughes, A. M. (2002). Clarification of advanced nursing practice: Characteristics and competencies. *Clinical Nurse Specialist, 16*(3), 147–152.

Dreyfus, H. L., & Dreyfus, S. E. (1986). *Mind over machine: The power of intuition and expertise in the era of the computer.* New York: Free Press.

Elstein, A. S. (1976). Clinical judgment: Psychological research and medical practice. *Science, 194,* 696–700.

Elstein, A. S., & Schwartz, A. (2000). Clinical reasoning in medicine. In J. Higgs and M. Jones (Eds.), *Clinical reasoning in the health professions* (2nd ed., pp. 95–106). Oxford: Butterworth-Heinemann.

Elstein, A. S., Shulman, L. S., & Sprafka, S. A. (1978). *Medical problem solving: An analysis of clinical reasoning.* Cambridge: Harvard University Press.

Facione, P. (1990). *Critical thinking: A statement of consensus for purposes of educational assessment and instruction.* Fullerton, CA: American Philosophical Association, California State University.

Fenton, M. V. (1983). Identification of the skilled performance of master's prepared nurses as a method of curriculum planning and evaluation. In P. Benner, *From novice to expert: Excellence and power in clinical nursing practice* (pp. 262–274). Upper Saddle River, NJ: Prentice Hall.

Hamm, R. M. (1988). Clinical intuition and clinical analysis: Expertise and the cognitive continuum. In J. Dowie and A. Elstein, *Professional judgment: A reader in clinical decision making* (pp. 78–105). New York: Cambridge University Press.

Hammond, K. R. (1964). An approach to the study of clinical inference in nursing: Part II. *Nursing Research, 13*(4), 315–319.

Hammond, K., Kelly, K., & Castellan, E. A. (1966). Clinical inference in nursing: Use of information seeking strategies by nurses. *Nursing Research, 15*(4), 330–336.

Hayes, B., & Adams, R. (2000). Parallels between clinical reasoning and categorization. In J. Higgs & M. Jones (Eds.), *Clinical reasoning in the health professions* (2nd ed., pp. 45–53). Oxford: Butterworth-Heinemann.

Higgs, J., Burn, A., & Jones, M. (2001). Integrating clinical reasoning and evidence-based practice. *AACN Clinical Issues, 12*(4), 482–490.

Higgs, J., & Jones, M. (1995). Clinical reasoning. In J. Higgs and M. Jones (Eds.), *Clinical reasoning in the health professions* (pp. 3–10). Oxford: Butterworth-Heinemann.

Higgs, J., & Jones, M. (2000). Clinical reasoning in the health professions. In J. Higgs and M. Jones (Eds.), *Clinical reasoning in the health professions* (2nd ed., pp. 3–14). Oxford: Butterworth-Heinemann.

Huch, M. H. (1995). Nursing science as a basis for advanced practice. *Nursing Science Quarterly, 8*(1), 6–7.

Kassirer, J. P., & Kopelman, R. I. (1991). *Learning clinical reasoning.* Baltimore: William & Wilkins.

Lauri, S., & Salantera, S. (2002). Developing an instrument to measure and describe clinical decision making in different nursing fields. *Journal of Professional Nursing, 18*(2), 93–100.

Lunney, M. (2009). Assessment, clinical judgment and nursing diagnosis: How to determine an accurate diagnosis. In North American Nursing Diagnosis Association, *Nursing diagnoses: Definitions and classification 2009–2011,* pg 1–17. Ames, IA: Wiley-Blackwell,

Narayan, S. M., & Corcoran-Perry, S. (1997). Line of reasoning as a representation of nurses' clinical decision making. *Research in Nursing & Health, 20*, 353–364.

Narayan, S. M., Corcoran-Perry, S., Drew, D., Hoyman, K., & Lewis, M. (2003). Decision analysis as a tool to support an analytical pattern-of-reasoning. *Nursing and Health Sciences, 5*, 229–243.

National Association of Clinical Nurse Specialists (NACNS). (2004). *Statement on clinical nurse specialist practice and education* (2nd ed.). Harrisburg, PA: Author.

National Organization of Nurse Practitioner Faculties (NONPF). (1995). *Curriculum guidelines and program standards for nurse practitioner education.* Washington DC: Author.

National Organization of Nurse Practitioner Faculties (NONPF). (2006). *Domains and competencies of nurse practitioner practice.* Washington DC: Author.

Newell, A., & Simon, H. A. (1972). *Human problem solving.* Englewood Cliffs, NJ: Prentice Hall.

Patel, V. L., & Kaufman, D. R. (2000). Clinical reasoning and biomedical knowledge: Implications for teaching. In J. Higgs and M. Jones (Eds.), *Clinical reasoning in the health professions* (2nd ed., pp. 33–44). Oxford: Butterworth-Heinemann.

Pyles, S., & Stern, P. (1983). Discovery of nursing gestalt in critical care nursing: The importance of the gray gorilla syndrome. *Image: The Journal of Nursing Scholarship, 15*, 51–57.

Rew, L. (1988). Intuition in decision making. *Image: Journal of Nursing Scholarship, 20*, 150–155.

Ritter, B. J. (2003). An analysis of expert nurse practitioners' diagnostic reasoning. *Journal of the American Academy of Nurse Practitioners, 15*(3), 137–141.

Sands, H. M. (2001). *Making the diagnosis: Factors shaping diagnostic reasoning among entry level nurse practitioners.* Unpublished doctoral dissertation, University of California, Los Angeles.

Scheffer, B. K., & Rubenfeld, M. G. (2000). A consensus statement on critical thinking in nursing. *Journal of Nursing Education, 39*(8), 352–359.

Simmons, B. (2002). *Clinical reasoning in experienced nurses.* Unpublished doctoral dissertation, Loyola University, Chicago.

Smith, M. C. (1995). The core of advanced practice nursing. *Nursing Science Quarterly, 8*, 2–3.

Smith, S. K. (1987). An analysis of the phenomenon of deterioration in the critically ill. *Image: Journal of Nursing Scholarship, 20*(1), 12–15.

Tanner, C. A., Padrick, K. P., Westfall, U. E., & Putzier, D. J. (1987). Diagnostic reasoning strategies of nurses and nursing students. *Nursing Research, 36*, 358–362.

Tanner, C. A., Benner, P., Chesla, C., & Gordon, D. (1993). The phenomenology of knowing the patient. *Image: Journal of Nursing Scholarship, 25*, 273–280.

Thompson, C. (2002). Human error, bias, decision making and judgment in nursing: The need for a systematic approach. nd. In C. Thompson and D. Dowding (Eds.), *Clinical decision making and judgment in nursing* (pp. 21–45). Edinburgh: Churchill Livingstone.

Thompson, C., & Dowding, D. (2002). *Clinical decision making and judgment in nursing.* Edinburgh: Churchill Livingstone.

Titchen, A., & Higgs, J. (2000). Facilitating the acquisition of knowledge and reasoning. In J. Higgs and M. Jones (Eds.), *Clinical reasoning in the health professions* (2nd ed., pp. 222–229). Oxford: Butterworth-Heinemann.

Tracy, M. F. (2009). Direct clinical practice. In A. B. Hamric, J. A. Spross, & C. M. Hanson (Eds.) *Advanced practice nursing An integrative Approach* (4th ed.), pgs. 123–158. St. Louis: Saunders Elsevier.

Tversky, A., & Kahneman, D. (1974). Judgment under uncertainty: Heuristics and biases. *Science, 185,* 1124–1131.

White, J. E., Nativio, D. G., Kobert, S. N., & Engberg, S. J. (1992). Content and process in clinical decision making by nurse practitioners. *Image: Journal of Nursing Scholarship, 24,* 153–158.

Health Care Policy: Implications for Advanced Practice

7

LINDA REIVITZ

One of the penalties for refusing to participate in politics is that you end up being governed by your inferiors.

—Plato

Issues related to health policy are frequently in the headlines today: a recall of peanut butter products, vaccination guidelines for children, a comparison of the U.S. health care system with that of the United Kingdom or Japan, the need for surveillance activities to determine whether bird flu is a threat, the projected shortage of nurses in 2025 and the bankruptcy of Medicare in 2019 or earlier. These are all vivid examples of the kinds of popular health policy issues in current public discourse. They are popular largely because of the immense implications they have on the greater U.S. community. However, health policy discussions are not always about such prominent or pressing national matters. Local health policy problems and solutions can be just as important to an affected community.

A great illustration of this point comes from a graduate nursing student who also served as the director of a county public health agency. The elected county board that funded her program had one decision left to make as they wrapped up their long discussion on the county's annual budget: Should they use the limited amount of money which had not yet been allocated to hire an additional public health nurse, or should

123

they purchase a new truck? This question, pressing to the public health director who had the best interests of a local health agency in mind, is also about health policy, if on a smaller scale.

No matter the scale of the health policy issue or the size of the community it affects, the process of creating health policies is basically the same on the local, state, and national level. Knowing how that process works and ways to influence it empowers the advanced practice nurse to stand up for and fight against health policies on any level. The purpose of this chapter is to help the APN understand and engage in that process.

Why should advanced practice nurses care? Policy makers at the federal, state, and local levels influence what nursing professionals can do, how they do it, and what they are paid. Public policies decide who has insurance and what insurance will pay. They set the standard of how often swimming pools and restaurants are inspected and whether smoking is allowed in the workplace. Public policies and how they are implemented also shape the direction of health care delivery. They affect the experience of providers as they practice and the experience of consumers as they attempt to receive care in an increasingly complex and expensive system.

The bottom line is that local, state, and national policies affect our daily and professional lives. Without the input of the people in the community they serve, policy makers will make decisions based on a narrower perspective. It is our job as community members to add our stories, ideas, and expertise to the decision-making process. It could mean the difference between investing in another public health nurse or purchasing a new truck.

PUBLIC POLICY: THE PROCESS

Creating public policy is a messy process. Ideally, there would be straightforward steps that would help decision makers define problems, consider solutions, choose the optimal solution, and then implement it. After that, the situation could be evaluated, and if the objectives were not met, there would be an opportunity to adjust or completely change the originally proposed solution to better address the issue at hand. However, for a variety of reasons, the process of policy making rarely if ever works that way.

First, there are too many problems for policy makers to solve. They have to prioritize and decide what to focus on. As a result, some

Ship To:

THERESA OBONYANO
3618 MUSTANG LN
MANVEL, TEXAS 77578-3575

Order ID: 104-1933087-5813817

Thank you for buying from Piney Oak Books on Amazon Marketplace.

Shipping Address:
THERESA OBONYANO
3618 MUSTANG LN
MANVEL, TEXAS 77578-3575

	Order Date:	Apr 23, 2014
	Shipping Service:	Standard
	Buyer Name:	Theresa Obonyano
	Seller Name:	Piney Oak Books

Quantity	Product Details
1	**Advanced Practice Nursing: Core Concepts for Professional Role Development, Fourth Edition [Paperback] [2009] Jansen PhD RN C GNP-BC NP-C, Dr. Michalene; Zwygart-Stauffacher PhD RN GNP/GC, Dr. Mary** **SKU:** 082610515775U **ASIN:** 0826105157 **Listing ID:** 0213OPF7ITX

Returning your item:
Go to "Your Account" on Amazon.com, click "Your Orders" and then click the "seller profile" link for this order to get information about the return and refund policies that apply.
Visit http://www.amazon.com/returns to print a return shipping label. Please have your order ID ready.

Thanks for buying on Amazon Marketplace. To provide feedback for the seller please visit www.amazon.com/feedback. To contact the seller, please visit Amazon.com and click on "Your Account" at the top of any page. In Your Account, go to the "Orders" section and click on the link "Leave seller feedback". Select the order or click on the "View Order" button. Click on the "seller profile" under the appropriate product. On the lower right side of the page under "Seller Help", click on "Contact this seller".

problems receive little if any attention. Second, even if someone has a solid solution, it may be very expensive or not technically feasible. Nuclear power plants, for example, may be an effective solution to help meet our energy needs, but they produce nuclear waste that is difficult to safely store or dispose of, creating a bigger problem than the one nuclear power would solve. Third, there are often notable disagreements over which solution is truly optimal. Experts generally do not agree with each other, and public opinion is rarely even close to unanimous on any issue. Finally, the most important problems of today may be far down the list of concerns tomorrow, and the problem that should be tackled today is something no one anticipated the week before.

With all these layers of complication, how might a person persuade the county board to consider hiring a public health nurse rather than buying a truck? In his book, John Kingdon (1995) sets forth a model that provides insight into the policy-making process, teaching readers how and when they can be most effective in influencing policy decisions. His model works equally well for policy making at the federal, state, and county levels.

Kingdon's Model: Agenda Setting and Specification of Alternatives

Kingdon (1995) states that public policy starts with two processes: (1) agenda setting, deciding which issue or problem policy makers and outside interests will pay attention to, and (2) the specification of alternatives, deciding which options they will seriously consider to solve the problems on the agenda.

There are many important issues that could be addressed when setting an agenda: increasing unemployment, international trade, education, public parks, transportation, energy conservation, or health care, to name a few. Within health care, policy makers can focus on a multitude of specific problems, including research funding for cancer or Alzheimer's disease, development of community-based programs for seniors, or a shortage of health providers. Moreover, as we have seen with Hurricane Katrina, the Virginia Tech shootings, and the events of September 11, 2001, the issues on the agenda for policy makers can rapidly change.

The second part of Kingdon's model—the specification of alternatives—focuses on the process of creating policies, or solutions, once the agenda has been set. In the 2008 presidential race, the almost 46 million Americans who were uninsured (U.S. Census Bureau, 2008) was a distinct item on the agenda for both Democrats and Republicans, serving as a major talking point for both candidates. Senators Obama and McCain had very different solutions, or policies, to address this issue. Senator Obama proposed an expansion of federal programs that provide insurance for children (State Children's Health Insurance Program [S-CHIP]) and a way for those under 65 to buy into the Medicare system, among other ideas. Senator McCain proposed giving tax credits to people who purchase insurance as a way of encouraging them to do so. In short, the two candidates had very different ideas about how to solve the same problem (Kaiser Family Foundation, 2008a).

Kingdon: The Important Actors

In Kingdon's model, there are factors that help answer the question: What problems will we attempt to solve and how do we intend to solve them? The first group of influential factors contains those involved in the policy-making process, namely, the actors. These actors come from different backgrounds, groups, and organizations, so not surprisingly they have different perspectives to bring to every part of the policy-making process.

The foremost actors in the policy-making process are elected officials. Kingdon (1995) tells us that at the federal level the president and members of Congress set the national agenda. A state's governor and legislature serve the same role on a state level. They decide which issues will be discussed and which will be set aside for possible consideration at a later time. Members of Congress decide what proposals or bills will be introduced, which will have public hearings, and which will be debated. No hearing and no debate means the legislation has little chance of becoming law. Information on how to influence which issues are addressed by policy makers will be provided later in this chapter.

Not only do the varying perspectives of elected officials influence which issues and policies will be on the agenda, their perspectives also inform how those issues and problems are defined. Once again using the 2008 presidential race as an example, many candidates and voters believed that health care reform was needed because millions of Americans are uninsured. However, health care reform means different things to different actors. To some, health care reform means encouraging the creation of health savings accounts, giving tax credits for those who purchase long-term care insurance or pushing for the expansion of community health centers. To others, it means changes in malpractice liability, expanded eligibility for medical assistance, or funding for electronic medical records. Each solution will solve a different problem, yet all fall under the heading "health care reform."

The public as a group of actors has a large role in deciding what policies are discussed and ultimately what policy changes occur. Voting is the first major way the public voices its opinion as certain candidates win over others, dictating which perspectives and values are brought to the agenda-setting and specification of alternatives table. The public voice is also heard when people send letters to legislators, attend hearings, testify at hearings on behalf of groups or organizations they are part of, e-mail their legislators, or go to local constituent listening sessions held by many legislators.

The media, another group of actors, may get an issue onto the policy-making agenda or shape the national discussion of issues or policies already being discussed. A series by the *Washington Post* about care for military personnel at Walter Reed Hospital is just one example of how the media can influence what is on the nation's agenda (Priest & Hull, 2007a; Priest & Hull, 2007b). Through the various media outlets, policy makers are able to hear a drumbeat for action of one kind or another.

So-called "experts," a fourth group of actors, are especially important in formulating policies to address issues on the agenda. There are experts in government agencies, universities, think tanks, congressional committees, and associations such as the AARP or the National Potato Council. Although the advice and counsel of experts is valued in policy making, such advice may or may not be taken by legislators. One reason expert advice may not be considered is that it may not be available in a timely manner. When legislators or members of Congress are looking for an answer, they are generally not able to wait 2 years for a study to be conducted to find the answer. A second reason is that experts often disagree.

Last, but certainly not least, are interest groups. For purposes of this chapter, the terms *interest group* and *advocacy group* are used interchangeably. Interest groups look after the interests of their constituents and advocate for preferred policy choices based on the preferences of their members. There are interest groups representing the Boy Scouts of America, steel manufacturers, and hospitals, to name a few. Certainly it is possible to become jaded and cynical about the power and influence of interest groups in policy making today; there are over 15,000 lobbyists in Washington, DC, and interest groups spent over $3 billion lobbying Congress in 2008 (Center for Responsive Politics, 2009a, 2009b).

Nevertheless, some theories have long held that all politics and all government decision making is the result of advocacy groups' activities and that "any other attempt to explain politics and government is doomed to failure" (Lemann, 2008). Whether groups are all-powerful or not, there is little question that the power of individuals is magnified when they form groups (Birkland, 2005), and the power of one group is magnified when it forms a coalition with others (Weissert & Weissert, 2002). Because of the power in numbers, interest groups can be an effective way for people to collectively express their desire for policy change (Birkland, 2005).

Interest groups work hard to get issues on the agenda and policies enacted that have the best interests of their constituency in mind. They work even harder to block policy changes they do not like. In health care alone, there are different interest groups representing the views of rural, urban, teaching, and all other kinds of hospitals. There are interest groups representing nurses, doctors, pharmacists, home care organizations, and nursing home aides. There are advocacy groups representing insurance companies, durable medical equipment companies, hospice organizations, and pharmaceutical firms. There are groups representing seniors, the uninsured, and people with diabetes, heart disease, and Alzheimer's disease. The list goes on and on.

All advocacy groups, of course, are not the same. Some have far more money than others. Some represent far more people than others. But money and size do not necessarily determine how much influence interest groups have over policy makers. Legislators, for example, may listen more sympathetically to small business owners trying to provide health insurance to their employees than to those working for an insurance trade group. Additionally, legislators may listen more sympathetically to an actual patient with kidney failure or to a nurse who cares for such patients rather than a lobbyist working for the American Medical Association (AMA) or National Kidney Foundation (NKF).

Kingdon: The Three Ps

In addition to agendas, alternatives, and actors, Kingdon (1995) lays out the importance of the "three Ps" in the policy-making process. He calls them the problem stream, policy stream, and political stream. One can think of them as problems, policies, and politics.

The problem stream. A policy maker must believe that a problem actually exists; otherwise, there is no need to act. Reaching agreement on what constitutes a problem can be a challenging task among policy makers. Think about this question: Are high gas prices a problem? Certainly elected policy makers received a lot of complaints from their constituencies about high prices in the summer of 2008 when gas was near $4 per gallon. On the flip side, those who believe we should reduce energy consumption or reduce our reliance on foreign oil may argue that high gas prices are not a problem, but part of the solution, because they lead to greater use of public transportation and reduced energy consumption.

Let's consider this question: Is tuberculosis (TB) a problem? It largely depends on whom you ask. If you posed this question to people walking down Main Street in your community, most would probably say no. Most legislators would echo that opinion because they likely have not seen or heard anything to the contrary. However, a nurse working in a public health agency, especially in a major city, will likely answer yes. What Kingdon teaches us here is that for policy change to occur, policy makers must be convinced or alerted about a problem first. If nurses or advocates want increased funding for TB prevention or treatment programs, they must convince policy makers, who control public funding, that TB is a problem.

Outside of other actors bringing issues to their attention through activism, policy makers can also recognize that a problem exists when there is a crisis, such as a TB or measles outbreak, a natural disaster, or a dramatic increase in mortgage foreclosures. For this reason, a crisis is not always bad if policy change is your goal. A crisis can create a sense of urgency or the desire to get something done. As Rahm Emanuel, President Barack Obama's chief of staff, said shortly before the new president's inauguration, "You never want a serious crisis to go to waste" (Seib, 2008).

Less dramatically, policy makers may also gain awareness about certain issues through their own lived experiences. They may read about problems in letters from constituents, reports from agencies, or newsletters from advocacy groups. They may also become acutely aware of a problem because of personal events, which is especially important for legislation on health care. For example, a legislator's wife has breast cancer, a daughter is an alcoholic, a parent develops Alzheimer's, or a neighbor's son has AIDS; these experiences may push legislators to be more passionate about an issue and to act more quickly on that issue than they would have done otherwise.

There are many instances in which legislators have become activists or leaders on health care issues when they have seen the problem personally. One example arose during the debate on the nearly $800 billion economic stimulus bill, which passed Congress in mid-February 2009. The Senate reduced spending in many areas compared to the amounts originally proposed by the House of Representatives but did not cut an additional $10 billion for medical research. This legislation was put into the bill by Senator Arlen Specter (R-PA), a survivor of two bouts of cancer, open-heart surgery, and a faulty diagnosis of Lou Gehrig's disease (Harris, 2009).

The policy stream. The policy stream contains ideas for policy change. Ideas can come from anywhere: experts, academics, interest groups, or students in a fourth grade class. Ideas may come from a policy group, such as AARP, the Heritage Foundation, or the American Hospital Association, or from an individual.

The National Health Service Corp (NHSC) is an example of the latter. The creation of this organization, to help place doctors in medically underserved areas, was an idea proposed to Senator Warren Magnuson (D-WA) by one of his constituents, a physician and activist named Dr. Abraham Bergman. The idea was drafted into a bill and in a relatively short period of time, marked by fits and starts, good and bad luck, chance, persistence, and passion, the bill became law (Redman, 1973). Since the early 1970s when the program began, over 27,000 primary care clinicians (including nurses) have been placed in health professional shortage areas. By 2004, the budget for the NHSC scholarship and loan repayment program was almost $170 million (United States Department of Health and Human Services [DHHS], Health Resources & Services Administration, 2008).

Although it sounds trite, there is a strong relationship between problems and the kinds of ideas that are proposed to solve them. How a problem is defined influences and limits the solutions that are proposed to address it. That is why two policy makers can look at the same problem and describe it differently. In part, they are defining the problem based on what *they* think the solution ought to be. As Thomas Birkland states in his book on the policy process, "the actual act of identifying a problem is as much a normative judgment as it is an objective statement of fact . . ." (Birkland, 2005, p 15). That is, whether something is really a problem is actually part of the debate itself.

An example of this relates to the simple question: How many people in the United States are uninsured? High numbers of people without insurance is a problem, but how *big* of a problem is it? The U.S. Census Bureau reported that almost 46 million Americans had no health insurance in 2007 (U.S. Census Bureau, 2008), a number that is expected to increase with the economic downturn that began in 2008 (Hewitt Associates, 2009). However, some policy analysts question whether those who have been uninsured for less than a year should count as uninsured. Others say the problem is exaggerated because many people without insurance have enough income to purchase insurance if they really wanted it (Shott, 2007). Either way, these analysts do not define the problem the same way the Census Bureau does, and they conclude that the problem of the uninsured is less serious than is commonly described.

Another example of the importance of problem definition can be seen in the issue of uninsured children. Approximately two thirds of uninsured children are eligible for public insurance programs such as Medical Assistance or S-CHIP. Policy makers reasonably assumed that the best way to solve this problem was to find those uninsured, eligible children and their families using aggressive and extensive outreach programs and enroll them. However, what if the problem was erroneously defined? Recent research concluded that if state Medicaid and S-CHIP programs simply *retained* all children who are enrolled and have no alternative coverage in a given year, the number of uninsured children in the United States would fall by one third (Sommers, 2007).

In this example, the way the problem is defined determines what solutions are considered to solve it. In one case, the real problem behind high numbers of uninsured children is defined as outreach, front-end solutions that focus on aggressively providing information and services to groups that might otherwise be neglected. The goal would be to get eligible people enrolled in the program. In the latter case, the problem is defined as retention, which could potentially be solved by simplifying the renewal process, creating shorter forms, making forms in multiple languages, or requiring less frequent renewals.

A final example, although there are many, is the issue of whether cell phones should be banned while driving. What is the problem in this case? Are drivers and their passengers unsafe because the driver's hands are not on the steering wheel of the car? If this is the problem, an effective solution may be to ban the use of hand-held cell phones while driving. This in fact is the solution chosen by many policy makers at the state, city, and county level (Insurance Institute for Highway Safety, 2009). However, research indicates that the real issue is that any talking on a cell phone distracts drivers from the task at hand, a problem that exists whether drivers are holding the phone or not (Insurance Institute for Highway Safety, 2005). For this reason, the National Safety Council has recommended a total ban on cell-phone use while driving (Parker-Pope, 2009).

The political stream. Whether or not policy change is possible depends on what is going on in the political stream. The political stream includes factors such as public opinion, the national mood, and election results. Opinion polls quantify feelings and tell policy makers whether the public is satisfied or dissatisfied, anxious or unconcerned. For example, findings from opinion polls over the years have told us that people lost confidence in the Food and Drug Administration, the public is willing to support many options to expand health insurance coverage, and adults see childhood obesity as a major problem (*The Wall Street Journal Online* [WSJO] & Harris Interactive, 2008, 2007, 2006). Specific to health care, the Kaiser Family Foundation, in partnership with others, has measured the public's opinions on health insurance, health care costs, AIDS, direct-to-consumer advertising for prescription drugs, Medicare, and views on long-term care (Kaiser Family Foundation, 2009).

The attitudes expressed in polls are played out on Election Day. Exactly what issues were discussed most often in campaigns? In polls, how did Americans respond when asked about the issues most important to them? Where did health care sit on their priority list? If it is not high on the list, policy makers could assume that issues other than health care require attention first. What beliefs and values does a new president bring to his or her position? Which party has the majority in Congress, and what do most members of Congress believe about the role and size of government? The answers to these questions can give a solid indication of what the national mood is at a particular point in history and what policy change the public prefers.

Elected officials read polls, of course, but they often can discern their constituency's mood from reading their mail, meeting with constituents at town hall meetings, and interacting with diners at the local eatery. They sense when their constituents are upbeat or gloomy and what they expect from government.

Kingdon: The Three Ps Combined

Although public sentiment may push policy makers to act, public opinion alone does not get policy change enacted; neither will election results or the national mood. For change to occur, according to Kingdon, all three Ps must be present (1995). When there is a recognized problem, a solution available in the policy community to solve that problem, and a favorable political environment, a policy window is open. This does not happen often. Kingdon writes, "Policy windows open infrequently, and do not stay open long. Despite their rarity, the major changes in public policy result from the appearance of these opportunities" (1995, p. 166). We will discuss one such opportunity later in this chapter. First, we will look at two other important factors critical to understanding how policy change occurs: incrementalism and coalition building.

Incrementalism. Many policy activists discover, to their chagrin, that most policy changes in the United States are small changes, not big ones. Policy makers identify a problem, enact relatively narrow policy changes to fix it, and then focus their attention on something else. In this sense, incrementalism is a description of the kinds of policy changes that are made: small ones. However, as Kingdon points out, incrementalism is also a strategy used to enact policy change, a little piece at a time (1995).

As policy debates are fought and it becomes clear that compromise is necessary to make change happen, advocates discuss whether they should accept "half a loaf." Will they accept funding for planning grants if there is not enough legislative support for implementation of a statewide program? Will they accept health insurance for all children if there is not enough legislative support for a national insurance system? If they cannot get support for 2 hours of mandated instruction about the benefits of organ donations in driver's education courses, will they accept a mandate of 30 minutes instead? Advocates may be told that compromise is the best method of achieving change and that they should not allow the ideal to become the enemy of the good (Hitt, 2009; Pear, 1987; Wangsness, 2009).

In 1993, during his first year in office, President Clinton decided he wanted the "whole loaf" as far as health reform was concerned. He proposed legislation that expanded coverage to all Americans, outlined a minimum level of benefits, and mandated that employers pay a significant portion of employee premiums (White House Domestic Policy Council [WHDPC], 1993a). His proposal also had provisions on improving access to care in rural and urban communities, helping academic health centers, bringing sense to medical malpractice (the administration's terminology), and requiring insurance plans to enroll everyone who applied regardless of their health status. He eliminated

Medicaid and provided incentives to increase medical research, among other things (WHDPC, 1993b).

The plan was anything but incremental. It was over 1,300 pages long, complex, and difficult to explain. The plan was unmercifully attacked by the insurance industry and others against it. Many who supported it were lukewarm in their support, wishing for a single-payer national system instead. In the context of this example, Kingdon writes, "there were sharp, fundamental differences among advocates, and no consensus in the policy community about which proposal to support" (1995, p. 219). The advocates for change could not agree on which approach to change they preferred.

Clinton's health reform legislation never passed Congress and was never even voted on by either the House of Representatives or the Senate. At the same time, the problems the president was trying to solve were still there, and small, incremental changes did occur. Congress did not enact universal health coverage but instead enacted legislation to provide insurance to increased numbers of lower-income, uninsured children through S-CHIP (Kaiser Family Foundation, 1997). Congress also enacted small group insurance reforms, including some restrictions on insurance exclusions for pre-existing conditions, (Litman & Robins, 1997) and took some early steps toward requiring insurance companies to cover mental illness on the same basis as medical illness (Hennessy & Goldman, 2001).

Those reflecting on the demise of Clinton's original legislation asked themselves whether "we come back to that first rule of American politics, . . . incrementalism rules, and those who seek more pay the price" (Zelman & Brown, 1998, p. 67). For her part, and as a result of the battle in 1993, Senator Hillary Clinton adopted what she called "the school of small steps" toward health care reform as she campaigned for president in 2007 and 2008 (Associated Press, 2007).

Even though it can succeed, the strategy of incrementalism is controversial. Although it can achieve results in the long run, it may seem as if not enough is being done in the short term to solve the big problems of the day. In 2009, it appears that the Obama administration will attain various goals that might have pleased health care activists in the past: an expansion of the S-CHIP program (Kaiser, 2009a) and additional funding for the National Institutes for Health, prevention programs, the National Health Service Corps, and COBRA subsidies for workers who lose their jobs and are in danger of losing their employer-sponsored health insurance (Steinbrook, 2009). Yet among health care activists who want the president and Congress to "think big on health reform immediately," the slow steps of incrementalism seem insufficient (Young, 2009).

Coalitions. Allies are needed to get policy changed, and this means coalition building. You must find others who agree with you and work collaboratively with them for the change desired. Coalition building is a dynamic process. Supporters on one issue may not agree on any other issue, yet these "strange bedfellows" come together when it is in their mutual interest to do so.

In the early 1980s, for example, the business community and children's advocacy groups were important allies in getting Congress to expand the medical assistance program. Advocacy groups wanted more children insured, and business groups were afraid that an increasing number of uninsured children would lead Congress to enact something like a national health insurance program. Both got what they wanted: More children became eligible for medical assistance, and the larger medical assistance program acted like a safety valve, keeping Congress from enacting broader policy change.

Coalitions can generate enough support to push legislation through Congress or a state legislature. They can also get issues onto the national agenda as we have seen in 2007 and 2008. In those years, a variety of large and deep-pocketed coalitions formed to make health care reform an issue in the presidential campaign. With names like Divided We Fail (DWF), Health Coverage Coalition for the Uninsured (HCCU), Better Health Care Together (BHCT), and the Coalition to Advance Health Care (CAHR) Reform, unlikely allies came together to advocate for action by Congress to increase health care coverage and moderate health care costs (Cummings, 2008).

One coalition, HCCU, which included the U.S. Chamber of Commerce, AARP, health provider associations, and a major advocacy group called Families USA, came together to announce a plan for universal coverage, starting with children (Hamburger & Alonso-Zaldivar, 2007). A second coalition, Better Health Care Together (BHCT), brought together the chiefs of Wal-Mart and the Service Employees International Union, two groups that prior to their joint campaign had "one of the fiercest rivalries in the American economy, attacking one another's organizations through dueling blogs, newspaper advertisements and news conferences" (Barbaro & Pear, 2007). DWF, a third coalition, brought together the Business Roundtable (representing large corporations), the Service

Employees International Union, AARP, and the National Federation of Independent Businesses, a group prominent in the defeat of the Clinton reform proposal of 1993. Their coalition was "a national effort designed to engage the American people, businesses, non-profit organizations and elected officials in finding bipartisan solutions to ensure affordable, quality health care and long-term financial security—for everyone" (Divided We Fail, www.aarp.org/issues/dividedwefail/get_involved/).

No one can predict how or even whether these coalitions will hold together once Congress begins debate on significant health reform legislation, but they have taken the first step. They have made sure that health care is on the nation's agenda, which is "a striking comeback for an issue deemed politically radioactive" since the Clinton reform proposal was defeated over a decade ago (Cummings, 2008).

The Policy Process and the Nursing Process

As nursing students have studied the steps of policy making that Kingdon offers, more than one has noticed the similarity between the policy-making process and the nursing process: assessment, planning, intervention, and evaluation. As one nursing scholar on policy and politics put it, "Nursing and politics are a good match" (Leavitt, Cohen, & Mason, 2002, p. 71).

The policy-making process, moving from a problem to the implementation of a program that aims to fix it, requires the separation of one problem from another. It requires us to understand that many solutions exist, to prioritize our needs, to interact and compromise with many other interests, and to be ready to respond to change, which is certain to come in a highly dynamic environment. But how can nurses and APNs use this model to change policy? What should they do if they want to change policy in the United States?

Mental Health Parity: A Policy Case Study

As we discussed earlier, Kingdon argues that policy change can occur if three requirements are met: there is a perceived problem, there are solutions to solve that problem, and the "right" political environment exists. The following case study is an illustration of Kingdon's model. It describes the "long, strange journey" (Rovner, 2007) of mental health parity legislation through Congress.

Defining the Problem

Mental health parity arose as an issue for two reasons. First, in most health insurance plans there was a lack of parity or equality between benefits for mental and physical diseases. Copayments were often higher for those receiving treatment for mental illness than for physical illness. Treatment for substance abuse was often not covered at all. The number of inpatient days covered by insurance was significantly less for mental illness than for cancer treatment, diabetes, or other physical ailments (Hennessy & Goldman, 2001).

Second, mental health parity had symbolic importance. To those with mental and addictive disorders, parity was civil rights legislation. Passage of mental health parity legislation represented an end to one kind of discrimination and a necessary step toward ending the stigma associated with mental illness (Hennessy & Goldman, 2001).

Mental health parity legislation would not only address the problems of disparate insurance coverage and discrimination for those with mental illness, but it would offer a solution. It was also expected to help tackle high rates of untreated mental illness, the fragmentation of the current system, and increased treatment costs paid by taxpayers.

According to the U.S. Surgeon General, one in five Americans has a diagnosable mental illness in any given year; yet, says the Surgeon General, "less than one third of adults with a diagnosable mental disorder receive treatment in one year" (U.S. DHHS, 1999, p. 18). Depression and other mental health problems prompted 156 million visits to doctors' offices and clinics in 2005 (Agency for Healthcare Research and Quality [AHRQ] & U.S. DHHS, 2008). Yet mental health services and programs are seriously fragmented. The federal government alone operates 42 different programs for people with mental illness, and additional programs that are available to help those with mental illness—programs associated with housing, education, criminal justice, and substance abuse, among others—each have their own eligibility rules and procedures (Iglehart, 2004).

Fragmentation is also a reason why many who suffer from mental illness go untreated for comorbidities. Research presented at meetings of the American Psychiatric Association indicated that patients with schizophrenia lose as much as 20 years of life to illnesses such as diabetes and heart disease because most are not being treated for those conditions. Undertreatment was attributed to the fact that psychiatrists assume that physical illness will be taken care of by a family doctor or physician, and this is not the case. The research also suggested that it was possible that health care systems that provide care for people with chronic mental illness are so fragmented that it is simply easy for patients to fall through the cracks (Smith, 2006).

The problems fragmentation poses in mental health programs are compounded by the increasing cost of treatment. Overall, the cost of mental health and substance abuse treatment has grown to over $105 billion per year, and it is increasingly being paid for with taxpayer dollars. In fact, Medicaid, a public insurance program, is the largest single payer of mental health care (Mark et al., 2005), and overall in 2005, mental disorders were the most costly medical conditions to treat in the United States (Roehrig, Miller, Lake, & Bryant, 2009).

Beyond the cost of treatment, even for those with insurance, stigma, shame, fear, and ignorance are external barriers to receiving and getting mental health care. That is why parity legislation was an acknowledgment for those with mental illness that they were not second-class citizens.

Finding a Solution

Congress took its first step toward equitable insurance coverage when it passed the Mental Health Parity Act (MHPA) of 1996. That legislation was a solution to the parity problem to a limited degree. It provided only that lifetime and annual dollar limits for mental health benefits must be the same as those for physical health (Hennessy& Goldman, 2001). As a result, many issues were left unaddressed:

- Policies could still exclude mental health coverage.
- No coverage was required for substance abuse treatment.
- Self-insured plans and individual policies were excluded.
- Businesses with 50 or fewer employees were excluded.
- Differential copayments or deductibles for mental and physical health were allowed as were different limits for inpatient days or outpatient visits per year.
- No help was provided for the uninsured.

Although the legislation was far from adequate, it was a small incremental change toward complete parity.

For the next 12 years, a variety of interested stakeholders for and against strengthening the 1996 law fought over this issue. Some sought to strengthen it, starting with those who lived daily with the inequity of the current system, such as patients, their families, and mental health providers. Many organizations were persistent in their advocacy for parity at both the federal and state levels, especially the National Alliance on Mental Illness (NAMI). NAMI advocates for parity, fairness, and an end to discrimination for those who are mentally ill (NAMI, 2007, 2008). Largely through their efforts, upwards of 40 state legislatures enacted parity legislation, ranging from comprehensive parity in Maryland and Oregon to laws in other states that require insurance parity only for treatment of specific disorders, such as bipolar disease or schizophrenia (NAMI, 2007).

Those opposed to true equity fought anything that served to strengthen the 1996 law. Some simply opposed government mandates of any kind. Those opposed to such mandates feel that government should not mandate insurance benefits because that is an individual decision that should be made by those companies or individuals who purchase insurance. Many were also concerned about cost. Insurance costs were increasing as high as 10% per year; and parity, it was feared, would increase insurance costs further for insurance companies who sold policies and for employers who purchased them. Although it could help some patients, they conceded, it would drive up the cost of insurance and increase the number of the uninsured (Matthews, 1999).

Exactly how much parity legislation would add to the cost of health care was unclear. Cost estimates in the first few years after the enactment of the MHPA in 1996 ranged from less than 1% to between 5 and 10% (Matthews, 1999). A study that looked at the cost of insurance for federal employees, who have had parity in benefits since 2001, concluded that parity legislation, when coupled with management of behavioral health care, improves insurance protection without an increase in total costs (Goldman et al., 2006). Later estimates from the Congressional Budget Office (CBO) reported that parity legislation would increase premiums by about .2% (2007).

Some supporters of parity even believed that parity in coverage could help reduce overall health insurance costs. As one state Blue Cross Blue Shield CEO put it: "Who are the people most likely to need parity? They're people in really tough shape. Where do they end up? In the emergency room," which is more expensive (Smith, 2007).

With all this variation in cost estimates, fear that mental health parity would increase costs remained. A common argument was that if legislation mandated comprehensive benefits, including coverage for all disorders listed in the diagnostic manual used by mental health professionals (the

Diagnostic and Statistical Manual of Mental Disorders [*DSM-IV*]), insurance would have to pay for treatment of disorders such as jet lag and caffeine addiction (Pear, 2008).

The Actors

Even though there were plenty of actors for and against mental health parity legislation, mental health parity was by no means a partisan issue. At the state level, parity legislation was signed by Republican George W. Bush when he was governor of Texas. As president, Mr. Bush established a commission to review the care of people with mental illness (Iglehart, 2004). At the federal level, mental health parity was championed by both Republicans and Democrats, the common thread being those who were personally touched by the issue.

Senator Peter Domenici, a Republican from New Mexico, was one of the authors of the 1996 legislation. He became aware of the parity issue after his daughter was diagnosed with schizophrenia (Lueck, 2008). The other author was Senator Paul Wellstone, a Democrat from Minnesota, who had a brother afflicted with a severe mental illness (Pear, 2008).

Building a Coalition

After the passage of limited parity legislation in 1996, Domenici and Wellstone continued their push for full mental health parity. When Senator Wellstone was killed in a plane crash in 2002, Domenici asked Senator Ted Kennedy of Massachusetts to become a cosponsor of parity legislation. Senator Kennedy accepted and was later joined in this effort by his son, Democratic Representative Patrick Kennedy from Rhode Island, who introduced parity legislation in the House of Representatives. Representative Kennedy had previously been diagnosed with bipolar disorder and treated for alcoholism and substance abuse. He was joined in sponsoring parity legislation by Republican Representative Jim Ramstad from Minnesota, a recovering alcoholic who often poignantly spoke of his addiction during legislative debate on parity (Rovner, 2008).

Despite their agreement on the need for full parity legislation, the two Kennedys disagreed on how to achieve the goal of full mental health parity. Representative Kennedy wanted a comprehensive bill whereas his father was more pragmatic. The senior Kennedy felt that the legislation would only pass if compromises were made in order to garner support from business and insurance groups that over the years had been able to defeat any improvements to the 1996 legislation (Pear, 2007).

A Change in the Political Environment

Over time, support for the concept of parity increased. As alluded to earlier, by executive order in 1999, President Bill Clinton implemented full parity for federal employees (Goldman et al., 2006). Many members of the U.S. Senate and nearly 60% of all members of the House of Representatives expressed support for parity legislation, at least in concept (Pear, 2007). In 2008, Congress established mental health parity in Medicare when it passed legislation reducing the copayments for outpatient mental health services from 50% to 20%, thus making them equal to the copayments for other types of Medicare benefits (Kaiser Family Foundation, 2008b). Yet mental health parity legislation that satisfied employers and insurance companies about the potential cost of parity legislation and that also satisfied advocates for full parity could not be found.

The key to compromise was a consensus process that began in 2004 under the leadership of Senators Kennedy, Domenici, and Michael Enzi, a Wyoming Republican. They brought together representatives from advocacy groups, such as NAMI; business groups, such as the U.S. Chamber of Commerce, National Retail Federation, and American Benefits Council; and insurance groups, such as America's Health Insurance Plans. All these very different perspectives came together in order to draft a parity bill that all interests could support. Each group had veto power over the specifics of what was in the legislation and over time each group gained a little bit more trust in the others (Pear, 2008).

Eventually this diverse group of interests came together to support one bill that had compromises on both sides of the issue (Zhang, 2007). By eliminating a requirement that insurers must cover treatment for any condition listed in the *DSM-IV*, the legislation gave employers the flexibility they wanted to design their own insurance plans. By stipulating that mental health treatment had to be as equally covered as physical treatment, the bill satisfied mental health parity advocates' desire to take from insurers the ability to impose arbitrary limits on mental health services.

Several other external factors were also important in the passage of mental health parity legislation. First, over time there was a deepening understanding about the brain and mental illness as well as an acknowledgment that treatment for mental illness was successful (U.S. DHHS, 1999). As Representative Jim Ramstad said during a congressional debate, "I am living proof that treatment works and recovery is real" (Pear, 2008).

Second, soon after the adoption of mental health parity in 1996, a close tie was established between parity and managed care. Daniel Gitterman, Roland Sturm, and Richard Scheffler called this tie a "policy bargain" (2001, p. 74). Advocates would get parity in benefits, but they must get the care in a way that would allow costs to be contained. This was often referred to as managed behavioral care. Advocates for parity acknowledged that mental health benefits would be delivered within a managed care framework specifically designed to control costs, encourage effective use of resources, and ensure that the care provided was appropriate. The result was that businesses and insurers became more comfortable that the cost of parity, their most central concern, could be controlled.

Third, in the decade after 1996, there were multiple tragic, catastrophic events including the attacks on September 11, 2001; Hurricane Katrina; wars in Iraq and Afghanistan; and shootings at Virginia Tech and other college campuses. These traumatizing events resulted in serious mental illness among those who experienced them. The issue of mental health parity became more salient to the public when they realized that they or their neighbors could someday be in need of mental health services.

By the end of 2008, 12 years after the passage of the Mental Health Parity Act, the process begun by Senators Kennedy and Domenici was about to bear fruit, and timing was everything. In October 2008, the Senate passed legislation providing a $700 billion bailout package for Wall Street. The Kennedy–Domenici proposal was included in that legislation (Hulse, 2008). The bailout package, including the mental health parity provisions, was then sent to the House of Representatives for consideration, but it was not clear the House would approve it. Similar bailout legislation had been defeated in the House a few days earlier (Hulse, 2008).

The mental health parity proposal was added to the larger bailout package specifically to persuade 51 members of the House, who had already voted against a bailout, to change their minds (Kaiser Family Foundation, 2008c). House members had to decide whether their support for mental health parity was greater than their opposition to the bailout package.

Advocacy groups became active once again (Kaiser Family Foundation, 2008c). Members of more than 200 advocacy organizations were encouraged to call their local representatives and urge them to vote for the bailout legislation because it would also provide mental health parity.

The legislation passed the House and was signed by the president the same day. Comprehensive mental health parity had finally become law (NAMI, 2009; Pear, 2008).

Kingdon's Model in Action

Riding on the coattails of a $700 billion bailout package for Wall Street may seem like an odd way to successfully end this 12-year journey for equal insurance benefits for mental and physical illness. Yet, by observing Kingdon's model, it is understandable.

Committed policy makers such as Senators Wellstone, Domenici, and Kennedy introduced parity legislation year after year. They never stopped advocating for what they considered equal rights for individuals with mental illness. Their commitment was matched by that of the advocates in NAMI and other organizations who fought for years to help individuals and families touched by serious mental illness. These senators had a solution to the inequity they saw, and a variation of that solution had been enacted in almost every state (NAMI, 2007). The state experiments with parity, and its "tie" with managed care, demonstrated that the costs associated with parity could be contained. Moreover, the coalition-building efforts by Senator Kennedy allowed opponents to gain trust in one another and to compromise.

The problem was known and acknowledged. The solution was clear. Then that last bit of good fortune surfaced. Days before Congress was expected to adjourn, the proponents of a Wall Street bailout package needed votes to pass that legislation in the House of Representatives. Was the need for support of the bailout legislation just good luck for those supporting mental health parity? Perhaps, but there is an adage that says you make your own luck. The proponents for mental health parity had been waiting for the window of opportunity to open, and when it did, they took full advantage.

In the case of mental health parity, the timing was especially fortunate for other reasons as well. At the end of 2008, Senator Domenici and Representative Ramstad both retired from Congress. Two strong voices in favor of parity would soon be gone. Senator Kennedy fell ill with a brain tumor, which not only sapped his prodigious amounts of energy but also robbed supporters of mental health parity of his considerable legislative influence and expertise. If parity had not been passed when it did, there is no telling when the window of opportunity may have opened again.

Where Do You Start?

There are many resources on the Internet for those who want information about policy issues. Table 7.1 contains a sample of such websites. Some of the organizations listed will connect you with government agencies and sources. Others are prominent policy and research organizations. Many other such sites can be found with ease.

There are also many how-to resources that can be accessed via the Internet if the goal is policy change. Getting involved by using resources online is fast and easy. For APNs, several websites make it exceedingly easy for you to be an advocate for advanced practice causes. Some of these organizations and websites are listed in Table 7.2.

Websites may provide a "toolbox" for you, which often includes tips for writing letters, e-mailing, calling, or meeting with legislators. They include ideas on how to make an impact. They might include a tutorial on the legislative process. After filling in your address, many will tell you who your legislators are and how to contact them. They will tell you whether and where there are local chapters of the organization and

Table 7.1

POLICY RESOURCES

U.S. government sources

THOMAS, legislative information from the Library of Congress	http://thomas.loc.gov
U.S. House of Representatives	www.house.gov
U.S. Senate	www.senate.gov
Centers for Disease Control and Prevention	www.cdc.gov
Centers for Medicare and Medicaid Services	www.cms.hhs.gov
Food and Drug Administration	www.fda.gov
National Health Service Corps	http://nhsc.bhpr.hrsa.gov
National Institute of Nursing Research	www.ninr.nih.gov
Substance Abuse and Mental Health Services Administration (SAMHSA)	www.samhsa.gov

Independent research and policy institutes

Cato Institute	www.cato.org
Center on Budget and Policy Priorities	www.cbpp.org
The Commonwealth Fund	www.commonwealthfund.org
The Heritage Foundation	www.heritage.org
Kaiser Family Foundation	http://kff.org
National Center for Policy Analysis	www.ncpa.org
National Conference of State Legislatures [State Legislative Tracking Web Resources]	www.ncsl.org/lrl/ 50statetracking.htm

ADVOCACY RESOURCES FOR APNs

Table 7.2

Organization	Mission	What is Available on the Website	Where to Find It
American Nurses Association (ANA)	Advances the nursing profession by fostering high standards of nursing practice, promoting the rights of nurses in the workplace, projecting a positive and realistic view of nursing, and lobbying Congress and regulatory agencies on health care issues affecting nurses and the public.	An RN activist tool kit allows you to sign up for the ANA grassroots action team (N-STAT), which contacts legislators when policy action that affects nurses is about to be voted on. Learn about the basics of lobbying and communicating with those on Capitol Hill and find out about specific issues of concern to the ANA in each state. Contact your congressman and sign up to stay informed.	www.nursingworld.org
American College of Nurse Practitioners (ACNP)	Ensures a solid policy regulatory foundation that enables NPs to continue providing accessible, high-quality health care to the nation.	Presents its public policy agenda and policy priorities. Provides "action alerts" on legislation of interest to APNs. Contains an advocacy toolbox, a legislative tracking chart (for members), information on state issues, and provides ways to get involved.	www.acnpweb.org
American Academy of Nurse Practitioners (AANP)	Promotes excellence in NP practice, education, and research; shapes the future of health care through advancing health policy; is the source of information for NPs, the health care community and consumers; and builds a positive image of the NP role as a leader in the national and global health care community.	Information on issues and legislation, including legislative alerts and updates, summaries of legislation key to NPs, and how your member of Congress voted on relevant legislation. Also features lobbying tips and detailed information on how to successfully communicate with your legislator.	www.aanp.org

provide a calendar of upcoming events. They will often ask you to share your story or make a donation.

Organization websites will tell you what their policy agenda is and may allow you to sign up for action alerts, so you receive notice when legislation of interest is being debated by the Congress or state legislature. They often provide a precomposed letter that you can simply sign or personalize and then easily e-mail to your congressman or senator. You can often make your views known easily in 5 minutes or less.

As you surf the Web, do not be surprised if a website only seems to provide you with one point of view. When you access a website, you should be a discerning consumer. Many are created to give you a biased, slanted, or self-serving point of view. There is nothing wrong with this. They are created to advocate for a specific point of view. As a consumer, it is your responsibility to beware.

Some sites are created to help you be a better advocate, regardless of what your specific area of interest is. One example is the Center for Health Improvement (http://healthpolicyguide.org). With sections on identifying opportunities for change, understanding the policy process, using data to state your case, joining forces in coalitions, and getting the word out, this site helps you to understand the policy process and gives information on how you can bring policy change to your community.

Other websites are created more to provide education than opportunities for policy activism. An example is the website for the United Network for Organ Sharing (http://unos.org). That site has a variety of tutorials and resources for clinicians and patients on organ donations and transplants. It has information on patient survival rates for various transplants and member tool kits, which have information on screening criteria for getting on a transplant waiting list. The purpose of the site is to improve the organ allocation process, and the information provided reflects that. It is not the place to go if you are mostly interested in learning about and influencing health policy.

Similarly, the American Cancer Society website (www.cancer.org) provides a considerable amount of educational material, including information on cancer facts and research programs, support services to survivors, and help for patients making treatment decisions. The website directs those most interested in advocacy to its American Cancer Society Cancer Action Network (www.acscan.org) for information on how to take part in state and federal advocacy campaigns.

Depending on a person's interests, there are many organizations that provide information and engage in policy advocacy, such as the American

Lung Association (www.lungusa.org), American Heart Association (www
.americanheart.org), American Diabetes Association (www.diabetes.org),
Ovarian Cancer National Alliance (www.ovariancancer.org), and Leukemia
and Lymphoma Society (www.leukemia-lymphoma.org). All of these
websites have a mix of information on family and patient support services, advocacy toolboxes, disease statistics, and information.

Is E-mail Advocacy Effective?

Members of Congress receive 200 million e-mails per year (OMB Watch,
2007), up from 80 million in the year 2000 (OMB Watch, 2002). Given
such volume, many questions arise regarding the effectiveness of this form
of communication. Do members of Congress pay attention to or acknowledge the e-mails they receive? Is it worth the time to send an e-mail to a
legislator; should you plan on writing a letter instead, knowing that you
may or may not have the time to do so? What kind of communication is
most effective? These issues have been studied for over a decade.

The studies have generally concluded that personalized communication with your elected representative, whether by e-mail, letter, or phone
call, is better than an identical message generated by a form (OMB
Watch, 2005). However, signing an e-mail that is identical to thousands
of others can also be effective (Hysom, 2008).

So send an e-mail, personalized if possible, or write a letter. Go to
a town hall meeting. Invite officials to meet with you and your members.
Meet your elected representative in his or her office or in a local diner
downtown if that is what they prefer. Phone their offices when an important
vote is coming up and thank them for acting on your behalf when they do
so. There are many ways to connect and communicate. The important
thing is that you do.

If you don't write that letter or send that e-mail, think about the
consequences. Millions of other people will send their letters or e-mails,
asking or advocating for *their* cause. You can't get what they want if you
never ask for it. Silence is inaction. An activated minority will always
trump a lazy, uninterested majority. The power is in advocacy, and advocacy
is just a click away.

Nurses and Future Policy

Policy makers have been "reforming" health care in the United States at
least since 1912 when Theodore Roosevelt proposed a national health

system in his presidential campaign. (Litman & Robins, 1997). In the past century, half a dozen major national health insurance proposals were considered—and defeated (Litman & Robins, 1997).

Leavitt & Mason (1998, p. 4) tell us that during the last major effort, early in the Clinton administration, nurses were ready "because nurses no longer questioned whether being professional included being political. It did." They knew the value of engaging in the process that determines what our health system looks like and determines how and where scarce financial resources are allocated.

As stated earlier, reform can take many different shapes. Sometimes if we can't get major reforms enacted, we have to settle for incremental change. Will nurses be ready for the next round of "reform" and the one after that? Will nurses get to the table where decisions are made, and will their point of view be taken into account? The answer should be: they did.

Acknowledgment

The author wishes to acknowledge Jorna Cychosz for her assistance in the preparation of this manuscript.

REFERENCES

Agency for Healthcare Research and Quality (AHRQ) & U.S. Department of Health and Human Services. (2008, March). *Mental health woes remain one of the top reasons for doctor visits: AHRQ news and numbers.* Retrieved February 9, 2009, from www.ahrq.gov/news/nn/nn030608.htm

Associated Press. (2007, June 25). Clinton adopts cautious approach on health care reform. *USA Today.* Retrieved March 8, 2009, from www.usatoday.com/news/politics/election2008/2007-06-25-health-reform_N.htm

Barbaro, M., & Pear, R. (2007, February 7). Wal-Mart and a union unite, at least on health policy. *New York Times.* Retrieved Jan 21, 2009, from www.nytimes.com/2007/02/07/business/07walmart.html?_r=2&oref=slogin&oref=slogin

Birkland, T. (2005). *An Introduction to the policy process: Theories, concepts and models of public policy making* (2nd ed.). Armonk: M. E. Sharpe.

Center for Health Improvement. (2008). *Bringing policy change to your community-development goals.* Retrieved January 22, 2009, from www.healthpolicyguide.org/advocacy.asp?id=5208

Center for Responsive Politics. (2009a). *Lobbying database.* Retrieved February 28, 2009, from www.opensecrets.org/lobby/index.php

Center for Responsive Politics. (2009b). *Washington lobbying grew to $3.2 billion last year, despite economy.* Retrieved February 28, 2009, from www.opensecrets.org/news/2009/01/washington-lobbying-grew-to-32.html

Congressional Budget Office. (2007, September 7). *H.R. 1424, Paul Wellstone Mental Health and Addiction Equity Act of 2007*. Retrieved January 17, 2009, from www.cbo.gov/ftpdocs/86xx/doc8608/hr1424.pdf

Cummings, J. (2008, June 10). A 2008 campaign flash point. *Politico*. Retrieved January 21, 2009, from http://dyn.politico.com/printstory.cfm?uuid=6FFC8A84-3048-5C12-00AD033BC51289A9

Divided We Fail. (2009). Retrieved January 22, 2009 from www.aarp.org/issues/dividedwefail/get_involved/

Gitterman, D., Sturm, R., & Scheffler, R. (2001). Toward full mental health parity and beyond. *Health Affairs*, 20(4), 68–76.

Goldman, H. H., Frank, R. G., Burnam, M. A., Huskamp, H. A., Ridgely, M. S., Normand, S. L., Young. A. S., Barry, C. L., Azzone, V., Busch, A. B., Azrin, S. T., Moran, G., Lichtenstein, C., & Blasinsky, M. (2006). Behavioral health insurance parity for federal employees. *The New England Journal of Medicine*, 354(13), 1378–1386.

Hamburger, T., & Alonso-Zaldivar, R. (2007, January 16). Unlikely allies push expanded healthcare. [Electronic version]. *Los Angeles Times*, A-1. Retrieved March 7, 2009, from http://articles.latimes.com/2007/jan/16/nation/na-health16

Harris, G. (2009, February 14). Specter, a fulcrum of the stimulus bill, pulls off a coup for health money. *The New York Times*. Retrieved February 15, 2009, from www.nytimes.com/2009/02/14/health/policy/14specter.html?_r=1&scp=1&sq=Fulcrum&st=cse

Hennessy, D., & Goldman, H. (2001). Full parity: Steps toward treatment equity for mental and addictive disorders. *Health Affairs*, 20(4), 58–67.

Hewitt Associates. (2009, March 4). Keeping employees healthy remains a priority for U.S. companies, despite short-term need to cut costs. *Hewitt*. Retrieved March 5, 2009, from www.hewittassociates.com/Intl/NA/en-US/AboutHewitt/Newsroom/PressReleaseDetail.aspx?cid=6389

Hitt, G. (2009, February 5). GOP wields more influence over the stimulus bill. *Wall Street Journal*. Retrieved February 6, 2009, from http://online.wsj.com/article/SB123376269235148125.html

Hulse, C. (2008, October 2). Pressure builds on house after senate backs bailout. *New York Times*. Retrieved March 10, 2009, from www.nytimes.com/2008/10/02/business/02bailout.html?hp

Hysom, T. (2008). *Communicating with Congress: Recommendations for improving the democratic dialogue*. Congressional Management Foundation. Retrieved January 31, 2009, from www.cmfweb.org/storage/cmfweb/documents/CMF_Pubs/cwc_recommendationsreport.pdf

Iglehart, J. (2004). The mental health maze and the call for transformation. *The New England Journal of Medicine*, 350(5), 507-514.

Insurance Institute for Highway Safety. (2005, July). [Press Release]. *1ˢᵗ evidence of effects of cell phone use on injury crashes: Crash risk is four times higher when driver is using a hand-held cell phone*. Retrieved March 9, 2009, from www.iihs.org/news/2005/iihs_news_071205.pdf

Insurance Institute for Highway Safety. (2009, March). *Cellphone laws*. Retrieved March 9, 2009, from www.iihs.org/laws/cellphonelaws.aspx

Kaiser Family Foundation. (1997). Children's health insurance: 1997 budget reconciliation provisions. Retrieved March 9, 2009, from http://kff.org/medicaid/2082-child.cfm

Kaiser Family Foundation. (2008a). *2008 presidential candidate health care proposals: Side-by-side summary.* Retrieved March 14, 2009, from http://pdf.kff.org/health08/compare_5_16.pdf

Kaiser Family Foundation. (2008b, July 17). *New law that delays Medicare physician payment cut also affects beneficiaries.* Retrieved March 9, 2009, from www.kaisernetwork.org/daily_reports/rep_index.cfm?hint=3&DR_ID=53349

Kaiser Family Foundation. (2008c, October 3). *Mental health advocates, lawmakers push for house to pass bailout bill that includes mental parity.* Retrieved March 9, 2009, from www.kaisernetwork.org/daily_reports/rep_index.cfm?DR_ID=54802

Kaiser Family Foundation. (2009). *Kaiser public opinion spotlight.* Retrieved Feb 15, 2009, from www.kff.org/spotlight/index.cfm

Kaiser Family Foundation. (2009a). *Children's Health Insurance Program Reauthorization Act of 2009 (CHIPRA).* Retrieved March 7, 2009, from http://kff.org/medicaid/upload/7863.pdf

Kingdon, J. W. (1995). *Agendas, alternatives, and public policies.* Boston: Little, Brown.

Leavitt, J., Cohen, S., & Mason, D. J. (2002). Political analysis and strategies. In D. J. Mason, J. K. Leavitt, & M. W. Chaffee (Eds.), *Policy & politics in nursing and health care* (pp. 71–91). St Louis: W. B. Saunders.

Leavitt, J. K. & Mason, D. J. (1998). Policy and politics: a framework for action. In D. J. Mason & J. K. Leavitt (Eds). *Policy and politics in nursing and health care* (pp. 4). Philadelphia: W. B. Saunders.

Lemann, N. (2008, April 11). Conflict of interests. *The New Yorker.* Retrieved August 15, 2008, from www.newyorker.com/arts/critics/atlarge/2008/08/11/080811crat_atlarge_lemann

Litman, T., & Robins, L. (Eds.). (1997). *Health politics and policy* (3rd ed.). Albany: Delmar Publishers, Inc.

Lueck, S. (2008, October 4). After 12-year quest, Domenici's mental-health bill succeeds. *Wall Street Journal.* Retrieved January 22, 2009, from http://online.wsj.com/article/SB122307644210303899.html

Mark, T. L., Coffey, R. M., Vandivort-Warren, R., Harwood, H. J., King. E. C., & the MHSA Spending Estimates Team. (2005, March 29). U.S. spending for mental health and substance abuse treatment, 1991-2001. *Health Affairs,* W5-133-W5-142. Retrieved February 9, 2009, from http://content.healthaffairs.org/cgi/reprint/hlthaff.w5.133v1

Matthews, M. (1999, June 30). Do we need mental health parity? *National Center for Policy Analysis.* Retrieved January 18, 2009, from www.ncpa.org/pub/ba297

National Alliance on Mental Illness. *Where we stand: Parity in insurance coverage.* Retrieved March 9, 2009, from www.nami.org/Content/ContentGroups/Policy/WhereWeStand/Parity_in_Insurance_Coverage_-_WHERE_WE_STAND.htm

National Alliance on Mental Illness. (2007). *State mental health parity laws 2007.* Retrieved March 9, 2009, from www.nami.org/Content/ContentGroups/Policy/Issues_Spotlights/Parity1/State_Mental_Health_Parity_Laws_20071.htm

National Alliance on Mental Illness. (2008). *Public policy platform of the National Alliance on Mental Illness (NAMI).* Retrieved March 9, 2009, from www.nami.org/Content/NavigationMenu/Inform_Yourself/About_Public_Policy/NAMI_Policy_Platform/ Policy_Platform.htm

OMB Watch. (2002, February 19). *Congressional attitudes towards constituent e-mail.* Retrieved March 14, 2009, from www.ombwatch.org/node/276

OMB Watch. (2005, July 12). *New study on Congress and advocacy.* Retrieved March 14, 2009, from www.ombwatch.org/node/5045

OMB Watch. (2007, October 10). *Conference focuses on e-mail frustration felt by Congress and advocacy groups.* Retrieved March 14, 2009, from www.ombwatch.org/node/3492

Parker-Pope, T. (2009, January 12). A problem of the brain, not the hands: Group urges phone ban for drivers. *New York Times.* Retrieved January 15, 2009, from www.nytimes.com/2009/01/13/health/13well.html?_r=1&ref=views

Pear, R. (1987, September 20). Medicare expansion imperiled by high costs. *New York Times.* Retrieved March 9, 2009, from http://query.nytimes.com/gst/fullpage.html?sec=health&res=9B0DE7DA173BF933A1575AC0A961948260

Pear, R. (2007, March 19). Proposals for mental health parity pit a father's pragmatism against a son's passion. *New York Times.* Retrieved January 20, 2009, from http://nytimes.com/2007/03/19/washington/19mental.html?ref=washington

Pear, R. (2008, October 6). Bailout provides more mental health coverage. *New York Times.* Retrieved January 18, 2009, from www.nytimes.com/2008/10/06/washington/06mental.html

Priest, D., & Hull, A. (2007a, February 18). Soldiers face neglect, frustration at army's top medical facility. *Washington Post.* Retrieved March 1, 2009, from www.washingtonpost.com/wp-dyn/content/article/2007/02/17/AR2007021701172pf.html

Priest, D., & Hull, A. (2007b, February 20). Recovering at Walter Reed. *Washington Post.* Retrieved March 1, 2009, from www.washingtonpost.com/wp-dyn/content/discussion/2007/02/16/DI2007021601020_pf.html

Redman, E. (1973). *The dance of legislation.* New York: Simon & Schuster.

Roehrig, C., Miller, G., Lake, C., & Bryant, J. (2009). National health spending by medical condition, 1996–2005. *Health Affairs*, 28(2), w358-w367. Retrieved March 8, 2009, from http://content.healthaffairs.org/cgi/content/full/28/2/w358

Rovner, J. (2007, January 8). Advocates renew push for mental health "parity" bill. *National Public Radio, Morning Edition.* Retrieved February 10, 2009, from www.npr.org/templates/player/mediaPlayer.html?action=1&t=1&islist=false&id=6740128&m=6740129

Rovner, J. (2008, October 6). Mental health parity approved with bailout bill. *National Public Radio, All Things Considered.* Retrieved February 11, 2009, from www.npr.org/templates/story/story.php?storyId=95435676

Seib, G. (2008, November 21). In crisis, opportunity for Obama. *Wall Street Journal.* Retrieved January 2, 2009, from http://online.wsj.com/article/SB122721278056345271.html

Shott, J. (2007, September 3). America's uninsured. *Spero News.* Retrieved September 7, 2007, from http://speroforum.com/site/article.asp?id=10869&t=America

Smith, M. (2006, May 24). Schizophrenia patients go untreated for comorbidities. *MedPage Today.* Retrieved January 14, 2009, from www.medpagetoday.com/MeetingCoverage/APA/3385

Smith, M. (2007, January 17). Mental health parity pursued: Ramstad, Kennedy sponsor legislation for equal medical coverage. *St Paul Pioneer Press.* Retrieved March 9, 2009, from St Paul Pioneer Press Archives.

Sommers, B. (2007). Why millions of children eligible for Medicaid and SCHIP are uninsured: Poor retention versus poor take-up. *Health Affairs*, 26(5), w560–w567.

Retrieved January 3, 2009, from http://content.healthaffairs.org/cgi/reprint/26/5/w560

Steinbrook, R. (2009, February 17). Health care and the American Recovery and Reinvestment Act. *The New England Journal of Medicine*, 360(11), 1057–1060. Retrieved on February 17, 2009, from http://content.nejm.org/cgi/content/full/NEJMp0900665

U.S. Census Bureau. (2008). *Income, poverty, and health insurance coverage in the United States: 2007*. Retrieved March 1, 2009, from www.census.gov/prod/2008pubs/p60–235.pdf

U.S. Department of Health and Human Services. (1999). *Mental health: A report of the Surgeon General*. [Electronic version]. Rockville: U.S. Department of Health and Human Services, Substance Abuse and Mental Health Services Administration, Center for Mental Health Services, National Institutes of Health, National Institute of Mental Health.

U.S. Department of Health and Human Services, Health Resources and Services Administration. (2008). *FY 2009 budget justification*. Retrieved January 3, 2009, from www.hrsa.gov/about/budgetjustification09/NHSC.htm

The Wall Street Journal Online & Harris Interactive. (2008). Confidence in FDA hits new low, according to WSJ.com/Harris Interactive Study: U.S. adults concerned about safety of prescription drugs. *Health-Care Poll*, 7(5). Retrieved January 22, 2009, from www.harrisinteractive.com/news/newsletters/wsjhealthnews/HI_WSJ_HealthCarePoll_2008_v07_i05.pdf

Wangsness, L. (2009, February 18). Doctors criticize Massachusetts health law. *Boston Globe*. Retrieved February 23, 2009, from www.boston.com/news/politics/politicalintelligence/2009/02/doctors_critici.html

Weissert, C., & Weissert, W. (2002). *Governing health: The politics of health policy* (2nd ed.). Baltimore: Johns Hopkins University Press.

White House Domestic Policy Council. (1993a). *Health security: The president's report to the American people*. New York: Simon & Schuster.

White House Domestic Policy Council. (1993b). *The president's health security plan: The Clinton blueprint*. New York: Times Books.

Young, J. (2009, January 26). Pelosi expects 'major step' on health reform in 2009. *The Hill*. Retrieved January 28, 2009, from http://thehill.com/leading-the-news/pelosi-expects-major-step—on-health-reform-in-2009-2009-01-26.html

Zelman, W., & Brown, L. (1998). Looking back on health care reform: "No easy choices." *Health Affairs*, 17(6), 61-68. Retrieved January 15, 2009, from http://content.healthaffairs.org/cgi/reprint/17/6/61

Zhang, J. (2007, February 13). Mental health nears 'parity'. *Wall Street Journal*. Retrieved February 22, 2009, from http://online.wsj.com/article/SB117133635176006784.html

Regulation, Certification, and Clinical Privileges

MICHAELENE P. JANSEN

8

As advanced practice nurses seek new or continued employment, they must consider what regulations will allow or limit their practice in their state. In doing so, they can choose a position that is congruent with their educational scope of practice. They should also know what credentials might be needed to practice in a certain state, institution, or organization. For example, if they choose to practice in a selected state, would they be able to prescribe medications, sign death certificates, admit patients to hospitals, sign workers compensation claims or disabled parking permits? Would they be required to be supervised by a physician or have restrictions placed on their billing? These are all issues that surround regulation, certification, and credentialing for advanced practice nurses.

The terms *regulation, certification,* and *credentialing* as they apply to advanced practice nurses (APN) can be very confusing to the public as well as health care providers. These terms are often used incorrectly, and they can cause misperceptions or confusion among the consumer. There are distinct differences in the meaning of each term and the things that advanced practice nurses are allowed to do. Understanding these terms will help APNs carry out their roles while avoiding any barriers that may exist. The purpose of this chapter is to define and discuss these terms so that all advanced practice nurses will obtain appropriate licensure, certification, and credentials to safely and optimally carry out their role.

REGULATION

A regulation is a law that has been passed by the state or federal legislature and signed by the governor of that state or the president of the United States. Nursing practice is regulated by each state in accordance with state statutes and interpreted through administrative rules. In most states, nurse practitioners (NPs) are regulated under the authority of a Board of Nursing. In a review of state APN regulation in 2008, two states, Nebraska and Illinois, had separate advanced practice boards; nurse practitioners from five states were controlled by Boards of Nursing and Medicine; and two states regulated nurse practitioners through their state's Education Department (Pearson, 2009; Phillips, 2009).

Regulation of NPs varies from state to state, and changes occur yearly. This variability inhibits advanced practice and often narrows the scope of practice for which advanced practice nurses are prepared (Lugo, O'Grady, Hodnicki, & Hanson, 2007). As of 2008, 23 states have enacted a Nurse Licensure Compact for registered nurses and vocational licensed nurses to increase mobility between states, but only two states, Iowa and Utah, have advanced practice registered nurse compacts (National Council of State Boards of Nursing, 2008). Two reports are readily available each year to provide updates to regulation, prescriptive authority, reimbursement, and other issues related to nurse practitioner practice. These reports are published by *The American Journal for Nurse Practitioners* (www.webnp.net) and *The Nurse Practitioner.*

The road to removing regulatory barriers for ANPs has been bumpy, to say the least. However, through perseverance and endless efforts on individual and professional nurse practitioner advocates, NPs can practice and prescribe medications in every state. That said however, much more work needs to be done to educate legislators, interprofessional groups, and the public in order to provide access to safe, competent care for all consumers.

Medical organizations have recently made a concerted effort to oppose nurses' and other health professionals' expansion or revision of state practice laws. Under leadership from the American Medical Association (AMA), the Scope of Practice Partnership (SOPP) was launched in 2006 to promote the following three principles regarding practice of health professionals who are not physicians:

(a)   As authorized by the medical staff, they function in a newly expanded medical support role to the physician in the provision of patient care.

(b) They participate in the management of patients under the direct supervision or direction of a member of the medical staff who is responsible for the patient's care.

(c) They make entries on patients' records, including progress notes, only to the extent established by the medical staff (American Medical Association, p. 2).

Clearly the language of the AMA/SOPP does not recognize that nursing is an autonomous profession with its own knowledge base. Because the AMA is actively promoting its supervision of providers such as nurse practitioners, a group has been formed to counteract SOPP. This group, the Coalition for Patient Rights (CPR), is a partnership of 37 professional organizations whose goal is to ensure that patients everywhere have access to quality health care providers of their choice (including APNs). The CPR seeks to ensure that physicians are not successful in passing laws, policies, and regulations that limit the APN's scope of practice. The SOPP and CPR are examples of recent increased turf-guarding and contentiousness between APNs and physicians. Running counter to this turf guarding are new partnerships with some physician groups. A monograph published by the American College of Physicians (2008) respectfully acknowledges the contributions of APNs and sets the stage for continuing collaboration between physicians and nurses to solve the immense access to care issues facing the United States. This very helpful document outlines principles for regulation of all health professionals and documents ways that groups can work together to jointly provide quality care while adhering to regulations and maintaining high standards for all providers (Association of Social Work Boards, Federation of State Boards of Physical Therapy, Federation of State Medical Boards, National Association of Boards of Pharmacy, National Board for Certification in Occupational Therapy, & National Council of State Boards of Nursing, 2007).

Title Protection

Title protection limits the use of a title unless the user meets the regulations mandated by state regulation. Currently 25 states have legislation that protects the title "nurse" (ANA, 2009). Restriction of the term "nurse" provides reassurance to the public that the individual using that title has met all the requirements mandated for licensure in that state. Please note that this does not mean there are 25 states that do not regulate professional nursing. It just means that persons can call themselves a nurse without meeting the requirements in those states.

All states have some form of title protection for nurse practitioners (Phillips, 2009), but they vary in who has the legal authority to regulate nurse practitioner practice. There is also variability as to the title for nurse practitioners in each state. Currently there are 11 titles associated with recognition of nurse practitioners by state regulatory boards. Table 8.1 provides a list of these titles. The APRN Consensus Workgroup and APRN Joint Dialogue Group (2008) identify nurse practitioners as certified nurse practitioners (CNPs), one of the four APRN roles.

Clinical nurse specialists are advocating among state legislators to promote title protection for their role (National Association of Clinical Nurse Specialists, 2004). Recent legislation in some states provided for CNS title protection (Duffy, Minarik, & Lyon, 2008). Title protection for nurse-midwives and nurse anesthetists also varies among states.

Title protection is not synonymous with autonomous or uniform regulation. APNs must continue to promote legislation to remove statutory restrictions that limit advanced practice nursing. The APRN Consensus Workgroup and APRN Joint Dialogue Group (2008) propose the title *Advanced Practice Registered Nurse* (APRN) as the licensing title for the four advanced practice roles.

Even as advanced practice education moves toward requiring the clinical doctorate for practice at the entry level, several states have statutory restrictions against doctorally prepared nurse practitioners being addressed as "doctor" (Pearson, 2009). Several advanced practice nursing

Table 8.1

NURSE PRACTITIONER TITLES RECOGNIZED BY STATE REGULATORY BODIES

ANP	Advanced Nurse Practitioner
APN	Advanced Practice Nurse
APNP	Advanced Practice Nurse Prescriber
APRN	Advanced Practice Registered Nurse
APRN-NP	Advanced Practice Registered Nurse—Nurse Practitioner
ARNP	Advanced Registered Nurse Practitioner
CNP	Certified Nurse Practitioner
CRNP	Certified Registered Nurse Practitioner
NP	Nurse Practitioner
NP-BC	Nurse Practitioner—Board Certified
RNP	Registered Nurse Practitioner

organizations developed a unified statement outlining Doctor of Nursing Practice certification, education, and use of the title "doctor" (Nurse Practitioner Roundtable, 2008). The unified statement acknowledges that a medical doctor or doctor of osteopathy may be title protected, but notes that recognition of the title "doctor" for nurse practitioners who are doctorally prepared facilitates parity within health care.

APRN Regulatory Model

Given the variability in scope of practice, what advanced practice roles are recognized, criteria for entry into advanced practice, and what certification exams are accepted, it can be difficult for advanced practice nurses to move between states. A model has been developed that includes four essential elements—licensure, accreditation, certification, and education (LACE)—as a means to protect the public and decrease barriers for advanced practice nurses who practice in multiple states (APRN Consensus Workgroup & APRN Joint Dialogue Group, 2008).

The APRN regulatory model includes registered nurse anesthetists, certified nurse-midwives, clinical nurse specialists, and certified nurse practitioners. The consensus group recognized that there are many nurses with graduate preparation such as nurse educators, informatics specialists, or administrators; however, their focus is not direct care to individuals. The model provides for advanced practice nurses to "be licensed as independent practitioners for practice at the level of one of the four APRN roles within at least one of the six identified population foci. Education, certification, and licensure of an individual must be congruent in terms of role and population foci. APRNs may be specialized but they cannot be licensed solely within a specialty area" (APRN Consensus Workgroup & APRN Joint Dialogue Group, 2008, p. 5).

The APRN Regulatory Model (Figure 8.1) illustrates the four advanced practice roles educated by an accredited academic program in at least one of six population foci: family/individual across the life span, adult/gerontology, neonatal, pediatrics, women's health/gender related, and psychiatric/mental health. Licensing would occur at the level of role and population focus, and certification will reflect the population focus. APRN specialties are areas of focus beyond the role and population. Implementation of the model will occur incrementally by state boards of nursing. Full implementation is anticipated by 2015 when the entry education level for advanced practice will be the Doctor of Nursing Practice. Figure 8.2 illustrates the relationship among educational

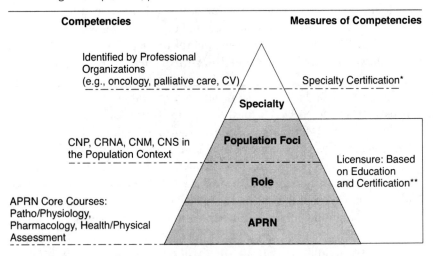

APRN REGULATORY MODEL

APRN SPECIALTIES
Focus of practice beyond role and population focus
linked to health care needs
Examples include but are not limited to: Oncology, Older Adults, Orthopedics,
Nephrology, Palliative Care

Population foci

Licensure Occurs at Levels of Role & Population Foci

Family/Individual Across Lifespan | Adult-Gerontology* | Neonatal | Pediatrics | Women's Health/Gender-Related | Psychiatric-Mental Health**

APRN roles

Nurse Anesthetist | Nurse-Midwife | Clinical Nurse Specialist++ | Nurse Practitioner+

+ acute or primary care certified nurse practitioners (CNPs)
++ clinical nurse specialist (CNS) is educated and assessed through national certification
process across the continuum from wellness through acute care

Figure 8.1 APRN Regulatory Model. *Source*: APRN Consensus Workgroup and APRN
Joint Dialogue Group (2008, p. 9).

Competencies   **Measures of Competencies**

Identified by Professional
Organizations
(e.g., oncology, palliative care, CV)   Specialty Certification*

Specialty

CNP, CRNA, CNM, CNS in
the Population Context   **Population Foci**   Licensure: Based
on Education
Role   and Certification**

APRN Core Courses:
Patho/Physiology,
Pharmacology, Health/Physical   **APRN**
Assessment

* Certification for specialty may include exam, portfolio, peer review, etc.
** Certification for licensure will be psychometrically sound and legally defensible
   examination by an accredited certifying program.

Figure 8.2 Relationship among educational competencies, licensure and certification in
the role/population foci, and education and credentialing in a specialty. *Source*: APRN
Consensus Workgroup and APRN Joint Dialogue Group (2008, p. 14).

competencies, licensure, and certification in the role/population foci and education and credentialing in a specialty.

CERTIFICATION

The introduction of the APRN Regulatory Model has put a greater emphasis on certification. Certification by a national board has been a requirement for regulatory processes and prescriptive authority. Certification differs from licensure in that certification is a process by which a nongovernmental agency or association certifies that an individual licensed to practice a profession has met certain predetermined standards specified by that profession for specialty practice. The purpose of certification is to assure various publics that an individual has mastered a body of knowledge and acquired skills for a particular population.

Historically, certification in nursing is murky with no uniform standards. Many specialty organizations certified nurses with varying educational backgrounds at one general level. Most certification agencies now require a master's or higher degree to be eligible for certification at an advanced practice level. As the APRN Regulatory Model is implemented, certification for licensing at an advanced practice level will reflect the six populations identified. Specialty certification will occur by the same or additional certifying bodies. Specialty certification will not suffice alone for licensing as an APRN.

Certifying Bodies

American Nurses Credentialing Center (ANCC)

The American Nurses Credentialing Center (ANCC) provides certification for the nursing profession, guaranteeing to the public that nurses have a certain level of knowledge or skill. The ANCC is an outgrowth of the American Nurses Association (ANA) certification program, which was established in 1973 to function as an independent center through which ANA would serve as its own credentialing program. ANCC certification "protects the public by enabling anyone to identify competent people more readily. Simultaneously it aids the profession by encouraging and recognizing professional achievement. Certification also recognizes specialization, enhances professionalism, and, in some cases, serves as a criterion for financial reimbursement. It may also foster an enlarged role within the employment setting" (ANCC, 2009).

ANCC offers certification for clinical nurse specialists in eight areas: (1) adult psychiatric and mental health, (2) child/adolescent psychiatric and mental health, (3) gerontology, (4) adult health, (5) home health nursing, (6) pediatric nursing, (7) community/public health, and (8) advanced diabetes management. In a collaborative effort with the National Association of Clinical Nurse Specialists, ANCC will offer a core clinical nurse specialist (CNS) exam that will address CNS competencies across the life span regardless of specialty. The core exam will address a need for national certification by state regulatory bodies for CNSs who do not fit the current specialty exams offered by ANCC.

ANCC also certifies nurse practitioners in nine clinical areas: (1) adult, (2) family, (3) gerontology, (4) pediatric, (5) acute care, (6) adult psychiatric and mental health, (7) family psychiatric and mental health, (8) school nursing, and (9) advanced diabetes management. It is anticipated that the adult and gerontology certification exam will become a combined examination, and that a gerontology specialty examination will be developed as the APRN Regulatory Model is implemented.

Over the years, ANCC has granted multiple credentials to designate certification at an advanced practice level. Over the past 15 years, APNs have seen multiple changes in the credentials. For example, prior to 1993, NPs certifying with ANCC were given the title "C" to indicate certification. CNSs were given the credential "CS." From 1993 to 2000 both CNSs and NPs were given "CS" as the certifying credential. Since 2000, NPs and CNSs were first given the credential APRN-BC, then APRN, BC, to indicate advanced practice registered nurse, board certified. Currently, NPs and CNSs have their own certification credential that reflects the clinical focus. For example, a family NP would have the following credentials: FNP-BC representing family nurse practitioner–board certified. An adult CNS would use the credentials ACNS-BC to signify board certification in this specialty.

American Academy of Nurse Practitioners— Certification Program

The American Academy of Nurse Practitioners (AANP) has an affiliated organization, AANP—Certification Program (AANPCP) that provides entry-level, competency-based examinations in three areas: adult, gerontology, and family. The purpose of this certification is "to provide a valid and reliable program for entry-level nurse practitioners to recognize their education, knowledge and professional expertise" (AANPCP, 2009). Certification by AANPCP is recognized in all 50 states, as well as by Medicare, Medicaid, the Veterans Administration, and private insurance companies. Nurse practitioners receiving certification by AANPCP use NP-C (nurse practitioner certified) as their credential.

American Association of Critical Nurses Certification Corporation

The certification arm of the American Association of Critical Care Nurses (AACN), the AACN Certification Corporation, began offering certification for clinical nurse specialists in 1999. The corporation offers CNS certification in adult, pediatric, and neonatal acute care. The credential indicating this certification for clinical nurse specialists is CCNS. Recently, the AACN Certification Corporation began to offer a certification exam for acute care nurse practitioner certification (ACNPC).

Other Certification Opportunities

Although most specialty organizations provide certification for professional nursing practice, few offer certification at an advanced practice level. The American Psychiatric Nurses Association (APNA) considered offering certification for advanced practice psychiatric mental health nurses, but currently the certification as a psychiatric/mental health clinical nurse specialist or nurse practitioner comes through ANCC. The National Certification Corporation (NCC) for the obstetric, gynecological, and neonatal nursing specialties offers certification for women's health care nurse practitioner and neonatal nurse practitioner. NCC also offers a subspecialty certification in gynecologic reproductive health along with the two core certifications. NCC was formerly known as the NAACOG Certification Corporation. NAACOG has been renamed the Association for Women's Health, Obstetrics and Neonatal Nursing and became an independent certification organization in 1991. Pediatric nurse practitioners can also be certified by the National Board of Pediatric Nurse Practitioners and Associates. The Oncology Nursing Society through the Oncology Nursing Certification Corporation offers certification for nurse practitioners (AOCNP) and clinical nurse specialists (AOCNS).

The Council for the Advancement of Comprehensive Care (CACC), established in 2000, is a consortium of academic and health policy leaders who are committed to ensuring high standards of doctoral nursing practice. In 2008, CACC collaborated with the Board of Medical Examiners to develop and administer a certification examination for doctors of nursing practice (DNP). The comprehensive care certification examination is comparable to performance standards as Step 3 (final) United States medical licensing exam (USMLE) for medical students. Although the exams are similar, the comprehensive care certification exam is only for graduates of DNP programs, and the candidate must be certified as an APRN. APRNs who pass this exam are designated diplomates in comprehensive care by the American Board of the Council for the Advancement of Comprehensive Care (CACC, 2009). ANCC released a statement in March 2009 to clarify that this exam is considered a specialty exam defined by Columbia University and is not a population-based exam (AACN, 2009). The CACC exam is an exam for DNP graduates from comprehensive care programs.

Criteria for Certification

Each certifying body has its own set of eligibility criteria. Certification corporations certifying nurse practitioners, clinical nurse specialists, and certified registered nurse anesthetists require the master's degree. Some of the early nurse practitioners and certified registered nurse anesthetists graduated from non-master's certificate programs and have been "grandfathered in." As 2015 approaches, eligibility criteria will require a practice doctorate to apply for certification.

Each certification area (family, adult, acute care, women's health, etc.) may have different practice or recertification requirements. Given the dynamic nature of certification and professional standards, the reader is referred to the specific certification website for the desired advanced practice role. Exhibit 8.1 provides a list of websites offering information on eligibility and the application process.

Accreditation of Educational Programs

Accreditation of educational programs for advanced practice nurses will become integrated with the APRN Regulation Model. Competencies for nurse practitioner and clinical nurse specialists have been developed by the National Association of Clinical Nurse Specialists (NACNS) and

Exhibit 8.1

CERTIFICATION WEBSITES

American Association of Critical Care Nurse Credentialing Corporation:
www.aacn.org/DM/MainPages/CertificationHome.aspx
American Nurses Credentialing Center: www.nursecredentialing.org/
Council on Certification of Nurse Anesthestists: www.aana.com/council
ACNM Certification Council: www.accmidwife.org
American Academy of Nurse Practitioners Certification Program: www
.aanp.org/certification
Oncology Nursing Certification Program: www.oncc.org
National Certification Corporation: www.nccnet.org

the National Organization of Nurse Practitioner Faculties (NONPF), respectively (NACNS, 2004; NONPF, 2006). NONPF has also developed criteria for evaluation of nurse practitioner programs (NONPF, 2008). The American Association of Colleges of Nursing (AACN) has developed an *Essentials* document that provides guidance to existing and developing DNP programs (AACN, 2006). The National Association of Certified Nurse Specialists (NACNS) is developing DNP core educational competencies for entry level CNSs.

Certified nurse-midwifery programs and certified registered nurse anesthetist programs must be accredited by the Division of Accreditation of the American College of Nurse Midwives and the Council on Accreditation of Nurse Anesthetist Educational Programs, respectively, in order for their graduates to be eligible for certification.

Credentials

One of the concerns related to certification is the multiplicity of acronyms that are used to indicate certification and that each certifying body uses its own credentials. The frequent change in credentials as well as the variety of terms used to indicate advanced practice nursing is confusing for the consumer as well as other health care professionals. As regulatory bodies become more uniform and as certification corporations align their exams with the APRN Regulatory Model, there may be more consistency and understanding of the titles that reflect advanced practice.

In the interim, APNs can facilitate common terminology within their organizations. For example, having a common format for name badges that is consistent with documentation signatures would be a first step. Smolenski (2005) provides guidance for listing credentials in the following order: degree, licensure, state designation or requirement, national certification, honor or awards, then other certification. An illustration of this titling is as follows: Jane Doe, DNP, APRN, ANP-BC, FAAN.

CLINICAL PRIVILEGES

Clinical privileges are "authorizations granted by the governing body of a hospital to provide specific patient care services within well-defined limits, based on the qualifications reviewed in the credentialing process" (Cooper, 1998, p. 30). The credentialing process ensures the protection of patients by providing a process for institutions to select competent practitioners (Klein, 2003). The Joint Commission on Accreditation of Health Care Organizations (JCAHO) specifies characteristics of a process for the delineation of clinical privileges. JCAHO's 2008 Critical Access Hospital and Hospital Standards state that medical staff must credential and privilege all licensed independent practitioners (LIP). The process and procedural detail must be outlined in medical staff bylaws. Nonlicensed independent practitioners such as physician assistants (PAs) and advanced practice registered nurses (APRNs) may be privileged through an established medical staff process that reflects the JCAHO credentialing and privileging standards.

Clinical privileges have been successfully obtained for certified nurse-midwives (CNM) and certified registered nurse anesthetists (CRNA). Set standards are processes typically established through the appropriate medical departments (i.e., obstetrics or anesthesia). Clinical privileges for clinical nurse specialists and nurse practitioners have been more difficult to obtain. The great diversity in qualifications for APNs, including CRNAs and CNMs, makes it difficult for agencies to develop uniform clinical privileging guidelines for all APNs.

Although there is some variability in the credentialing process, JCAHO recommends a series of steps for medical staff. Credentialing is the first step in the process that leads to privileging. Typically, the credentialing process includes the application, verification of credentials, evaluation of applicant-specific information, and a recommendation to the governing medical board for appointment and privileges. The medical staff has the

9

Practice Issues, Prescriptive Authority, and Liability

MICHAELENE P. JANSEN

Advanced practice nurses (APNs) encounter a variety of professional issues in their practices. Most questions focus on what APNs can or cannot do within the scope of nursing practice. Although advanced practice nurses have made progress in terms of removing barriers to practice, many barriers continue to exist. As health care reform evolves in individual states or on a national level, it will be critical for APNs to be fully cognizant of legislative or regulatory activity that may impede their ability to perform within their full scope of practice. At the same time, APNs are expanding their educational focus, bringing forth new issues and challenges. Chapter 8 discusses some of the regulatory issues that face APNs. This chapter will focus on other aspects of care, including selected practice issues, prescriptive authority, and liability.

PRACTICE ISSUES

There are many practice issues that can be discussed; some have definitive answers, and some do not. Most practice issues have safety, legal, or ethical implications. Some practice issues may resolve as new legislation is passed or new policy is put in place, but other issues may persist and new practice issues will emerge. This section will discuss selected practice issues related to innovative technology, billing and reimbursement, blurred practice boundaries, and professional accountability. There are many "gray" areas in advanced nursing practice; therefore, knowing your legal responsibility, scope of practice, and prescriptive authority is extremely important.

Innovative Health Technology

As health care technology grows exponentially, several issues arise. First, with advancement in treatment modalities, many patients are surviving beyond their prognostic time frames. As these patients survive, unantici-pated consequences of their treatment may arise. For example, Zakak (2009) raises the possibility of fertility issues in childhood cancer survivors. Therapies used to treat the cancers were successful in terms of curing or remitting the cancer but may have eliminated the patient's ability to conceive and thus achieve the developmental milestone of parenthood. Anticipating consequences of therapies is essential in providing informed consent and in allowing patients to choose alternative treatments.

Another issue related to innovative technology is the choice of test that is needed to diagnose or follow up on a condition. Perhaps the clini-cal practice guideline suggests a computerized tomography (CT) scan for evaluation of a mass, but a newer technology is developed that may provide better diagnostic information. However, the new technology is much more expensive and puts the patient at a greater radiation risk. Innovative technology might also allow a parent to choose not to treat a child's condition or terminate a pregnancy based on the probability that the child or fetus would not survive (Williams, 2006). Elderly patients may choose not to undergo expensive diagnostic tests or treatment because they have lived a healthy productive life and are prepared for death. APNs will face many similar situations that conflict with personal ethical beliefs and must determine whether to support the patient's choice based on the ethical, regulatory, and legal boundaries of their practice.

Off-label use of pharmacologic agents is another example in which the original research submitted to the Food and Drug Administration (FDA) was for one indication and, through its use, another indication arose. The manufacturer often decides not to go through the process of gaining FDA approval for a second indication. If APNs were to prescribe the medication for a use other than the approved indication, would pre-scribing that medication put them at risk for malpractice, even though the use of that medication for the nonapproved indication is common among health care providers?

Billing and Reimbursement Issues

Accurate billing and coding is difficult to learn, but it is extremely important to ensure that the APN obtains the appropriate reimbursement and does not overbill or underbill the patient. Although APNs historically underbill for services provided, both underbilling and overbilling are considered fraud. Chapter 10 provides an excellent overview of the reimbursement process, billing, and coding. Ongoing review and continuing education on reimbursement cannot be overemphasized. Some practice issues related to billing and reimbursement arise from shared billing practices or pressure from organizations to bill "incident to" for higher reimbursement.

Along the lines of reimbursement is the choice of pharmacologic agents. Pharmacy formularies adopted by insurance companies may insist on a certain pharmacologic agent for a certain diagnostic code. That particular drug may not be the most beneficial for the patient. Prior authorizations can be requested, but they are denied if the generic or formulary equivalent has not been tried for a certain amount of time. If the medication is approved, it is often approved at a higher copay for the patient. The time spent obtaining approval or the time the patient has to spend trying and failing an alternative agent diminishes the quality of care.

Blurred Boundaries

APNs may be placed in situations in which there is not a clear delineation of role. The APN needs to feel comfortable when making any decision or engaging in any procedure. For example, a nurse practitioner (NP) whose practice is limited to adults provides care for a 32-year-old mother. The mother asks the NP to assume care for her 10-year-old daughter because she has confidence in the NP and the closest provider for the daughter is 30 miles away. You might argue that when the adult-care NPs care for 10-year-olds, they are clearly out of their scope of practice. However, if that 10-year-old was in a life-threatening situation, would the NP be liable for not initiating care?

APNs may encounter other situations that stretch the limits of educational preparation or that are not clearly defined within the regulatory realm. Hudspeth (2007) discusses balancing the need for adequate educational preparation with the needs of behavior health services. For example, an adult nurse practitioner or a clinical nurse specialist may have a large percentage of patients with behavior health issues. APNs will need to determine if they have adequate preparation to care for these patients or if more education and/or certification is required. Brekken (2008) addresses balancing the need to provide adequate pain management yet following regulatory guidelines for controlled substances.

Professional Accountability

Advanced practice nurses are continually faced with situations that have implications for accountability. Snyder (2005) describes the accountability that occurs when there is failure to accurately assess diminished driving skills in patients with dementia that result in premature or delayed driving cessation. Inaccurate assessment of driving skills can have adverse effects on the patient, family, and on public safety. For example, if a patient is seen by an APN for evaluation of progressive visual loss and the APN does not address driving skills, is the APN accountable or liable for injuries that occur if that patient is involved in a motor vehicle accident following that evaluation?

Another area of accountability relates to identifying incompetence or fraud. If APNs encounter fraud or an unethical situation, they are faced with "blowing the whistle" or choosing not to take action (Hannigan, 2006). As we will discuss later in this chapter, the APN is responsible for ensuring safe, competent care.

Accountability issues are not limited to advanced practice in the United Sates. Wiseman (2007) examines accountability of advanced practice nurses as they expand their role within the United Kingdom. As new roles develop, it is important to examine them closely within a framework that takes education, legal, and ethical issues into account. This often provides a challenge in health care systems that are beginning to incorporate advanced nursing practice.

The scenarios discussed in this section are laden with ethical, fiscal, and legal implications. The APN must be adequately prepared to address these issues and have a solid ethical, legal, and professional foundation to make appropriate decisions for the protection and safety of the public.

LIABILITY

As advanced practice nurses assume more autonomy and independence, liability issues arise. It is critical that APNs work within their scope of practice; maintain certification, including continuing education requirements; and maintain adequate liability coverage.

To practice within their scope of practice, APNs must comply with state regulatory statutes. Laws are interpreted through administrative rules as discussed in Chapter 8. The law's interpretation determines whether APNs are practicing within their scope of practice.

An example of the importance of administrative rules in interpreting state statutes is illustrated in the following case. A pediatric nurse practitioner became interested in pain management and was hired by a pain clinic. After working there for some time, it was requested that she obtain prescriptive authority to allow her to prescribe pain medication, including controlled substances for all age groups. Based on the administrative rule that allows prescription orders appropriate to the advanced practice nurse's area of competence as established by education, training, or experience, the Board of Nursing deemed the advanced practice nurse eligible to obtain prescriptive privileges because of her experience in the pain clinic. However, the APN believed that it was in her best interest to return to school and obtain post-master's certification as an adult nurse practitioner to expand her scope of practice to include all the populations to which she provided care.

There has been an increase in malpractice claims filed against NPs in recent years, because more NPs are employed than ever before. Some people believe that attorneys often name anyone associated with the case as a way to increase their client's award or recovery costs. Overall, however, NPs have had fewer adverse claims against them compared to doctors of osteopathy (DOs) or physicians (MDs). Pearson (2009) performed an analysis to further examine adverse actions taken against nurse practitioners. She used data from the National Practitioner Data Bank (NPDB) and the Healthcare Integrity and Protection Data Bank (HIPDB) to evaluate the number of accumulated malpractice actions, regulatory or civil judgments, and criminal convictions submitted by NPs, DOs, and MDs (p. 9). The NPDB data revealed 1 in 173 accumulated malpractice and adverse actions for NPs, compared to 1 in 4 for DOs and MDs (p. 9). In the HIPDB, the occurrence ratios were 1 in 226 for NPs, 1 in 13 for DOs, and 1 in 23 for MDs.

One question that many advanced practice nurses raise is whether they should carry their own malpractice insurance in addition to their employer's liability coverage. Some legal experts recommend that APNs do so because often there may be a conflict of interest within a given claim. The other side of the argument is that APNs may be named in a claim because they carry their own insurance (Wright, 2004).

Buppert (2008) advises APNs who are thinking about how much liability insurance to carry, to buy "as much as you can get and afford" (p. 406).

Malpractice occurs when an APN fails to exhibit expected skills and competence based on professional standards and practices (Buppert, 2008a) and when negligence on the part of the practitioner is identified. Most malpractice claims against advanced practice nurses are related to diagnostic errors (Buppert, 2006). Negligence can occur when an APN fails to follow up with a patient appropriately, refer the patient when necessary, disclose information to a patient, or provide appropriate care. This would include failure to monitor or observe a patient's health status; diagnose or delay diagnosis; perform procedures safely and competently; treat a patient appropriately, including prescribing and minimally administering medications; communicate patient information in a timely manner; protect a patient from avoidable injuries; and practice within the scope of the APN's nursing education and position description. For further in-depth discussion and information related to liability and legal issues, the reader is referred to Buppert's excellent legal reference (2008a).

During the last decade, the United States has experienced an increase in the frequency and severity of medical malpractice claims. Malpractice premiums have risen significantly, and many firms that have provided malpractice insurance in the past have discontinued offering coverage (Thorpe, 2004). Medical liability premiums increased greatly during the 1980s, particularly in obstetrics (Yeo & Edmunds, 2004), and increases in insurance premiums prompted many hospital and clinic closings in the early 2000s.

APNs must become familiar with legal terminology to avoid committing unintentional acts of negligence. Table 9.1 briefly outlines terms that are often unfamiliar. One term, intentional tort, meaning that an APN commits an act that brings about an intended result, may be confusing

Table 9.1

LEGAL TERMINOLOGY

Tort	an injury or wrongdoing
Tort liability	the right of an injured individual to be made whole again
Intentional tort	an individual (APN) commits an act with intent to bring about the result in question
Negligence	a failure to fulfill a responsibility that subsequently results in injury to an individual

for the APN. Intentional torts can include assault and battery (forcing an individual to take a medication), invasion of privacy (breaking confidentiality), and defamation (slander or libel) (Wright, 2004).

Malpractice is covered under tort law. Klutz (2004) has called for state or federal tort reform to decrease the skyrocketing cost of malpractice insurance premiums. States that have set caps on liability awards have not experienced the insurance crisis. One of the contributing factors to high insurance premiums is that some insurance companies underwrite cost of malpractice policies in investments, and when the stock market is unstable as it has been in recent years, insurance companies either fail or increase the cost of their premiums significantly. Once a rare occurrence, providers are increasingly leaving their practices due to the high cost of insurance premiums. Another response to increased malpractice litigation is the tendency to practice defensive medicine rather than use evidence-based practice guidelines. Defensive practices, i.e., ordering unnecessary tests to rule out all possible diagnoses, only contribute to increasing health care costs (Klutz, 2004).

APNS should learn what type of insurance policy best fits their needs. The two most common types of insurance available are "occurrence" and "claims made." An occurrence policy covers an APN for any incident that occurs during the time insured. For example, an APN is covered following employment for any claims that occur during the employment period. A claims policy covers the APN only during the time that the policy is in effect (Wright, 2004). For example, a claim made after employment has ended is not covered by this type of policy. APNs who change employment should purchase a "tail" policy to cover any claims that occur after the APN has left that place of employment.

APNs can protect themselves from potential malpractice claims in several ways. First and foremost, advanced practice nurses must practice within their scope of practice and the legal scope as determined by their individual state. Second, APNs should carry professional liability insurance either through their employer, through personal professional liability insurance, or both. Arguments can be made both ways for whether an APN should carry both employment and personal liability insurance. For example, if the APN only carries professional liability insurance through the employer, the policy may not cover private duty, volunteer, or off duty incidents. Buppert (2006) advises that APNs read the policy very closely to answer these questions before they arise and recommends that they carry at least one million dollars per occurrence in coverage.

An advanced practice nurse can take several preventive measures to avoid legal or malpractice claims. The importance of thorough and accurate documentation cannot be overemphasized. If ethical or legal issues arise, the APN should report concerns to the proper persons or authorities. It is also important that APNs know the roles and responsibilities within their scope of practice. Negligence or malpractice can occur if the APN does not keep current on standards of practice or treatments. Also, a good patient–client relationship is important. APNs must also delegate appropriately to avoid claims of negligence. Buppert (2008, p. 406) offers the following suggestions to avoid malpractice claims:

- do not offer services or advice to individuals outside of clinical practice setting
- do not offer advice, diagnose or treatment outside your scope of practice or expertise
- base diagnosis and therapy on evidenced based practice guidelines (if available)
- refer patient if differential diagnosis includes one with high mortality that has not been ruled out
- conduct all standard of care screening tests for patient's age, gender or risk factors and follow through if results positive
- document your actions and process of medical decision making
- leave work setting if unable to practice safely in current environment
- purchase your own "occurrence" malpractice insurance policy (p. 406)

In summary, legal issues related to negligence and malpractice can be a cause of concern and stress for health care providers, including advanced practice nurses. APNs should take preventative measures to limit the risk of having claims filed against them.

PRESCRIPTIVE AUTHORITY

Historically, the issue of prescriptive authority has been a barrier to autonomy in advanced nursing practice. The ability to prescribe medications allows the APN more flexibility in implementing holistic care for patients. Although great strides have been made legislatively to allow full prescriptive authority in each state, there continues to be inconsistency among states. To review or learn the prescriptive authority for advanced practice nurses in individual states, the reader is referred to two reports published annually that provide current information in each state (Pearson, 2009; Phillips, 2009).

Prescriptive authority can be granted in several ways. The greatest independence is in those states where APNs are allowed to prescribe medications, including controlled substances, independent of any required physician involvement. Some states allow APNs to prescribe medications, including controlled substances, but require some degree of physician involvement or delegation. Other states allow APNs to prescribe medications but exclude controlled substances and require some degree of physician involvement or delegation (Pearson, 2009; Phillips, 2009).

The first states to provide legislation granting prescriptive authority were Washington, Oregon, and Alaska during the 1970s. As prescriptive authority has expanded into all 50 states, only Alabama, Florida, and Hawaii do not allow APNs to prescribe controlled substances. Several other states limit the schedules of controlled substances that APNs can prescribe.

Another issue surrounding prescriptive authority is the language used in regulations and legislation. Some rules and regulations specify "nurse practitioner," excluding clinical nurse specialists, certified nurse-midwives, and certified registered nurse anesthetists. Increasingly, legislation is written to reflect the expanded advanced practice title. Terms that have been used include midlevel practitioner, midlevel provider, advanced practice nurse, and advanced practice registered nurse. Terms such as "midlevel provider/practitioner" often refer to nurse practitioners, clinical nurse specialists, and physician assistants. Active participation in the political process by professional nursing lobbyists and individuals has resulted in positive legislative benefits for all advanced practice nurses.

Once legislation is passed, most laws go to an administrative rules committee comprised of legislators that develop rules for interpreting the law. Administrative rules committees often seek input from professionals, consumers, and parties affected by the law. It is extremely important for advanced practice nurses to be "at the table" during these discussions. Special interest groups can influence whether rules are broadly or literally interpreted. One such example is how states define collaboration or supervision in their administrative rules.

Other trends serve to restrict or limit prescriptive practice. These include a movement toward joint regulation (a joint board with representatives from pharmacy, medicine, and nursing); reluctance to "grandfather" in nurses with existing prescriptive authority; ignoring state boards of nursing actions by other governmental agencies; restricting drug utilization review boards to pharmacists and physicians; and reluctance by insurance companies to fill prescriptions written by APNs. Inconsistencies among states related to prescriptive authority contribute to the frustration of APNs whose authority to prescribe medications is called into question.

In 1991, the Drug Enforcement Agency (DEA) proposed rules for affiliated practitioners (i.e., nurse practitioners, physician assistants) that would have imposed restrictive regulations for advanced practice nurses that superseded state laws. The DEA rules did not acknowledge the existing prescriptive regulations in states. Nurses in independent practice would have been affected by the ruling. However, the DEA withdrew these proposed rules subsequent to huge protest from the nursing community. A second ruling entitled Definition and Registration of Mid-Level Practitioners was proposed in 1992 (Federal Registrar, 1992). The 1992 ruling is less restrictive as regards prescriptive authority for advanced practice nurses. Drug Enforcement Agency (DEA) registration is required to prescribe controlled substances. The national provider identification number (NPI) is required on all noncontrolled substance prescriptions. APNs can apply for DEA registration online at www.deadiversion.usdoj.gov/drugreg/index.html, and NPI numbers can be obtained or accessed online at www.nppes.com.hss.gov. A practitioner prescribing manual is also available through the DEA (2006) at www .deadiversion.usdoj.gov/pubs/manuals/pract/pract_manual012508.pdf.

Drug Utilization Review programs mandated by the Omnibus Budget Reconciliation Act of 1990, effective January 1, 1993, were designed to reduce fraud, abuse, overuse, or unnecessary care among physicians, pharmacists, and patients. Currently, no state specifically provides for the inclusion of nurses or other health care members of the review program board. The exclusion of APNs from these boards is a concern because prescriptive practice by APNs will be evaluated by individuals lacking a nursing perspective.

Prescriptive authority of medications, including controlled substances, is not only a privilege; it is a responsibility that advanced practice nurses cannot take lightly. The provider is fully responsible for understanding the regulatory parameters for prescribing these drugs. Ongoing continuing pharmacotherapeutics education is essential in safe prescribing practices. All prescribers should avoid any prescribing practices that would put their prescriptive privileges at risk.

SUMMARY

This chapter addresses professional issues that influence advanced practice. APNs may encounter situations that place them at risk for liability claims or regulatory misconduct. It is the responsibility of advanced practice nurses to have a full sense of their scope of practice, maintain adequate liability coverage, and prescribe within the legal authority for their state.

REFERENCES

Brekken, S. A., & Sheets, S. V. (2008). Pain management. *Nursing Administration Quarterly, 32*(4), 288–295.

Buppert, C. (2006). Questions and answers on malpractice insurance for nurse practitioners. *Medscape.* Retrieved on April 5, 2009, from www.medscape.com/viewarticle/520660.

Buppert, C. (2008). Frequently asked questions and answers about malpractice insurance. *Dermatology Nursing, 20*(5), 405–406.

Buppert, C. (2008a). *Nurse practitioner's business practice and legal guide* (3rd ed.). Boston: Jones & Bartlett.

Drug Enforcement Agency (2006). *Practitioner's manual.* Washington, DC: United States Department of Justice Drug Enforcement Agency, Office of Diversion Control. Retrieved March 31, 2009, from www.deadiversion.usdoj.gov/pubs/manuals/pract/pract_manual012508.pdf

Federal Register. (1992). Definition and registration of mid-level practitioners 21 CFR Parts 1301 and 1304. *Federal Register, 57*(146), 33465.

Hannigan, N. S. (2006). Blowing the whistle on health care fraud: Should I? *Journal of the American Academy of Nurse Practitioners, 18*(11), 512–517.

Hudspeth, R. (2007). Balancing need, preparation and scope of practice: Issues impacting behavioral health services by advanced practice registered nurses. *Nursing Administration Quarterly, 31*(3), 264–265.

Klutz, D. L. (2004). Tort reform: an issue for nurse practitioners. *Journal of the American Academy of Nurse Practitioners, 16*(2), 70–75.

Pearson, L. J. (2009). The Pearson report. *The American Journal for Nurse Practitioners, 13*(2), 4–82. www.webnp.net

Phillips, S. J. (2009). Legislative update 2009. *The Nurse Practitioner, 34*(1), 19–41.

Snyder, C.H. (2005). Dementia and driving: autonomy versus safety. *Journal of the American Academy of Nurse Practitioners, 17*(10), 393–402.

Thorpe, K. E. (2004, January 21). The medical malpractice "crisis": Recent trends and the impact of state tort reform. *Health Affairs,* Web Exclusive.

Williams, C. (2006). Dilemmas in fetal medicine: Premature application of technology or responding to women's choice. *Sociology of Health and Illness, 28*(1), 1–20.

Wiseman, H. (2007). Advanced nursing practice—the influences and accountabilities. *British Journal of Nursing, 16*(3), 167–173.

Wright, W.L. (2004). *Liability and malpractice: Everything the NP needs to know.* Presentation given at the National Conference of Gerontological Nurse Practitioners, September 29–October 3, 2004. Phoenix, AZ: Author.

Yeo, T. P. & Edmunds, M.W. (2004). What to expect from medical liability tort reform. *Nurse Practitioner, 29*(5), 7.

Zakak, N. N. (2009). Fertility issues of childhood cancer survivors: Role of pediatric nurse practitioners in fertility preservation. *Journal of Pediatric Oncology Nursing, 26*(1), 48–59.

10

Reimbursement Realities for Advanced Practice Nurses

LINDA LINDEKE

ACCESS, QUALITY, AND COST

Health care costs are rising worldwide as expensive technology is incorporated, life expectancy increases, and infant survival rates reach lower gestational levels (Keegan, Sisko, Truffer, Smith, Cowen, et. al., 2008). Employers continue to raise employee cost sharing for health care by increasing the deductible amounts and co-payments for care. Health care spending in 2007 rose more than 6% from 2006 to $2.2 trillion, or $7,500 per person in the United States (Hartman, Martin, McDonnell, Catlin, & the National Health Expenditure Accounts Team, 2009). In 2008, those with employer-sponsored health insurance paid $12,680 for family coverage, with an average of $3,354 out-of-pocket expenses for co-payments, medications, and other health-related costs (Kaiser Family Foundation, 2008). Rising health care costs are one of the key causes of the current economic downturn.

Although health care costs continue to increase worldwide, the American health care system remains the most expensive in the world. For example, health care spending as a percentage of the U.S. gross domestic product (GDP) is expected to exceed 16% of the nation's gross domestic product (GDP) in 2009, far more than in any other developed country (Kaiser Family Foundation, 2008). This rate is in striking contrast to that of other countries providing a similar quality of health care. For instance, Canada spent 10.7% of its 2008 GDP on health care (Canadian Institute for Health Information, 2008). Factors contributing to higher U.S. costs include a fragmented payer system creating weakness on the demand side of the market, high administrative costs (almost 25% of health care expenditures), and resistance to the idea of putting limits on health care (Reinhardt, Hussey, & Anderson, 2004).

Health care reform efforts are focusing on cost containment, disease prevention, and evidence-based practice as means to address the economic realities. However, there is no "quick fix" for long-standing issues related to health care access, quality, and cost-effectiveness (Baicker & Chandra, 2008). Health care is costing patients, employers, and payers more each year and has become a very closely watched economic indicator. Advanced practice nurses (APNs) must be well informed about the context and specifics of reimbursement to be successful in practice.

The fiscal structure of health care is affected by multiple forces, many of which are political. Federal and state actions influence health care reimbursement in many ways, such as by regulating health care systems, by supporting research, and particularly by financing and delivering health care services. There are 50 different state-specific configurations of health care because most reimbursement laws and policies are developed at the state level. Reimbursement politics are played out in Congress, state legislatures, and within county governments. Political processes may also take place at APN work sites as employment agreements and organizational policies are negotiated. APNs must understand the various health care forces and players, particularly issues related to access, quality, and cost.

Access to care is complex in the United States and is directly related to cost issues. In 2007, about 45.7 million individuals (15.3%) in the United States lacked insurance coverage and access to health care (U.S. Census Bureau, 2008). Approximately 58.3% of individuals with insurance in 2007 were covered by private insurance plans, a decline from 63.2% in 2001; this number is expected to continue to decrease because the economic downturn causes employers to be less likely to provide health insurance for their employees (Sherman, Greensteen, & Parrott, 2008). Some people either choose to or are forced to self-insure, some are unable or unwilling to negotiate the bureaucracy necessary to obtain coverage from public programs for which they are eligible, and others are ineligible for public or employer-based coverage (frequently because of part-time employment). Access to care for the uninsured, as well as the underinsured, remains one of the most pressing issues facing American society today.

Even Americans with insurance have concerns as co-payments increase and benefits become more and more limited. Many health plans require referrals and prior authorizations for the more costly health care components. Additionally, some health plans limit patients to only seeing the providers on their salaried staff (staff-model health maintenance organizations or HMOs), or to a contracted list of specialists and agencies (preferred provider organizations, or PPOs). Thus, Americans with and without health care coverage have concerns about access to needed care. Although there are no "stated" limits on health care (often termed "rationing"), there are de facto limits in many systems. "Triage" or "tiering" of clients according to the types and price of coverage offered by employer plans and insurance carriers is a way of limiting health care services. HMOs, self-insured companies, and small businesses may have high deductibles, co-payments, and prior authorization procedures that limit choices of providers, procedures, and referrals.

Quality of health care in the United States is also a continuing public concern. Supreme Court deliberations about the rights of patients to sue managed care organizations (MCOs) and attempts to pass a Patient Bill of Rights in Congress (so far unsuccessful) are expressions of this concern. The Patient Bill of Rights initiative is based on a public perception that health care quality has declined as a result of the MCOs' quest for a profitable bottom line. Cuts in Medicare and Medicaid benefits have also increased the public's concern that the quality of care may be further reduced in the future.

Many programs attempt to monitor and improve health care quality. One example is the Agency for Healthcare Research and Quality (AHRQ), a federal agency devoted to tracking trends, providing model programs, and researching outcomes. Partnerships of public and private agencies such as the Consumer Assessment of Healthcare Providers and Systems program (CAHPS) work together to assess care, report system performance, and recommend or fund improvement efforts. A myriad of reports of care outcomes of hospitals, nursing homes, and individual providers is available for comparison. The Commonwealth Fund, the Institute of Medicine, the Robert Wood Johnson Foundation, the National Committee for Quality Improvement, and National Quality Forum are just a few of the organizations very active in quality improvement efforts. Nurses working toward care improvement are active in all those entities as well as in many professional nursing organizations.

APNs can contribute to these efforts by membership and leadership in these organizations.

U.S. REIMBURSEMENT TRENDS

The U.S. health care delivery system hardly resembles the system in place just a decade ago, and a whole new language has developed that APNs must understand (Table 10.1). Congress failed to pass the 1993 Clinton health care reform initiative ostensibly in the effort to develop systems to control rapidly increasing health care costs. Repercussions of this failed legislation included: (1) rapid mergers of health care systems, (2) formation of integrated service delivery networks, and (3) competitive contracting between employers and service providers. As a result, the U.S. health care industry has wholeheartedly adopted the bottom-line–oriented, profit–loss mentality of the business world. As this trend pervades American health care, APNs can offer ways of ensuring access and quality of care while keeping costs reasonable for consumers.

Capitated systems (that replace fee-for-service payments) are the norm; payers contract with provider groups to pay a per-member amount to cover the cost of member health care services over a certain time period. Capitated care in MCOs now dominates the industry. Many MCOs, in turn, have undergone multiple mergers to form large provider organizations (PPOs) and networks. Services are increasingly delivered in outpatient clinics that contract with payers for coverage of client groups. Hospital stays (regulated by federally administered diagnostic-related group regulations, or DRGs) have been shortened because of the cost, and patients are discharged earlier and sicker than in the past. The amount of health care delivered in outpatient settings has increased to over 60% in 2008, compared to 40% in 1980 (Farrell, Jensen, & Kocher, 2008). Home care services may or may not be available upon discharge, often putting burdens on families and communities to provide care that used to occur in hospitals. Medicare regulations have become more complex, and employer-paid health care benefits, not surprisingly, have become a very contentious issue in labor negotiations.

Prescription drug use has increased, partly due to direct-to-consumer advertising that urges patients to contact their health care providers for the latest "miracle" drug. In an attempt to provide medications while controlling costs, the federal government implemented a voluntary program called Part D of Medicare in 2006 to subsidize prescribed medications for those covered by Medicare who apply for this special program. Part D is a very complex program that is a public–private partnership; it offers the elderly many different plan choices, and the application process is very complex. Opinions are mixed regarding its effectiveness as prescription drug costs continue to be a large part of Medicare expenditures and much lobbying occurs from the pharmaceutical industry. Americans appear to take more prescription medications than people in other countries do with comparable conditions (Schoen, Osborn, Doty, Bishop, Peugh, & Murukutla, 2007)

APNs can now be directly reimbursed for their services and must be knowledgeable about trends, developments, and proposed payment systems and reimbursement schedules. APNs will be successful in their practices to the extent that the value of their services is recognized by payers and employers and is equitably rewarded. APNs must be cost-effective and must track their productivity within complex systems; however, the rapid pace of change in reimbursement legislation, policies, and procedures makes this a daunting task.

APNs were not always reimbursed for their services by public and private payers. A series of lobbying efforts at national and state levels occurred over time to make this possible. Federal and state legislation

Table 10.1

REIMBURSEMENT VOCABULARY

Terminology	Definition
Actual charge	The amount of money a provider charges for a particular service, which may be more than the amount payers approve
Additional benefits	Health care services not covered by Medicare. Additional benefits are subject to cost sharing by plan enrollees.
Adjusted community rating	Premium rates based on regional differences in health care costs; leads to great regional differences in Medicare payment rates to providers
Advanced beneficiary notice (ABN)	A notice that a provider must give Medicare beneficiaries to sign when providing a service that Medicare does not consider medically necessary. If the patient does not get an ABN to sign before the service is provided and Medicare does not pay for it, the patient does not have to pay for the service.

(Continued)

Table 10.1 (Continued)

Terminology	Definition
Affiliated provider	A health care provider or facility that is paid by a health plan to give service to plan members (i.e., a credentialed provider).
Ancillary services	Professional services by a hospital or other inpatient facility (i.e., X-rays, drugs, laboratory services)
Appeal	A formal complaint made to a health plan
Approved amount (or approved charge)	The fee a payer sets as reasonable for a covered service (may be less than the amount charged by the provider)
Balance billing	A situation in which private fee-for-service providers can charge and bill Medicare patients 15% more than the plan's payment
Beneficiary	The name for a person who has health insurance through the Medicare or Medicaid program
Capitation	A per-member amount paid to providers to cover the cost of member health care services for a certain time period
Carrier	A private company that has a contract with Medicare to pay Medicare Part B bills
Catastrophic limit	The highest amount of money patients have to pay out of pocket during a certain time period for certain charges
Center for Medicare and Medicaid Services (CMS)	Federal agency that runs Medicare and works with the states to run Medicaid programs
Consolidated Omnibus Budget Reconciliation Act (COBRA)	A law that makes an employer continue to cover an employee for a period of time after spousal death, job loss, divorce, or hours/benefits reduction; typically requires payment of both employee and employer shares of the premium
Coordination of benefits	Process in which two or more health plans share costs of a claim
Cost sharing	The cost for medical care that patients pay (co-payment, co-insurance, deductible)
Covered benefit	A service that is paid for (partially or fully) by a health plan
Diagnosis-related group (DRG)	A payment system begun in 1983 to pay hospitals for health care based on patients' diagnosis, age, gender, and complications; DRGs affect length of hospital stay
Durable medical equipment/ goods	Reusable equipment that is ordered for use in the home (walkers, etc.) and paid for under Medicare

(Continued)

Table 10.1 (Continued)

Terminology	Definition
Facilities charge	A charge billed to a health plan or provider for the facility in which the service was received; results in two bills (provider bill and facility bill)
Fiscal intermediary	A private company that contracts with Medicare to pay Part A and some Part B bills; located in various regions of the United States
Fraud and abuse	Fraud: To purposely bill for services that were never given or to bill for a service at a higher reimbursement rate than the service produced Abuse: Payment for items or services that are billed by mistake
Health maintenance organization/ network	A health plan that contracts with group practices of providers to give services in one or more locations
Managed care plan with point-of-service (POS) option	A managed care health plan that lets patients use providers and hospitals outside the plan for an additional cost
Medically necessary services	Services deemed by Medicare to be proper and needed for a medical diagnosis or specific treatment
Medical savings account (MSA)	A Medicare health plan option made up of two parts: (1) Medicare MSA Health Insurance Policy (has a high deductible); (2) Special savings account in which Medicare deposits money to help patients pay their own medical bills
Preferred provider organization (PPO)	A managed care plan in which hospitals and providers belong to a network and contract together with payers/ employers to provide services at predetermined rates
Prior authorization	MCO approval that is necessary prior to receiving care from providers who are out of the PPO or not on staff list (can be verbal or is a written form from the MCO)
Referral	A written document that must be received by a provider before giving care to a health plan beneficiary
Resource-based relative value scale (RBRVS)	A Medicare fee schedule established in 1989 to reimburse providers based on relative work value units (RVUs)

currently regulates APN reimbursement. For example, the 1997 federal Balanced Budget Act (PL 105-33) provides direct Medicare reimbursement for nurse practitioners and clinical nurse specialists, effective January 1, 1998. Rules to implement this law were written by the Center for Medicare and Medicaid Services (CMS, formerly known as the Health Care Financing Administration, HCFA) and were finalized in November 1998. These Medicare laws and rules influence the policies of nongovernmental payers, although there is a great deal of variability from state to state. APNs must carefully monitor CMS activities to ensure that the policies continue to favor APN reimbursement. The goal is to have "provider-inclusive language," meaning that laws and policies do not specifically designate payment to physicians but use the term *providers,* which is inclusive of nurse practitioners and clinical nurse specialists. Terminology in policy and law is an extremely important issue for APN practice.

The Health Insurance Portability and Accountability Act (HIPAA), a law passed in 1996 (also sometimes called the "Kassebaum–Kennedy" law), began the practice of implementing provider-inclusive language in federal law and policy. It expanded health care coverage related to job loss or transfer and provided some patient protection by limiting ways that insurance companies could use preexisting medical conditions to deny health insurance coverage. Although HIPAA generally guarantees the right to renewal of health coverage, it did not supersede states' roles as the primary regulators of health insurance. It standardized health care billing and payment mechanisms across systems, a move that promised to reduce costs once it was fully implemented. As part of that standardization, stringent patient privacy regulations were also instituted. The anticipated cost and quality improvements from HIPAA have not yet been realized, though it has certainly had many positive results. Electronic health records (EHRs) have rapidly been introduced since HIPAA was passed, and there are predictions that in time EHRs will bring about cost savings and quality improvements.

A recent development is retail-based health care, which debuted in the early 2000s. Retail-based clinics are called by many names, including convenient care clinics and in-store clinics. Their numbers increase yearly, and they lower the cost of care because of their low overhead expenses (Thygeson, Van Vorst, Maciosek, & Solberg, 2008). Medical associations such as the American Academy of Pediatrics have questioned the quality of care in retail-based clinics (Corwin, Francis, McInerny, Ponzi, Reuben, et al., 2006). These clinics typically employ nurse practitioners and have given new visibility to APN practice (Miller, 2009). They appear to offer consumers a good quality alternative to care in ambulatory clinics and emergency rooms for commonly occurring complaints.

Another model of care and reimbursement being introduced is termed "medical home," sometimes referred to as "healthcare home." This payment mechanism aims to reimburse designated practices for care coordination activities. The goal is to deliver community-based, continuous, comprehensive, culturally appropriate health care (Duderstadt, 2008). Originally developed in pediatrics for children with chronic conditions, this model has been increasingly advocated for all primary care practices. A nurse practitioner-delivered medical home demonstration project demonstrated feasibility, excellent care outcomes, and patient satisfaction (Palfry, Sofis, Davidson, Liu, Freeman, & Ganz, 2004). It is essential that APNs track medical-health-care home models of care and reimbursement policies to ensure that they all contain provider-inclusive language. If not, this model of care will benefit physician practices and either exclude or make invisible the work of APNs.

Pay-for-performance (also called P4P) is another health care trend that APNs must carefully track and utilize to their best advantage. Reimbursement is linked to outcome measures by public and private payers, including CMSs. The goal is to provide incentives for quality care, a worthy aim. However, clinical performance is not easily measured due to multifactorial patient outcomes (Johnson, Harper, Hanson, & Dawson, 2007), and P4P has had mixed reviews as a strategy to decrease costs and increase care quality.

REIMBURSEMENT STRUCTURES

Third-party Payers

APNs must understand many issues about health care regulation (Figure 10.1), including the relationships between entities that pay for and provide services. For example,

1. For-profit insurance companies known as "indemnity providers" (e.g., Aetna, Prudential, etc.)
2. Government payment programs (e.g., Medicare, Medicaid, Tricare/CHAMPUS, the military health system)
3. Nonprofit corporations (e.g., Blue Cross/Blue Shield)
4. Self-insuring corporations or coalitions (e.g., union health care plans)

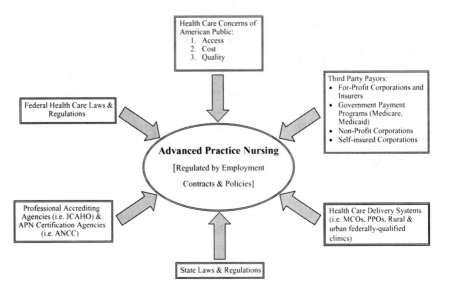

Figure 10.1 Reimbursement regulation for advanced practice nurses.

Although payer policies and procedures differ greatly, most are influenced by CMS Medicare regulations. Payers pay fee-for-service bills, the traditional way that health care has been funded. More recently they pay for health care delivered under service contracts with HMOs and PPOs; provider systems must compete and bid for those contracts, unions participate in the negotiations, and contracts are re-bid every few years. Employers typically offer their employees a choice of approved health system plans with which they can contract. Other employers self-insure by directly contracting with provider networks for their employees' care. These competitive contracts are frequently renegotiated in response to rising health care costs. Health care finance is complex and volatile, and provider system costs are under constant review by payers and regulators.

APNs must be individually identified through payer credentialing to obtain reimbursement under their own names. Payer credentialing makes APNs visible because their contributions can be specifically identified. Although many payers allow APNs to bill individually, others refuse to reimburse APN services, even in states with laws that mandate third-party APN reimbursement. Medicare and Medicaid have moved many clients from fee-for-service payment systems into managed care reimbursement systems, in which case MCO policies overlay CMS regulations. Therefore, APNs must be cognizant of the many layers of reimbursement policies and procedures in their state, region, and organization.

Provider Systems

U.S. health care is delivered by many types of providers, each with its own policies and practices affecting APN reimbursement. These types of providers include

1. Managed care organizations (MCOs)
2. Managed care networks
3. Health maintenance organizations (HMOs)
4. Preferred provider organizations (PPOs)
5. Nurse-managed centers (NMCs)
6. Fee-for-service private practices
7. Home health care agencies
8. Public health agencies
9. Community health centers
10. Federal qualified health centers (FQHCs)
11. Migrant health clinics
12. Indian Health Board (IHB) clinics and hospitals
13. Rural health clinics (RHCs)
14. Retail-based clinics

Some types of federally funded clinics (FQHCs) have policies that mandate NPs be employed in order for the clinic to receive funding dollars. These regulations were passed based on federal studies that demonstrated NP safety and cost-effectiveness. FQHCs credential NPs for reimbursement and hospital privileges, provide them membership on provider panels, and validate their scope of practice. In most other systems, however, APNs must negotiate for their place and power. APNs must strive to obtain leadership positions in provider systems so that their contributions to patient outcomes are identified and valued by administrators and payers. Examples of leadership roles include performing administrative functions, participating on policy committees, and conducting research projects.

One way that APNs have shown leadership and achieved independence is through the creation of nurse-managed centers (NMCs). Often serving underinsured and uninsured populations with the associated limitations in funding, NMCs have had mixed results in terms of longevity. They have organized for mutual support through the Institute for Nursing Centers (INC) that is a partnership between the Michigan Academic Consortium, the American Association of Colleges of Nursing, the Nursing

Centers Research Network, the Michigan Primary Care Association, the National Nursing Center Consortium, and the National Organization of Nurse Practitioner Faculties (NONPF). Successful NMCs must have low administrative overhead costs, low fixed costs, and the ability to generate sufficient patient volume. Nurses have evaluated NMC outcomes and have published their results (INC, 2008), and those outcomes have enabled them to obtain further grants to expand. The analysis of NMC outcomes that combine both cost analysis and cost-effectiveness measures demonstrate the benefits of APN practice overall and benefit all APNs.

SELECTED ENTITIES AND PROVIDER SYSTEMS

Medicare

Medicare was established in 1965 as part of President Lyndon Johnson's Great Society initiative; its programs are primarily oriented to acute care for the elderly. The goal was to create a safety net for the nation's elderly who had endured hardships in the world wars and the Depression during the 1930s. Medicare is a two-part, federally funded health care program; approximately 95% of the nation's elderly are enrolled in Medicare Part A. Part A provides hospital insurance that covers inpatient services, up to 100 days in a skilled nursing facility following hospitalization, and some home health care. Although there are no premiums for Part A Medicare, patient cost sharing is required. Cost sharing consists of an annual deductible as well as a payment percentage. Medicare does not cover eye examinations, medications, or long-term nursing care. Medicare Part B pays for physician visits, services and supplies, outpatient services, and home health care, all at rates set by the federal government.

The 1997 Balanced Budget Act (PL 105–33) allows Medicare reimbursement of services provided by nurse practitioners and clinical nurse specialists if the services are reimbursable when provided by a physician and if the services are within the APN scope of practice. The law removed all restrictions on the practice setting and permitted NPs and CNSs to submit fees for services rendered in hospitals, skilled nursing facilities, nursing homes, comprehensive outpatient rehabilitation facilities, community mental health centers, and rural health centers. Payments for NP and CNS services are discounted, compared to physician reimbursement, to 80% of the lesser of either the actual charge or 85% of the physician fee schedule amount.

NPs and CNSs billing under their own names must complete claim forms (called Form 1500) using their unique national provider identifier (NPI) numbers. These numbers are obtained from the Center for Medicare and Medicaid Services (CMS). Established as part of the 1997 legislation, this provider-specific tracking number is used by all systems for administrative and financial transactions.

Some APNs do not submit claims under their own names, although this practice is typically discouraged by nursing leaders and professional organizations because it implements a system of physician supervision of APN practice. Medicare has a payment system for nursing and physician assistant services rendered under physician supervision called "incident-to billing." Incident-to billing allows APNs to bill under physician names for services that are provided as "incident to" physician services. Payment then equals 100% of the physician fee schedule.

Although incident-to billing increases the revenue that APNs can generate under current reimbursement rates, this billing practice raises red flags for fraud and abuse because it is governed by a tangle of federal regulations. APN billable activities must be integrated into daily physician practice. Incident-to billing is typically interpreted as implying direct supervision of APNs by physicians. Supervising physicians must be physically present (although not in the patient examination room) at all times when APNs are providing billable services, and physicans must perform all the initial patient visits and must establish the plans of care that APNs then follow. Incident-to billing limits APN autonomy and may also be very impractical. For example, if the physician leaves the building for lunch or vacation, the APN could not bill "incident-to" for patients seen during that time frame. (Note: APNs could, however, bill for this care under their own names if they were individually credentialed as providers with the payer; the practice would receive 85% of the physician fee if they did so, rather than the 100% "incident-to" payment.) "Incident-to" billing makes the contribution of APNs to the fiscal output of organizations invisible. Billing under their own provider numbers (NPIs) is now strongly encouraged to increase productivity, to avoid the potential for billing fraud, and to permit full utilization of the legal APN scope of practice.

Another Medicare billing practice incorporates a system that reimburses providers based on relative work value units (RVUs). Established in 1989, the Resource-Based Relative Value Scale (RBRVS) is a system aligned with Current Procedural Terminology (CPT) codes. Each CPT code is assigned a relative dollar value by CMS based on practice research about work and practice expenses and professional liability insurance costs. Allowable service charges are determined annually by multiplying this RVU by a standard dollar amount conversion factor established by CMS, based on CMS's determination of regional cost variations (the geographic adjustment factor, GAF). CMS publishes its RBRVS annually in the Federal Register, and practices then use the RBRVS to determine their fees.

The goal is to have a logical system of national fees set annually in relationship to actual costs and ongoing research. The result is that New York practitioners will have higher Medicare payments than practitioners in Iowa, for example, because it costs more to run a practice in New York than it does in Iowa. With support from the American Nurses Association (ANA), Sullivan-Marx and Maislin (2000) carried out a study comparing NP and family physician RVUs; there was no significant difference between the provider groups. The ANA continues to work with the American Medical Association's Health Professional Advisory Committee on reimbursement issues, including ways to fairly integrate NP billing practices into the RBRVS structure.

The 1997 Balanced Budget Act (BBA) (PL 105–33) provided both access and barriers to Medicare reimbursement for APNs. During the rule-writing process for this act, the definition of "collaboration" was debated. The primary debate was about the impact of regulatory collaboration language on APN practice in states where physician collaboration is not required and advanced practice nurses practice independently. This contentious issue continues to be closely monitored federally and in each state by APN professional groups. Because state APN practice laws by and large determine APN practice, collaboration is a continuing and important issue for all APNs. Most contentious was the language in the 1997 BBA that set APN reimbursement at 85% of the physician rate; this was a compromise, and the bill would not have passed had APNs not agreed to this requirement.

PL 105–33 regulations require that in order to be credentialed as Medicare providers NPs or CNSs must be master's-prepared registered nurses authorized to practice as NPs or CNSs by the state in which the services are furnished and be certified as NPs or CNSs by recognized national certifying bodies that have established standards. The requirements have been problematic for many clinical nurse specialists because national certification has not been highly pursued by CNSs in the past, and in many cases no national certification examination exists to reflect their practice specialty. Although CNSs meet the master's degree requirement, certification continues to be an issue of debate within their ranks. CNSs in psychiatry and mental health are an exception because they have pursued reimbursement since the early 1970s and typically are nationally certified.

The rules also contained a time-limited "grandfather" clause to allow certified NPs without master's degrees to obtain provider numbers if they applied prior to January 1, 1999. In general, PL 105–33 was a victory for NPs and CNSs and met the intent of the law, which was to increase greater consumer access to NPs and CNSs. The legislation lifted some of the barriers to APN reimbursement.

Medicaid

Medicaid expanded the 1965 federal Medicare system by providing funds for states to pay for health care of low-income groups. Federally supported and state administered, Medicaid covers costs of care for vulnerable groups through programs such as Aid to Families with Dependent Children (AFDC). Low-income elderly persons and some individuals with disabilities are also covered under this program. Medicaid is different from Medicare in that it is a vendor program, meaning that providers offering services to these individuals or families must accept the Medicaid reimbursement as full payment and cannot request co-payments from patients. Because Medicaid payments are low (typically less than 50% of submitted bills), many providers (including dentists) restrict the number of Medicaid clients that they serve. Some states enroll Medicaid patients in MCOs by establishing contracts with MCOs in programs called "prepaid medical assistance programs (PMAPs).

Section 6405 of the Omnibus Budget Reconciliation Act (OBRA 1989, PL 101–239) authorizes Medicaid payment for services of certified pediatric nurse practitioners and certified family nurse practitioners. Requirements necessary for reimbursement include possession of a current RN license in the state in which services are provided, compliance with state APN legal requirements, and certification by a national APN certification board. APN Medicaid reimbursement rates vary between 70 to 100% of physician fees, depending on the state.

Indemnity Insurers

Indemnity insurers are traditional insurance companies that pay for but do not deliver health care. They typically require an annual deductible that members self-pay; once this deductible is reached, the company will pay 80% of their members' health care costs on a per-person, per-procedure basis. Reimbursement rates are based on "usual and customary charges," which vary between regions and companies. If provider charges are more than the indemnity insurer allows, patients are responsible to pay the balance. Some indemnity insurance companies will pay for APN services. APNs can contact these companies to negotiate for recognition as reimbursable providers.

Managed Care Organizations (MCOs)

Capitated managed care developed rapidly in the 1990s in response to many economic and political forces. One factor was that the U.S. post-World War II baby-boom generation is transitioning into middle age, increasing the aging population who will be high consumers of health care. This trend is projected to greatly increase costs, particularly for expensive, emerging technologies. MCOs sell health service packages to employers, individuals, or governmental agencies. Services are provided by the MCO panel of health care providers who may or may not be MCO employees. APNs can apply to become primary care providers (PCPs) on MCO provider panels, but this recognition has been slow in coming. MCOs reimburse PCPs using fee-for-service, a capitated or fee-per-member basis, or a combination of fee-for-service and capitation.

MCOs are growing rapidly in the United States and are typically large, complex organizations. They stress the importance of health promotion, chronic care management, and patient education, and they typically provide their members with preventive services. They have so far been unable to demonstrate the expected cost savings. Some managed care strategies, such as employing economies of scale in purchasing, centralizing services such as emergency care, and developing systems for referrals and after-hours care have been cost-effective. However, administrative costs are very high.

Managed care is frequently interpreted as "managed costs." Efforts by CMS to uncover fraud in Medicare/Medicaid billing has added to the negative light in which many providers and consumers view MCOs. APNs are also voicing their discomfort with MCO policies, particularly about the expectations that limit the length of patient visits to 10 to 15 minutes. RVU billing in MCOs is also a system that concerns APNs who value time and care continuity with their clients. In high-production managed care models, APNs may not be able to fulfill their responsibilities to prevent illness, coordinate care, and teach patients about their treatment plans.

CNM and CRNA Reimbursement

Certified nurse-midwives (CNMs) successfully obtain third-party reimbursement for their services based on their cost-effectiveness and high level of consumer satisfaction. Excellent research about CNM outcomes is compelling to payers seeking safe care at reasonable cost. In 1973, Washington was the first state to enact laws permitting CNM reimbursement by private and public benefit plans; currently 33 states have such language in their statutes. Seven other states have "any willing provider" laws that include midwives. The American College of Nurse-Midwives (ACNM) provides its members with excellent resources for billing, coding, and reimbursement through its website and publications. State laws and regulations must be in place to support CNM activities, including reimbursement. CNMs and all APNs must be active in public policy formulation in order to establish favorable legal and regulatory practice climates.

Although few of their clients qualify for Medicare, CMS Medicare regulations restrict midwifery payments to 65% of the physician fee schedule. ACNM is currently lobbying to increase Medicare reimbursement to 97%; in part, because Medicare regulations affect all payers in setting this precedent of establishing a widely used payment process. ACNM is also lobbying to have freestanding birth center facility costs covered in state Medicaid regulations. In some systems, CNMs work in "incident-to" relationships with physicians, which raises the potential for fraudulent claims if all the aspects of incident-to regulations are not strictly followed. Billing under their own names is strongly recommended for all APNs, including CNMs, so that autonomous practice can provide the best possible care to clients and families.

Despite many difficulties, certified registered nurse anesthetists (CRNAs) have been successful in obtaining third-party reimbursement. The Omnibus Budget Reconciliation Act (OBRA) of 1986 granted CRNAs the right to be directly reimbursed for their services to Medicare recipients. CRNA services are also reimbursed directly by Medicaid and a number of commercial carriers. When both a CRNA and an anesthesiologist participate in the same case, the services of both anesthesia providers can be billed according to the extent of their involvement in the case. Independently billing CRNAs provide savings for government programs and for private payers because they typically charge less than their physician counterparts. Many complex issues regarding CNRA working relationships with physicians (including anesthesiologists) affect their work environments and billing practices. The American Association of Nurse Anesthetists offers CRNAs many reimbursement resources.

DOCUMENTATION AND CODING TO GAIN REIMBURSEMENT

Documentation is the key to reimbursement and must be sufficient to support the level of charge being requested. In addition, APNs must understand their billing process and be able to use several types of diagnostic and procedure codes. One type of code is called the Health Care Common Procedure Coding System (HCPCS), which assigns a dollar amount to patient care activities. For example, there are HCPCS codes for immunization and wound suturing. Each patient visit is also coded using Current Procedural Terminology (CPT) codes, another part of the uniform coding language. The CPT coding directory covers all possible types of patient–provider interactions. It is owned and updated annually by the American Medical Association and has been adopted by Medicare and other third-party payers (AMA, 2004).

A subgroup of CPT codes includes the Evaluation and Management Codes (E&M Codes), the CPT codes most used by APNs (typically CPT codes 99201 through 99456). These five-digit codes are based on the levels of history taking and physical examination, complexity of decision making, counseling, and minutes of face-to-face time in each patient encounter. APNs must distinguish between new patients and established patients in their choice of codes because new patients are reimbursed at a higher rate than established patients. A new patient is considered to be one who has not received professional services within the past 3 years from a provider in the same specialty in the same practice. Telephone communication, however, is considered a professional service.

In addition to assigning a CPT code on the standard claim forms (Form 1500), APNs must select appropriate diagnostic codes from the International Classification of Diseases, Ninth Revision, Clinical Modification (ICD-9). ICD-9 is based on the World Health Organization disease classification. Its periodic modification is the responsibility of the National Center for Health Statistics and CMS. It classifies symptoms and diseases into six-digit numerical codes. A new version, ICD-10, is currently under development and will be implemented in 2013 (Center for Medicare and Medicaid Services, 2009).

Documentation begins with a concise statement of the chief complaint, usually stated in the patient's own words in the medical history (Table 10.2). The classic seven variables should be used to document the chief complaint (location, quality, severity, duration, timing, context, modifying factors, signs/symptoms). For billing purposes, there are four categories of history-taking: problem-focused, expanded problem-focused, detailed, and comprehensive. Each level expands the history according to the level of history taking required to investigate the chief complaint. A problem-focused history consists of the chief complaint and brief history of the present illness (HPI) or problem. An expanded problem-focused history adds a problem-pertinent review of systems (ROS). The ROS has data categories including constitutional, ear/eye/nose/throat, cardiac, respiratory, gastrointestinal, genitourinary, musculoskeletal, skin, breast, neurological, psychiatric, endocrine, hematology/ lymphatic, and allergic/immune. The detailed level extends the HPI and ROS and adds a pertinent past/family/social history (PFSH). The PFSH consists of three components: past history with illnesses, operations, injuries, and treatments; family history of relevant diseases; and an age-appropriate review of past and current social activities. If a PFSH is on the chart from an earlier encounter, it does not need to be restated, but it must be documented that the PFSH was reviewed with the patient and updated. The comprehensive history involves an extended HPI, complete ROS, and complete PFSH.

The physical examination follows a similar pattern with the same names for the four levels. The problem-focused examination is limited to the affected body area or organ system. The expanded problem-focused examination adds examination of other symptomatic or related systems. The detailed examination is similar but more detailed, and the comprehensive examination is a complete single-system or multisystem examination.

The levels of decision making refer to the complexity of establishing the diagnosis or treatment plan and are influenced by the number of possible diagnoses or management options, the size and complexity of the medical record, tests or other information that must be reviewed and analyzed during the visit, the risk of significant complications, morbidity or mortality, and the diagnostic procedures and management options.

There are four categories of decision making: straightforward, low complexity, moderate complexity, and high complexity. Straightforward decision making, the first level, involves a minimal number of diagnoses

Table 10.2

DOCUMENTATION FOR REIMBURSEMENT

Component	Level 1	Level 2	Level 3	Level 4	Level 5
History	Minimal	Problem-focused; 1–3 elements in History of Present Illness (HPI); no Review of Systems (ROS); no Patient/ Family/ Social History (PFSH)	Expanded problem-focused; 1–3 HPI elements; ROS for 1 related system; no PFSH	Detailed; 4+ HPI elements; 3+ chronic conditions; ROS for 2–9 systems; 1+ items of PFSH	Comprehensive; 4+ HPI elements; 3+ chronic conditions; ROS for 10+ systems; 1+ items from 2+ of 3 PFSH areas
Exam	Minimal	Problem-focused; 1–5 elements of body or organ system exam	Expanded problem-focused; 6–12 exam elements of body or systems	Detailed; 12–18 exam elements of body or systems	Comprehensive; 18+ exam elements in at least 9 systems of body areas
Decision-making examples	Minimal	Straightforward	Low complexity (i.e., routine meds; OT/PT; IVs)	Prescribed meds; MRI; closed reduction of fracture	Meds; monitor meds; resuscitate; refer for major surgery
Risk	Minimal	Minimal	Low	Moderate	High
Time	5 min.	10 min.	15 min.	25 min.	40 min.

or options, minimally complex data, and a minimal risk of complications. Low complexity increases those components to a limited level from the minimal level. The moderately complex level involves multiple diagnoses or options, moderate complexity of data, and a moderate risk of complications. The high complexity level is an encounter that deals with an extensive number of diagnoses or options, extensive complexity of data, and a high risk of complications.

Four additional components can be used to alter the coding, which include counseling, coordination of care, complexity of the presenting problem, and amount of time spent with the patient. To use those elements, careful documentation is necessary. The time category can include face-to-face time, plus review of the patient chart, writing of notes, and communicating with other professionals and patient family members. Time is the key billing factor to use if counseling and coordination of care exceeds 50% of the total visit time.

APNs can bill for services rendered in nursing homes and skilled nursing facilities. They can also bill for hospital services as long as they are not employees of the hospital. There are three levels of encounters in those settings: detailed, detailed-comprehensive, and comprehensive, each with corresponding required components. Another way to bill is using three categories of subsequent nursing facility care (one-problem history, expanded focus, and detailed). Physicians are allowed to bill Medicare for 12 nursing home client visits per year; NP/physician teams are allowed 18 visits per year. APNs also can bill for their services in emergency rooms, using special codes that are appropriate to that setting.

Some specific pointers regarding documentation are important. When a diagnosis is uncertain, coding the presenting symptom is advisable, such as "pain" or "fever." Listing "rule out" differential diagnoses on the encounter form is not acceptable, nor are the terms "possible" or "suspected." "Abnormal" is not an acceptable term without further description; however "normal" and "negative" are allowed. A checklist with positive items further explained is also acceptable. All laboratory test and radiographic requests must be justified to Medicare in terms of the medical necessity of their charges.

An example of a satisfactory way to document with billing based on time would be: "total time, 25 minutes; counseling, 15 minutes; discussed results of tests, provided 3 options for treatment; follow-up in 3 months." To document care coordination, chart notes might say: "Spent 25 minutes reviewing medications with family and explaining laboratory tests; appointments coordinated for return visit in 3 months;

public health nurse contacted regarding need for medication supervision." An APN can list multiple codes for a single visit and can bill for both an E&M visit and a procedure (e.g., examination with suture removal). In complex patients, APNs can bill for two visits in one day (a general examination and a special teaching/counseling session, for example) if a special modifier is used in addition to the two sets of coding and documentation; patients might have to pay two co-payments in that circumstance.

Organizations must submit bills quickly because there is typically a 3-month turnaround time from the payers, which affects the revenue flow. It is important to remember that the amounts billed out may be very different from the amounts collected from payers. For example, in many states Medicaid pays less than 50% of typical billed amounts.

Health care organizations employ coding specialists and hire consultants to conduct audits and teach staff about these important issues. Consultants often find that organizations are undercoding for their services. Coding too high (called upcoding) can trigger Medicare fraud investigations. Medicare carriers expect to see a bell-shaped curve with most visits at the CPT code 99213 level (problem-focused history, expanded problem-focused examination, low-complexity decision making). However, this is problematic for practices that provide a great deal of care to patients with complex or chronic illnesses.

Most organizations design a "superbill" for processing claims that incorporates all of the coding information in one place, including procedures, facility charges, vaccines, E&M codes, ICD-9 codes, and any other relevant information. The document trail must be available for internal and external audit purposes. APNs must communicate regularly with billing, coding, and audit staff and participate in regular revision of the "superbill." The increasing use of computer-based charting is leading to more standardization of these processes and forms.

Inadequate documentation and coding result in loss of revenue to organizations and therefore to providers, inability to track outcomes of care, and possible penalties if audits turn up discrepancies. Inadequate documentation also leaves APNs vulnerable in legal investigations. Thorough, accurate documentation provides an auditable evidence trail for reimbursement.

Documentation also is used to audit care quality. Some MCOs and PPOs reward practices and providers for complying with established practice protocols and standards as part of their quest to implement best-practice, evidence-based care. APNs must be cognizant of coding requirements and provide documentation that reflects the excellence of their care.

CONCLUSION

U.S. health care has undergone tremendous change during recent decades. For example, DRGs were put in place to control costs as part of a prospective payment system. That decreased hospital stays, causing an explosion in the need for skilled nursing facilities (SNFs), home health care programs, and increased patient visits to outpatient clinics. With health care costs burgeoning, APNs are cost-effective providers of quality patient care. To prove the affordability and quality of their care, however, APNs must be visible to payers and consumers. Visibility is enhanced when APNs obtain their own provider numbers, lobby for direct reimbursement from insurance companies, document appropriately, and accurately speak the language of coding and billing. Furthermore, APNs become visible as they develop strong relationships with administrators and billing staff and track their billing and collections outcomes. APNs must share their reimbursement expertise with each other in order to raise the performance of all advanced practice nurses. APNs who are not well informed about their practice revenue generation are at a great disadvantage in determining their fiscal impact on systems.

APNs typically individually negotiate their own employment contracts, a process greatly strengthened by having productivity and financial data. Additionally, tracking APN cost-effectiveness, productivity, and fiscal outcomes is essential to the entire nursing profession as it makes nurses' work visible in the bottom line of organizations. The ANA and other nursing professional organizations have long lobbied for direct reimbursement for health care and continue to pursue the goal of making nursing's contribution visible in overall cost analyses. Measuring care outcomes is one of nursing's highest priorities.

APNs were traditionally educated to provide care closely aligned to specific settings. Now they face the additional challenge of understanding multiple systems that change rapidly and reimbursement policies that constantly evolve. APNs must not only practice competently, they must also understand health care economics. Therefore, basic and continuing education of APNs is essential, and nurse educators and administrators must understand and teach about APN reimbursement. Educational content on leadership, financial management, politics, and health policy is essential to keep APNs' place at the table where decisions are made, policies are developed, and systems are designed.

Lobbying at various legislative levels is also crucial for APN reimbursement. There is a pressing need for consistent payment policies across states that are reflected in federal laws and regulations. Legislative and regulatory goals include

- legislation requiring APN payments that are on par with physicians (the "equal pay for equal work" principle)
- laws that ensure public access to APN care (i.e., changes to the Employee Retirement Income Security Act of 1974 [ERISA] that exempts self-insured organizations from state regulation and allows them to be more restrictive than regulated organizations)
- laws requiring payers to credential and list APNs as licensed independent providers (LIPs), thus placing APNs on MCO provider panels as specialty and primary care providers (PCPs). Research must continue to examine the characteristics, quality, and cost–benefit ratio of APN care. APN care that is evidence-based should be carefully studied to document its specific components and outcomes, including fiscal outcomes
- regulatory compliance could be studied as could the effectiveness of various methods of educating APNs about these vital issues

REFERENCES

American Medical Association (AMA). (2004). *The official industry CPT® code book.* Chicago: Author.

Baicker, K., & Chandra, A. (2008). Myths and misconceptions about U.S. health insurance. *Health Affairs, 27,* w145–155.

Canadian Institute for Health Information (CIHI). (2008). *National health expenditure trends 1975–2008.* Ottawa, Canada: Author.

Center for Medicare and Medicaid Services. (2009). *HHS modifies HIPAA code sets (ICD-10) and electronic transactions standards.* Retrieved January 16, 2009, from www.cms.hhs.gov/apps/media/press/factsheet

Corwin, R., Francis, A., McInerny, T., Ponzi, J., Reuben, M., et al. (2006). AAP principles concerning retail-based clinics. *Pediatrics, 120,* 1123–1125.

Duderstadt, K. (2008). Medical home: Nurse practitioners' role in health care delivery to vulnerable populations. *Journal of Pediatric Healthcare, 22,* 390–393.

Farrell, D., Jensen, E., & Kocher, B. (2008). *Why Americans pay more for health care. McKinsey Quarterly (December)*, 1–11. Retrieved January 17, 2008, from www.mckinseyquarterly.com/PDFDownload.aspx?L2=12&L3=63&ar=2275

Hartman, M., Martin, A., McDonnell, P., Catlin, A., and the National Health Expenditure Accounts Team. (2009). National health spending in 2007: Slower drug spending contributes to lowest rate of overall growth since 1998. *Health Affairs, 28*, 246–261.

Institute for Nursing Centers. (2008). National Data Warehouse third annual aggregate survey report: 2006–2007. Retrieved January 17, 2008, from www.nursingcenters .org/PDFs/INC%20Highlight%20Report%2010_6_08.pdf

Johnson, J., Harper, D., Hanson, C., & Dawson, E. (2007). Forging a quality agenda. *American Journal for Nurse Practitioners, 11*, 10–19.

Kaiser Family Foundation. (2008). *Employee health benefits: 2008 annual survey*. Retrieved January 13, 2009, from http://ehbs.kff.org/

Keegan, S., Sisko, A., Truffer, C., Smith, S., Cowan, C., Poisal, J., & Clemens, M. (2008). Health spending projections through 2017: The baby-boom generation is coming to Medicare. *Health Affairs, 27*, w-145–155.

Miller, K. (2009). Consumer-driven health care: Nurse practitioners making history. *Journal for Nurse Practitioners, 5*, 31–34.

Palfrey, J., Sofis, L., Davidson, E., Liu, J., Freeman, L., & Ganz, M. (2004) The Pediatric Alliance for Coordinated Care: Evaluation of a medical home model. *Pediatrics, 113* (suppl), 1507–1516.

Reinhardt, U., Hussey, P., & Anderson, G. (2004). U.S. health care spending in an international context. *Health Affairs, 23*, 10–25.

Schoen, C., Osborn, R., Doty, M., Bishop, M., Peugh, J., & Murukutla, M. (2007). Toward higher-performance health systems: Adults' health care experiences in seven countries, 2007. *Health Affairs, 26*(6), w717–w734.

Sherman, A., Greensteen, R., & Parrott, S. (2008). *For poverty rate and non-elderly median income, worst performance on record for any six years of economic growth*. Center on Budget and Policy Priorities. Retrieved January 17, 2009, from www.cbpp .org/8-26-08pov.htm

Sullivan-Marx, E., & Maislin, G. (2000). Comparison of nurse practitioner and family physician relative work values. *Journal of Nursing Scholarship, 32*, 71–76.

Thygeson, M., Van Vorst, K., Maciosek, M., & Solberg, L. (2008). Use and costs of care in retain clinics versus traditional care sites. *Health Affairs, 27*, 1280–1292.

U.S. Census Bureau. (2008). *Income, poverty, and health insurance coverage in the United States: 2007*. Retrieved January 13, 2008, from www.census.gov/prod/ 2008pubs/p60-235.pdf

Ethical Issues in Advanced Practice Nursing

KAREN S. FELDT

Advanced practice nurses (APNs) are active in a wide variety of clinical, educational, and executive roles with varying degrees of involvement in and influence on clinical practice. As part of their professional role, APNs must be able to recognize ethical conflicts and serve as a mediator or resource for patients, families, or other nurses who are struggling with ethical dilemmas. The new doctor of nursing practice (DNP) requirement for APNs will expand the knowledge required and role of APNs in a variety of settings. Understanding the application of ethical constructs and theories is essential for APNs and DNPs as they address complex health issues and manage ethical conflicts in research and business arenas (Peirce & Smith, 2008).

Advanced practice nurses are confronted with a variety of everyday ethical conflicts, including

1. Patient or family conflicts when the prognosis or goals of care are unclear (Laabs, 2005; Wiegand, 2003)
2. Family conflicts when surrogates are not honoring the patient's advance directives or when there is uncertainty over the aggressiveness of care in pediatric or terminally ill incompetent patients (Laabs, 2005; Volker, Kahn, & Penticuff, 2004; Peirce & Smith, 2008)

3. Clients whose care is compromised because of inadequate funding by insurers, or inadequate personal or public resources (Baum, Gollust, Goold, & Jacobson, 2007; Browne & Tarlier, 2008; Laabs, 2005; Ulrich, Soeken & Miller, 2003)
4. Concerns about privacy and confidentiality of information in the electronic medical record era (Demiris, Oliver, & Courtney, 2006; Peirce & Smith, 2008)
5. Conflicts between insurer/payer system guidelines and the perceived most appropriate care (Laabs, 2005; Ulrich, Soeken, & Miller, 2003; Ulrich & Soeken, 2005)
6. Uncertainty over demands for coding or billing practices that may be questionable or fraudulent (Peirce & Smith, 2008; Laabs, 2005; Hannigan, 2006)
7. Undue influence or conflict of interest in prescribing because of pharmaceutical promotions or use of pharmaceutical samples (Crigger, 2005; Erlen, 2008)
8. Struggles with pain management and opiate prescribing practices for patients in chronic pain (Fontana, 2008)

An emerging area of research exploring nursing ethics for APNs is beginning to address areas such as respect for human dignity (Kalb & O'Connor-Von, 2007) and the ethical problems encountered by APNs related to client care and organizational–industrial issues (Laabs, 2005; Laabs, 2007; Hannigan, 2006; Ulrich, Soeken, & Miller, 2003; Ulrich & Soeken, 2005). This chapter will review basic ethics definitions, discuss keys to application of ethical guidelines for APN challenges, and briefly critique the current ethical decisional frameworks.

ETHICAL CONCEPTS AND DEFINITIONS

The term *ethics* is used broadly to understand and examine the moral life, and the norms, social customs, and rules that define society's conceptions of "right" and "wrong." Ethical theories organize concepts or principles into a framework that can be used to approach ethical conflicts. Consequentialist theories identify an action as right or wrong based on the outcome or consequences of that action (Beauchamp & Childress, 2002). The ends (or consequences, if they are good consequences) justify the means (or the action taken). The action considered morally right is the action that produces the best overall result. Utilitarianism, perhaps the most well known of the consequentialist theories, identifies the principle of utility as the fundamental and only principle of ethics (Beauchamp & Childress, 2002). Nurses who follow this theory would take the action that produces the greatest good for the greatest number. For example, APNs who embrace this theory might work to shape public funding to address preventive measures or access to basic health care issues for larger populations rather than high-cost interventions for individuals (Baum, Gollust, Goold, & Jacobson, 2007; Browne & Tarlier, 2008).

Deontological theories differ widely from consequentialist theories. These theories, based on the works of Immanuel Kant, identify actions as morally right or wrong in relation to underlying moral principles (Frankena, 1988). Kant requires that all actions meet this categorical imperative: one ought never to act except in such a way that one can also will that action to become a universal law (Beauchamp & Childress, 2002; Frankena, 1988). In other words, actions must be reasoned through to determine if we would want all others to take that same action in all cases of that kind. Kantian ethics require the test of universalizability in all ethical decisions. For example, an APN would perceive that lying to a patient would be wrong in every case (universalizable veracity) even though the family of one patient requests that the APN hide the truth because of their concern over the patient's emotional status.

In health care, application of bioethical theories arose out of the field of acute care medicine when advances in medical technology increased enough to preserve life but conflicted with the quality of life preserved (Moody, 1992; Dierckx de Casterle, Roelens, & Gastmans, 1998). These bioethical theories focused on principles as a way to examine ethical conflicts. The deontological approach to ethical problem solving focused on the specific bioethical principles of autonomy, beneficence, nonmaleficence, justice, and rules of veracity, confidentiality, and fidelity (Table 11.1). This principle and rule-oriented framework encouraged specific decisional strategies to apply the theory to clinical practice. Advanced practice nurses soon discover competing ethical principles are the basis for ethical dilemmas in clinical situations. For example, a client may refuse to follow up by getting a necessary diagnostic test (autonomy) even though obtaining an accurate diagnosis and appropriate treatment for a recurring problem may benefit the client's health (beneficence) (Laabs, 2005).

Table 11.1

PRINCIPLES OF BIOMEDICAL ETHICS

Principle	Definition	Corresponding Virtue
Respect for autonomy	Self-determination	General respectfulness
Nonmaleficence	Avoiding harm	Nonmalevolence
Beneficence	Doing good	Benevolence
Justice	Treating people fairly	Fairness
Rules		
Veracity	Telling the truth	Truthfulness
Fidelity	Keeping promises	Faithfulness
Confidentiality	Respecting privileged information	Respect for privacy

Source: Beauchamp & Childress (2002). Reprinted with permission from author.

Other ethical theories are also emerging as relevant and helpful guides to health care practitioners. Virtue ethics offers a framework that provides a warmer interpersonal view of ethical decisions when compared with the calculated reasoning that Kantian principles require. Virtue ethics examines the character traits that affect a person's judgment and actions and dispose them to act in accordance with professional guidelines (Beauchamp & Childress, 2002; Gillon, 2003). The American Nurses Association (ANA) Code for Nurses (ANA, 2001) is a good example of incorporating virtue ethics into the ethical and legal obligations of the nursing profession (Exhibit 11.1). Respectfulness and integrity are identified in this code and have been examined as an important part of ethics education for advanced practice nurses (Kalb & O'Connor-Von, 2007; Peirce & Smith, 2008).

Beauchamp and Childress (2002) refer to virtues of compassion, discernment, trustworthiness, faithfulness, and integrity as character traits that would produce correct actions in health professionals. Cameron (2003) based a model of ethical decision making on virtue ethics, which focused on the behaviors and attributes of a morally good person. These virtues are supported in her research in which she interviewed nurses about the ethical and spiritual values that guided their practice. Nurses included the following ethical values: beneficence, honesty, justice, integrity (which nurses described as excellent, sound, incorruptible character),

Exhibit 11.1

AMERICAN NURSES ASSOCIATION CODE FOR NURSES

1. The nurse provides services with respect for human dignity and the uniqueness of the client unrestricted by considerations of social or economic status, personal attributes, or the nature of health problems.
2. The nurse safeguards the client's right to privacy by judiciously protecting information of a confidential nature.
3. The nurse acts to safeguard the client and the public when health care and safety are affected by the incompetent, unethical, or illegal practice of any person.
4. The nurse assumes responsibility and accountability for individual nursing judgments and actions.
5. The nurse maintains competence in nursing.
6. The nurse exercises informed judgment and uses individual competence and qualifications as criteria in seeking consultation, accepting responsibilities, and delegating nursing activities to others.
7. The nurse participates in activities that contribute to the ongoing development of the profession's body of knowledge.
8. The nurse participates in the profession's efforts to implement and improve standards of nursing.
9. The nurse participates in the profession's effort to establish and maintain conditions of employment conducive to high-quality nursing care.
10. The nurse participates in the profession's effort to protect the public from misinformation and misrepresentation and to maintain the integrity of nursing.
11. The nurse collaborates with members of the health care professions and other citizens in promoting community and national efforts to meet the health care needs of the public.

Source: ANA (2001), Reprinted with permission.

nonviolence (resolving issues peacefully), respect for the environment, and respect for human rights. They identified seven spiritual values: compassion, happiness, meaning (seeing one's life as part of a bigger picture), meditation, peace, sacredness, and spirituality (Cameron, 2003). Laabs (2007) describes a theory of maintaining moral integrity in the face of moral conflict as the key process that nurse practitioners use to manage the ethical issues encountered in primary care practices.

ETHICAL ISSUES VERSUS LEGAL ISSUES

Before discussing a decisional framework for ethical issues, it is important to identify the difference between ethical and legal issues. Ethics can guide the development and enforcement of laws. However, ethics and legal issues can conflict. For example, there are some actions that are perfectly legal, but they are considered immoral or unethical by some people (for example, capital punishment). Other actions are illegal in most states but are viewed as moral by some people (for example, physician-assisted suicide or voluntary euthanasia for terminally ill patients). Ethical concepts or principles are not black and white. Ethics reflect social customs and rules and are influenced by them. Ethical principles may be applied differently as scientific advances and social mores alter the way society views these norms.

Advance practice nurses should be aware of the legal rules that govern professional practice so that they can act in an ethical manner (Peirce & Smith, 2008). For example, laws concerning patient referrals (the Stark Act) and whistle blowing (False Claims Act of 1863) provide a legal basis or framework for professional behavior while clearly defining behavior that is fraudulent and illegal. APNs should understand and follow the laws on scope of professional practice within their state; legal guidelines regarding professional courtesy, kickbacks, and noncompetition agreements; and the Health Insurance Portability and Accountability Act (HIPAA) (Peirce & Smith, 2008). Although these laws guide professional ethical behavior, APNs must recognize that there are situations in which an action is legally correct but still creates a moral conflict. If ethical issues are confused with legal issues, APNs may only seek to understand the legal liability of a situation without fully exploring its ethical implications (see Cases 1 and 2). As this case indicates, the community had addressed the legal aspects of the case; however, the advanced practice nurse will need to resolve her approach to the ethical conflict between the confidentiality of the resident and her obligation for beneficence or the protection of other vulnerable adults.

In Case 2, the practice had addressed the legal aspects of billing; however, the advanced practice nurse will need to resolve her approach to the ethical conflict between her obligation for beneficence for her elderly clients and the financial accounting that is required to maintain the business aspects of the practice.

Nurses who are strongly influenced and focused on the legal aspects of an ethical conflict may come to a premature solution or conclusion about which actions to take. This approach may leave the underlying ethical conflict unresolved and create internal misgivings about how to approach ethical situations.

KEYS TO APPLYING ETHICAL GUIDELINES

In order to function in today's practice world, advanced practice nurses must have the foundation to understand, identify, and work through issues that affect all the aspects of practice. APNs should embrace both the reasoned, decision-making approaches, virtues, and relational guidelines that help them sort through the multitude of complex ethical issues that confront them in practice (Leino-Kilpi, 2004). Several nurse ethicists have developed decisional tools to assist nurses in applying bioethical principles. Two examples of these decision-making frameworks are Crisham's Moral Framework, (Crisham, 1981) and Calabro and Tukoski's (2003) Participative Ethical Decision Making approach. In Crisham's Model, nurses are encouraged to identify the dilemma, the stakeholders, the underlying values, the conflict, and the decision maker, and to work through a process using bioethical principles to reach a consensus.

This approach has been modified and updated by Calabro and Tukoski (2003) to assist nurse practitioners in resolving ethical conflicts. They identify several steps to participative ethical decision making. These include: (1) identifying the ethical dilemma; (2) delineating the variables in the dilemma (persons involved, time frame for decision); (3) assessing the NP's perspective; (4) assessing the patient's perspective; (5) sharing the assessment and exchanging goals in a participative way; (6) identifying a mutually acceptable ethical framework; and (7) identifying a potential solution.

Unfortunately, both of these decisional models are fraught with problems related to their underlying assumptions. First, both of these models assume that there can be a shared style of analysis and problem solving to an ethical issue between health care professionals and patients (Botes, 2000). The real world of clinical care can be marked by cultural or educational differences and language barriers that can create huge gaps in comprehension and can preclude any reasoned discussion. Calabro and Tukoski's model actually requires the professional and the patient

Exhibit 11.2

PROPOSAL FOR A CODE OF ETHICS FOR APNS

1. The APN should provide competent advanced practice nursing care with compassion, confidentiality, and respect for the individual, regardless of social, economic, or health status.

2. The APN has a primary commitment and responsibility to the patient, whether that patient is an individual, family, group, or community.

3. The APN shall support access to care for all patients and should strive to effect public policies that will result in equal access.

4. The APN shall support the patient's efforts toward an optimal level of health through education, self-care promotion, consultation, and collaboration with other health care team members.

5. The APN shall maintain and be accountable for accurate medical records for each patient. The NP shall not engage in fraud or deception and shall report any other health care provider that engages in such activities.

6. The ANP shall advocate for and strive to protect the rights, health, safety, and privacy of all patients. The ANP should collaborate with other professionals and the public on local, national, and international levels to promote this effort.

7. The ANP shall continue to advance personal and professional development through practice, education of the public, and lifelong continuous study, research, and activity in professional organizations.

8. The ANP shall in the provision of patient care responsibly choose whom to serve, with whom to associate, and the environment in which to provide that care [which reflects the scope of practice for the ANP].

Source: Peterson & Potter (2004).

---

to identify a mutually acceptable ethical framework. This step assumes that somehow the patient and the professional will eventually come to an agreed ethical philosophical approach. Given that many ethical dilemmas arise because the health professional and the patient have different beliefs, this assumption is particularly onerous.

A second common problem with decisional models based on bioethical principles is that they tend to prioritize individual autonomy (a deeply embedded Western cultural principle). Gillon (2003) argues that autonomy is a necessary component of all of the basic biomedical principles and must be the guiding principle for all ethical decisions. However, this principle takes on far less importance in some Asian cultures, where the good to the family or community may be more valued than individual autonomy (Gillon, 2003). Principle-oriented frameworks ignore the role of individual character in ethical deliberations and leave out the texture of the lived experience of each of the individuals. The principle-oriented framework in its assumption of a rational, reasoned approach neglects the importance of the style of communication, personal attributes of the nurse, the nonverbal connections, and the interpretation of the meaning of the problem (Cameron, 2003; Dierckx de Casterle, Roelens, & Gastmans, 1998; Gadow, 1989; Moody, 1992; Volker, 2003).

Third, these decisional models assume that there is some certainty regarding the treatment possibilities or outcomes in health care. Nurse practitioners and clinical nurse specialists will continuously be faced with the uncertainties of treatments and outcomes. For example: will this cancer treatment put the patient into remission, or will it weaken their immune system so that they cannot recover? Many patients and families seek information as they sort through tough treatment decisions, only to find that the patient responds physiologically completely differently than was expected. Sometimes sharing uncertainties of treatment outcomes assists the patient or family member in deciding to opt out of treatment instead of trying to please the specialist who is offering hope. Ruddick (1999) states that, although hope is a powerful force in bioethics, it can be deceptive in making ethical decisions and can change patient–health-provider decision making.

Fourth, principled decision-making frameworks assume that ethical decision making is a reasoned process made within a structured group by participants who are well informed about ethical principles. It is just as likely that ethical dilemmas are resolved in a moment of uncertainty with less than adequate information, leaving advanced practice nurses and patients to sort through the process at a later date or not at all. In today's health care systems, acute changes in status happen quickly; sometimes they are completely unanticipated. Clinical nurse specialists and nurse practitioners often deal with families who must struggle with making a decision for a sick family member who lacks decisional capacity for the first time in that family member's life. These families need a supportive presence and reminders of the personhood of the patient. Families often are afraid of making a "wrong" decision for a loved one and thus decide to do many things that the person may not have done (Laabs, 2005). These overwhelming crises make reasoning through an ethical process unlikely or difficult at best.

Finally, the decisional frameworks assume that health care organizations or working conditions allow time and supportive resources for a participatory, reasoned model of decision making (Botes, 2000; Moody, 1992; Peirce & Smith, 2008). In some settings, advanced practice nurses may be left out of the decision-making loop at a critical time. Not all APNs are able to quickly identify the process required for ethical decisions. In nonhospital care settings, ethics committees and ethics experts are less common. Practitioners with ethical concerns are more likely to get referred to a risk manager (who will identify legal concerns, not ethical processes) for assistance with ethical conflicts.

REST'S FOUR-COMPONENT MODEL

Rest identified four integrated abilities that determine moral behavior in health professionals. These conditions or components offer guidelines that allow for more than application of bioethical principles and include the virtue ethics and interpersonal qualities that can assist in resolving ethical conflicts.

The first condition is ethical sensitivity, or the ability to see things from the perspective of others. Rather than focusing on one's own views, a person with greater ethical sensitivity can interpret a situation from other points of view and show sensitivity to the feelings and reactions of others. This sensitivity includes a knowledge of legal, professional, and institutional codes and norms. Peirce & Smith (2008) state that DNP advanced practice nurses must demonstrate ethical sensitivity and knowledge of research ethics, clinical ethics, business ethics, and laws that influence practice. On a clinical level, an advanced practice nurse who is ethically sensitive seeks information and listens carefully. Cameron (2004) identifies ethical listening as paying full attention in order to hear an ethical problem in what someone says. This active ethical listening involves compassion, establishing rapport, using open-ended statements, and encouraging the person to examine the conflict on a deeper level. Ethical listening requires the professional to avoid lecturing, giving advice, or correcting comments so that the person feels free to talk openly and move closer to a resolution. Advanced practice nurses who use ethical listening skills become skilled at uncovering underlying ethical conflicts that require resolution.

The second component of the Four-Component Model is moral judgment. Moral judgment requires knowledge of concepts, codes of conduct, and ethical principles, and helps to identify the guidelines that support a decision for a right action. Advanced practice nurses should be familiar not only with the ANA Code for Nurses (ANA, 2001) and ethical theories and principles, but should also be aware of the research that helps to guide clinical decisions. Peterson and Potter (2004) reviewed and compared the nurse's code of ethics with the code of ethics for physicians formulated by the American Medical Association (AMA). They propose a code of ethics for nurse practitioners that addresses the unique aspects of this expanded role of nurses (see Exhibit 11.2). Part of this expanded role is for APNs to assist patients in decision making, which includes ensuring that they are fully informed and not coerced. Advanced practice nurses thus need to develop teaching skills that allow them to present the potential risks and benefits of treatments in an unbiased manner.

The third component of Rest's model is moral motivation, that is, the difference between knowing the right thing to do and making it a priority. Moral motivation has to do with the importance given to competing choices. Deficiencies in moral motivation occur when personal values compete with concerns for doing what is right. A nurse practitioner who decides to spend less time with each patient so that she can have the highest number of patients billed per month may be overlooking important clinical needs at the patient's expense (Ulrich, Soeken, & Miller, 2003). A nursing administrator who decides to staff short without agency staffing so that her department will exceed budget goals (giving her an administrative bonus) has a problem with moral motivation.

The fourth component of Rest's model is moral character. This component requires APNs to persist and have courage in implementing their skills. Bebeau writes, "A practitioner may be ethically sensitive, may make good ethical judgments, and place a high priority on professional values; but if the practitioner wilts under pressure, is easily distracted or discouraged, or is weak willed, then moral failure occurs (Bebeau, 2002, p. 287). Nurses in advanced practice roles should identify how they would carry out a specific moral action in the clinical setting. Clinical situations will expose them to a variety of problems that may require a necessary ethical action. For example, a clinical nurse specialist identifies a clinically incompetent or negligent performance of a staff nurse but decides not to report it because she is not the nurse's direct supervisor. She is missing the final important ingredient in ethically sound advanced practice.

SUMMARY: ETHICAL DECISION MAKING

Three ethical decision-making frameworks have been discussed as guides for advanced practice nurses. Although nurses may be most familiar with the bioethical principles, the principle-oriented frameworks are not as well equipped to address the many everyday ethical issues in health care that are not about life-and-death decisions. These day-to-day decisions may be best served by Rest's Four-Component Model that identified the need to ensure heightened ethical sensitivity and ethical implementation.

Advanced practice nurses are entering an ever more complex world of practice. They should be aware of the role of ethical behavior and choices not only in their clinical world but also in the research and business aspects of their practices (Peirce & Smith, 2008). They should work to improve their awareness of ethical clinical issues by active ethical listening. They should be educated about ethical theories and principles and should be aware of codes of conduct that will affect their moral judgment. They should examine their own professional conduct and the choices that compete with the ethical decisions they must make.

APNs must be aware of the ethical implications of information technology on patient privacy and confidentiality. The consideration of ethics is essential to the financial accounting and billing practices of clinical practices. Advanced practice nurses who work in research settings should conduct themselves ethically in the management of research data, privacy, and confidentiality, and be aware of the potential for conflict of interest in industry-supported research. Most important, APNs should have the tools to work through ethical dilemmas in all areas so that they can make appropriate ethical decisions.

Legal Issues Versus Ethical Issues

Case 1

Frank Jones lives independently in retirement housing. His wife has recently been discharged from the dementia unit of the assisted living section of the same community to a local nursing home that provides skilled care. Staff notes that Mr. Jones has continued to visit the dementia unit after his wife's discharge and has made suggestive sexual comments to other residents in the dementia area. He was found nude in a female resident's room making advances that were clearly distressing and unwanted by the female resident. Police were called, the incident was reported to adult protection, and Mr. Jones was discharged from the community. The victim's family decided not to press charges against the man if this were done. A week after discharge, the director of the assisted living community received a call from another retirement community indicating they were admitting Mr. Jones and had questions about his background, including his reason for moving. Mr. Jones and his daughter had not signed a release of records form.

The ethical obligation to respect resident confidentiality conflicted with the ethical obligation to warn a new community about potential risks to other vulnerable adults. The assisted living facility's lawyer said that since no charges were pressed against the man, it was "as if the incident didn't occur" and the community had no legal obligation to disclose. The APN who visited the residents on the dementia unit was uncomfortable with the lack of disclosure. Discuss her ethical obligations versus her legal obligations.

Case 2

J.R. is an adult nurse practitioner in a rural clinical practice attached to a small hospital that serves a lot of elderly clients. She frequently finds that her clients are in need of a procedure, for example, cerumen removal from ear canals, as she does her basic exam for the clinic visit. However, the business manager for the clinic requires that the patients be rescheduled for a separate day for procedures so that they can be billed separately for their primary concern (hypertension management) and the procedural issue (cerumen removal). That way the clinic is able to capture greater income for two visits. The rationale is, "We need to generate enough visits to justify keeping this clinic going." Although J.R. understands that it is perfectly legal to bill the visits in this manner, she is conflicted about the undue pressure to create more bills and the costs and time that are required for her elderly clients to return to the clinic.

REFERENCES

American Nurses Association. (2001). *Code of ethics for nurses with interpretive statements.* Washington DC: American Nurses Association.

Baum, N. M., Gollust, S. E., Goold, S. D., & Jacobson, P. D. (2007). Looking ahead: Addressing ethical challenges in public health practice. *Global Health Law, Ethics and Policy* 35(4), 657–667, 513.

Beauchamp, T., & Childress, J. (2002). *Principles of biomedical ethics* (5th ed.). New York: Oxford University Press.

Bebeau, M. J. (2002). The Defining Issues Test and the Four Component Model: Contributions to professional education. *Journal of Moral Education, 31*(3), 271–295.

Botes, A. (2000). An integrated approach to ethical decision-making in the health team. *Journal of Advanced Nursing* 32(5), 1076–1082.

Browne, A. J., & Tarlier, D. S. (2008). Examining the potential of nurse practitioners from a critical social justice perspective. *Nursing Inquiry, 15*(2), 83–93.

Calabro, M. D., & Tukoski, B. (2003). Participative ethical decision making. *Advance for Nurse Practitioners, 11*(6), 83–89.

Cameron, M. E. (2003). Our best ethical and spiritual values. *Journal of Professional Nursing, 19*(3), 117–118.

Cameron, M. E. (2004). Ethical listening as therapy. *Journal of Professional Nursing, 20*(3), 141–142.

Crigger, N. J. (2005). Pharmaceutical promotions and conflict of interest in nurse practitioner's decision making: The undiscovered country. *Journal of the American Academy of Nurse Practitioners, 17*(6), 207–211.

Crisham, P. (1981). Measuring moral judgment in nursing dilemmas. *Nursing Research, 30*(2), 104–110.

Demiris, G., Oliver, D. P., & Courtney, K. L. (2006). Ethical considerations for the utilization of telehealth technologies in home and hospice care by the nursing profession. *Nursing Administration Quarterly, 30,*(1) 56–66.

Dierckx de Casterle, B., Roelens, A., & Gastmans, C. (1998). An adjusted version of Kohlberg's moral theory: Discussion of its validity for research in nursing ethics. *Journal of Advanced Nursing* 27, 829–835.

Erlen, J. A. (2008). Conflict of interest. *Orthopaedic Nursing, 27*(2), 135–138.

Fontana, J. S. (2008). The social and political forces affecting prescribing practices for chronic pain. *Journal of Professional Nursing, 24*(1), 30–35.

Frankena, W. K. (1988). *Ethics* (2nd ed.). Englewood Cliffs, NJ: Prentice Hall.

Gadow, S. (1989) An ethical case for patient self-determination. *Seminars in Oncology Nursing, 5,* 99–101.

Gillon, R. (2003). Ethics needs principles: Four can encompass the rest, and respect for autonomy should be "first among equals." *Journal of Medical Ethics, 29,* 307–312.

Hannigan, N. (2006). Blowing the whistle on healthcare fraud: Should I? *Journal of the American Academy of Nurse Practitioners, 18,* 512–516.

Kalb, K. A., & O'Connor-Von, S. (2007). Ethics education in advanced practice nursing: Respect for human dignity. *Nursing Education Perspectives* 28(4), 196–202.

Laabs, C. A. (2005). Moral problems and distress among nurse practitioners in primary care. *Journal of the American Academy of Nurse Practitioners, 17*(2), 76–83.

Laabs, C. A. (2007). Primary care nurse practitioners' integrity when faced with moral conflict. *Nursing Ethics, 14*(6), 795–809.

Leino-Kilpi, H. (2004). We need more nursing ethics research (editorial). *Journal of Advanced Nursing, 45*(4), 345–346.

Moody, H. R. (1992). *Ethics in an aging society.* Baltimore: The Johns Hopkins University Press.

Peirce, A. G., & Smith, J. A. (2008). The ethics of curriculum for doctor of nursing practice programs. *Journal of Professional Nursing 24*(5), 270–274.

Peterson, M., & Potter, R. L. (2004). A proposal for a code of ethics for nurse practitioners. *Journal of the American Academy of Nurse Practitioners, 16*(3), 116–124.

Rest, J., & Narvaez, D. F. (Eds.). (1994). *Moral development in the professions: Psychology and applied ethics.* Hillsdale, NJ: Lawrence Erlbaum Associates.

Ruddick, W. (1999). Hope and deception. *Bioethics, 13*(3–4), 343–357.

Ulrich, C. M., Soeken, K. L., & Miller, N. (2003). Ethical conflict associated with managed care: Views of nurse practitioners. *Nursing Research, 52*(3), 168–175.

Ulrich, C. M., & Soeken, K. L (2005). A path analytical model of ethical conflict in practice and autonomy in a sample of nurse practitioners. *Nursing Ethics 12*(3), 305–315.

Volker, D. (2003). Is there a unique nursing ethic? *Nursing Science Quarterly, 16*(3), 207–211.

Volker, D. L. Kahn, D, & Penticuff, J. H. (2004). Patient control and end of life care, part I: The advanced practice nurse perspective. *Oncology Nursing Forum, 31*(5), 945–953.

Wiegand, J. (2003). Treatment dilemmas in neonatology. *Advance for Nurse Practitioners, 11*(5), 59–61.

12

Translating Research into Practice: Barriers and Solutions

KATHRYN BLAIR

Excellence in clinical practice requires not only a competent practitioner but one who is a lifelong learner with a desire to foster clinical expertise by becoming a consumer of research. Not all advanced practice nurses (APNs) will actively participate in research; however, all APNs should engage in translating research into practice.

With an average of 1,800 research papers and 55 randomized control trials published daily (Meats, Brassey, Heneghan, & Glasziou, 2007), translating research into practice is viewed as a time-consuming and daunting task. The end results are twofold: fewer than 14 % of published research actually reaches clinical practice (Tierney, Oppenheimer, Hudson, Benz, Finn, Hickner, Lanier, & Gaylin, 2007) and there is a significant delay, approximately 15 to 20 years from bench research to implementation into practice (Tierney, et al., 2007; Wilson & Fridinger, 2008).

The translation of research into practice also requires the integration of three processes: diffusion of research evidence to the clinician, critical analysis of such evidence, and applying such evidence to practice. The latter two steps are embedded in evidence-based practice and will be discussed within that context.

The dissemination of evidence to clinicians is the first step in the transfer of research into practice. Transitioning from research to practice, however, can suffer interruption at various points in the process. For example, sometimes information acquired in the laboratory (i.e., new methods for diagnosis and treatment) does not reach the practicing clinician. Another point of interruption can occur because of failure to incorporate evidence found in clinical trials into clinical practice or practice guidelines (Werch, Grenard, Burnett, Watkins, Ames, & Jobli, 2006).

MODELS FOR TRANSLATING RESEARCH INTO PRACTICE

Historically, there have been several models (diffusion, systematic reviews, industrial commodity, system engineering, and social innovation) that were developed to explain how research evidence reaches the clinician and to identify how this evidence translates into practice (Scott, 2007). The early *diffusion model* depicts information from journals and conferences as being transferred by "osmosis." The stronger the evidence, the more likely it was that research would filter down to the practitioner and find its way into practice. Unfortunately, this method did not assist the clinician in applying the evidence to the clinical arena.

Systematic reviews, meta-analyses, and clinical guidelines were developed to simplify the process. Experts would analyze and summarize the research and make recommendations, thus facilitating the application of the evidence into practice. Some practitioners resisted the application of guidelines because there was not always consensus among experts and some clinicians felt the guidelines were prescriptive and did not allow for patient variability.

The industrial commodity approach, like clinical practice guidelines, was an effort to distribute information and improve its use in clinical practice. Health care industry stakeholders (such as regulatory and insurance agencies) used case reviews, audits, and educational outreach programs to change clinical practice. Change was avoided because providers felt they were no longer in control of health care decisions.

Recently, *systems engineering*, the utilization of electronic information systems to improve access to information, has received a great deal of attention (Lang, Wyer, & Haynes, 2007). Unfortunately, as earlier systems did not interface well with clinical practices, their reliability came into question. Further, the individual adoption of this methodology was limited because of cost or resistance to change.

The most recent approach, social innovation, examines the motivators of behavior change within social systems, utilizing the characteristics of change and social learning to distribute new information and facilitate its application to practice. In essence, this model assesses the provider's readiness for change and tailors an educational program and materials with this variable in mind. Additionally, opinion leaders, peer networks, and key players in social networks (i.e., patients, insurers, administrators, etc.) are used to influence provider behavior. Interestingly, there is strong evidence that patient-mediated interventions or patient/consumer education is a powerful motivator for change. For example, when women were educated about the importance of mammograms, the incidence of mammograms performed, as ordered by their provider, increased (Weingarten, 2000).

In general, though, the failure of these models to change practice may be related to the "disconnect" between research and practice. Some research is not clinically relevant, and other research is preliminary or done with unsound methodology (Col, 2005). When the research is clinically relevant and methodologically sound, there can still be separation between research and practice. Several variables such as sample characteristics, the lack of comparisons, and the feasibility of the interventions contribute to the failure of adopting and applying research evidence to practice. From a clinician's viewpoint, "the right patients," or representative patients (i.e., ethnic and racial minorities, underserved, etc.), are often excluded from clinical trials, and most intervention trials are all-or-none (e.g., treatment versus placebo) rather than comparisons of less expensive alternatives. In many cases, the "feasibility" of a treatment is not addressed. For example, if a particular intervention is very costly or requires specialized equipment, the intervention will not gain widespread acceptance even when the evidence supports utilization (Claxton, Cohen, & Neumann, 2005; Glasgow, Magid, Beck, Ritzwoller, & Estabrooks, 2005).

To facilitate the transfer of information and lessen the perceived gap between researcher and clinician, the flow of information should be bidirectional (Werch et al., 2006). Practitioners should not only translate research into practice but should also be active in identifying salient issues associated with clinical practice that researchers should address. Researchers should seek input from clinicians to design research studies to address relevant questions and models for implementation.

In 2000, Congress charged the Agency for Healthcare Research and Quality (AHRQ) with assisting in the development of primary care practice–based research networks (PBRNs) to close the "reality gap" between the clinical evidence and what clinicians and patients want to know (Helfand, 2005). Although PBRNs are primarily comprised of physician networks, APN networks also exist (American Academy of Nurse Practitioner Network for Research, Advanced Practice Nurse–Ambulatory Research Consortium, and Advanced Practice Nurse Research Network, www.ahrq.gov).

PBRNs are a source for ongoing health services research, clinical research, and prevention research that is specific to a community or state (Tierney, et al., 2007). These forums for research improve its relevance to patients and clinicians and ease the transfer of clinical data into clinical practice.

The literature suggests that clinical decision making information rarely is on scientific data but on personal expertise or colleagues' experience to answer clinical questions (Genius & Genius, 2006; Spenceley, O'Leary, Chizawsky, Ross, & Estabrooks, 2008). If APNs believe that the best evidence should be available for the patients who seek care, these practitioners must assume the responsibility for engaging in evidence-based health care delivery and not rely solely on others for the answers.

EVIDENCE-BASED PRACTICE

Evidence-based practice (EBP) is the integration of research and clinical judgment that is used to evaluate and manage patient issues (Sackett, Rosenberg, Gray, Haynes, & Richardson, 1996). The key elements of EBP are clinically relevant research that is patient-centered and clinical judgment that includes not only clinical expertise but incorporates the patient-specific characteristics and preferences. The term evidence-based practice is used in this chapter rather than evidence-based medicine because it is broader in scope and more inclusive.

The practitioner must understand not only what EBP is but also what it is not. EBP is not a "cookbook" approach to care nor was it designed as a health care cost-cutting tool (Sackett et al., 1996). It goes without saying that EBP does not replace clinical judgment.

EBP has been reviewed and discussed in health care delivery systems for several decades, yet it is still shrouded in controversy. Some argue that the best evidence is not always relevant to a given patient or practice and that it cannot replace clinical decision making (Miser, 2006a). This argument is flawed: EBP is the template for making clinical decisions. Clinical experience is not usurped by research; rather the research evidence serves as a complement or adjunct to the clinician's judgment.

Assimilating EBP into health care delivery, the practitioner incorporates five steps: (1) ask the question, (2) collect data, (3) critically assess the research, (4) integrate the findings into practice, and (5) evaluate the outcomes of the decision that was made (Cleary-Holdforth & Leufer, 2008; Glasziou, 2006).

Therefore, the process of integrating EBP into health care services begins by addressing the following three questions: (1) What is the question or clinical problem? (2) Where is the answer? (3) Is the answer supported by research that is relevant, valid, and useful? (Miser, 2006a).

Characteristics of the Question or Clinical Problem

Identifying the problem or defining the question is the beginning of the exploratory process. Although several models exist to formulate the question with clarity, the simplest approach is PICO (population, intervention, comparison, and outcomes) (Cleary-Holdforth & Leufer, 2008). Population refers to the patient or condition of interest. As clinicians begin to formulate the question, they must identify the most important characteristics of the patient (i.e., age, race, gender, etc.) or the attributes of the condition that will be examined in the research. Intervention searches for the answers to what the clinician desires to do, such as identifying prognostic indicators, drug therapy, or diagnostic tests to be performed. Comparison addresses alternative therapies (i.e., differences between two drugs) or approaches (i.e., diagnostic test options), although in some cases there is no need for comparisons or alternative options. Outcome answers what is to be accomplished and what the effect (positive or negative) of the intervention will be.

Sources of Answers

When the practitioner has clearly articulated the question and the specific characteristics of the patient/problem, the next step is to look for answers. Several electronic databases such as the Cumulative Index of Nursing and Allied Health Literature (CINAHL), Medline, Database of Abstracts of Review of Effects (DARE), the Cochrane Library, and others can be useful tools in searching for information.

The value of the Internet cannot be understated. There are several reliable sources of clinical guidelines and systematic reviews. Please refer to Exhibit 12.1 for a listing of these resources and Web addresses.

Table 12.1

SYSTEMATIC REVIEWS AND CLINICAL GUIDELINES

AHRQ	www.ahrq.gov/clinic/epcix.htm
Bandolier	www.medicine.ox.ac.uk/bandolier/
Clinical evidence	http://clinicalevidence.bmj.com/ceweb/index.jsp
Cochrane Database of Systematic Reviews	www.cochrane.org/reviews/
Database of Abstracts of Review of Effects (DARE)	www.crd.york.ac.uk/crdweb/
Turning Research into Practice (TRIP)	www.tripdatabase.com/index.html
U.S. National Guideline Clearinghouse	www.guideline.gov
U.S. Preventive Services Task Force (USPSTF)	www.ahrq.gov/clinic/uspstfix.htm

---

Evaluation of Research

After locating "the answers" or the evidence that addresses the question as defined by the clinician, the final step is a critical assessment of the research. This step is probably the most difficult element of the process.

In order to understand the relevance and validity of research, the practitioner must be familiar with the levels of research studies. The hierarchy of research for interventions moves from randomized control trials (RCTs), often viewed as providing the best evidence, to expert opinion, the least favored, or lowest on the continuum. (Refer to Exhibit 12.1: Hierarchy of Intervention Studies.)

The RCT-N of one (each subject is studied in both the intervention and control groups and therefore serves as his or her own control) is the gold standard for clinical research (Miser, 2006b). The next level includes integrative studies, which summarize and draw conclusions from a series of primary studies. These integrative studies can be nonsystematic (written by an "expert" in the area of interest; the least favorable approach), or the more precise systematic reviews that include meta-analyses and clinical practice guidelines. The third and fourth levels include RCT conducted at multiple centers and a single center, respectively. Cohort, case control, cross-sectional, case report, case series, and finally expert opinion are the remaining levels of research (Miser, 2006b).

Exhibit 12.1

HIERARCHY OF INTERVENTION STUDIES

RCT°-N-of 1   Highest
Integrative studies
Meta-analysis
Systematic reviews
Multicenter RCTs
One-site RCT
Observational studies
      Cohort studies (longitudinal)°°
      Case control studies (retrospective)
      Cross-sectional studies (prevalence)
Case reports/series
Expert opinion   Lowest

  ° Randomized control trials
 °° Cohort studies can also be prospective or retrospective.

This hierarchy may not be appropriate for questions that are focused on diagnosis or screening, prognosis or causation. For example, if the practitioner is interested in the prognosis, the most appropriate study design would be a longitudinal cohort study. If causation is the issue, then a cohort or case control study would be the preferred design (Miser, 2006a).

Although RCTs are viewed by many as the gold standard in clinical decision making, the contributions of qualitative studies should not be devalued. Qualitative data are needed to answer questions of why, how, and when and are seldom included in RCTs in enough detail to apply an intervention consistently (Wilson & Fridinger, 2008).

The internal validity of the research depends on a critical analysis of the intent of the research and the methodology used to examine the results; external validity, in contrast, is assessed by answering the question of generalizability to a larger population (Miser, 2006a). From this analysis, the clinician can then discern the relevance of the evidence as it relates to a specific patient, population, or problem.

BARRIERS TO TRANSLATING RESEARCH INTO PRACTICE

The obstacles that prevent the translation of research into practice are many and complex. These barriers can be summarized into two categories: (1) individual characteristics that include sociological features (Lang et al., 2007) and (2) systems or organizational factors.

Individual barriers that have been reported include insufficient knowledge about the research process, lack of competence in reading and evaluating research or scientific articles and reports, lack of time, and lack of knowledge of statistical analyses (Bostrom, Kajermo, Nordstrom, & Wallin, 2008; Lang et al., 2007; McCloskey, 2008; Smith-Strom & Norvetvedt, 2007; Mendelson & Carino, 2005). Organizational or system barriers that have been described are lack of access to research, lack of authority to change practice, inadequate resources to implement change, and lack of support from staff and colleagues (Bostrom et al., 2008; Lang et al., 2007; McCloskey, 2008; Smith-Strom & Norvetvedt, 2007).

Individual Characteristics

APNs prepared at the master's level are taught to critique research, initiate EBP initiatives, and translate findings into practice (McCloskey, 2008); however, educational preparation alone does not seem to be sufficient to result in the translation of research into practice. One study suggests that attitudes may be more important than educational preparation (Munroe, Duffy, & Fisher, 2008).

Sociological variables that may influence attitudes about new research are pre-existing beliefs and values, personal experience, interpersonal relationships, and the opinions of colleagues (Genius & Genius, 2006). These factors must be altered if new information is to replace old information and be assimilated into practice.

Clinical information must filter down to individual clinicians and cross disciplines (Newhouse, 2008). The lack of interprofessional collaboration compromises research efforts between disciplines (i.e., biological sciences and physical sciences) and prevents the transmission of research data from one discipline to another. Although the different interests among various health care disciplines are justified, the artificial boundaries and turf issues created by different professions impede the flow of information (Zwarestein, & Reeves, 2006) and obscure the one commonality or unifying factor that should be improving patient care.

System/Organizational Barriers

Many health care institutions, whether they are hospitals or primary care clinics, frequently spend resources on acquiring and utilizing new and innovative medical equipment and developing new procedures to improve patient care. Failure to invest in human technology such as the development of behavioral interventions, prevention strategies, or quality improvement programs (Bradley, Schlesinger, Webster, Baker, & Inouye, 2004) or the failure to develop processes that support nurses and others in the evaluation of interventions and policy development (Newhouse, Dearholf, Poe, Pugh, & White, 2005) are examples of how organizations fail to contribute to the translation and implementation of research into patient care or clinical services. Without infrastructure support, nurses, particularly APNs, may perceive that they do not have the authority or organizational support to develop or evaluate new models of care.

Although many larger institutions have adopted electronic technology in their medical records with the intent of consolidating patient information and reducing errors, little technology is incorporated into the systems that directly access the clinical research or clinical practice guidelines that may improve patient care. Computer information systems that are integrated into electronic medical records are often underutilized, in part because practicing clinicians are often not engaged in the development of these systems. As computer information systems develop, best practices are becoming integrated into some of these systems. As clinical doctoral programs develop, APNs will be more knowledgeable about information systems and can participate in their development.

SOLUTIONS: A ROLE FOR ADVANCED PRACTICE NURSES

The solutions for translating research into practice are as diverse and multifaceted as the barriers. Proposed solutions can be examined at three levels: the micro level (individual clinician and patient), the meso level (systems or organizations), and the macro (economic and political) solutions (Scott, 2007).

Micro Level Solutions

Possible solutions for addressing the barriers to translating research into practice on the micro level require an examination of patient and clinician perspectives. Although much of the previous discussion has focused on the practitioner, a brief discussion of the patient's interface with the clinician's decision making is in order.

Implementation of research into practice requires engagement with the patient population (Col, 2005). Without patient involvement, the translation and application of research into practice will not occur or succeed.

Patient Perspective

From the patient's perspective, the clinician is a repository of information, and the underlying assumption is that the clinician's expertise is based on current and accurate information. The role of the clinician is to present the relevant information, risks, and benefits of interventions so that the patient can make an informed decision. Often this information is complex and is presented in a way that does not empower the patient to participate in the decision-making process (Col, 2005). Ultimately, the result of this type of interaction leads to miscommunication and withdrawal of the patient from active participation.

APNs are skilled in the art of communication and have a fundamental understanding of adult learning principles. With this skill set, APNs can reduce the flow of misinformation by serving as interpreters of information from lay media sources or other health care professionals. Informed patients can make appropriate health care decisions and can become participants in their own health care.

Practitioner Perspective

From a practitioner's perspective, the failure to utilize research to guide practice is governed by attitudes about research and its relevance to clinical practice. To increase the relevance of research, patient population needs should be the driving force for the research agenda. As articulated earlier, the flow of information should be bidirectional between the researcher and clinician. APNs should be the link between the researcher and the patient population. They could assist the researcher design studies that answer clinical questions that are relevant to patients and clinicians. APNs play a vital role in implementing new interventions or guidelines; therefore, they should be active participants in constructing and testing implementation models and delivery systems (Kottke et al., 2008).

Another way to increase the relevance of research to practice and promote attitude change begins with the educational experience of APNs. The traditional research course that is taught at the graduate level gives the APN the skills to evaluate and construct research projects. Perhaps the missing piece is the significance of the research to clinical practice. For APN students, the research course may not have clinical meaning; therefore, much of the information that is taught is forgotten and not used. Restructuring these courses in the context of EBP, making the connection between theory and practice, and reinforcing the knowledge and skills throughout the APN's educational experiences will affect attitudes and encourage the utilization of research (Coopey, Nix, & Clancy, 2006; Munroe et al., 2008). Research courses in current and developing clinical doctoral programs will emphasize utilization of research to strengthen this thread.

Clinical faculty or preceptors who are often practicing APNs can have a profound influence on APN students' opinions about research and its relationship to practice (Jeffers, Robinson, Luxner, & Redding, 2008). When EBP is incorporated into clinical experiences, attitudes are changed, and the APN students' skills in research translation and utilization are increased (Singleton, 2008; Singleton & Levin, 2008).

Personal and Professional Accountability

The change in educational experiences does not address personal and professional accountability. APNs who do not feel they are equipped to engage in EBP should then focus on professional development so that they acquire the tools for research evaluation, utilization, and implementation. APNs who possess this knowledge and these skills should have enhanced visibility and credibility with other members of health care delivery systems. This visibility and credibility should enable them then to gain the authority to create an environment that fosters EBP through research (Richardson, Turnock, & Gibson, 2007).

Professional and personal accountability demand that clinicians stay abreast with current research. To manage the flood of medical and nursing information, APNs can enlist the support of a medical librarian. The majority of providers do not know how to search for information that supports clinical decision making (Meats et al., 2007). Generally, clinicians will use a single term that does not uncover comparators or outcomes data sources. These searches often fail to uncover high-quality evidence that might be useful (Meats et al., 2007). Developing collaborative relationships with medical librarians can enhance this skill so that retrieval of evidence is easy and the accumulation of useless information and wasted time is avoided. Other strategies to manage the overwhelming amount of new evidence include obtaining subscriptions or access to evidence-based journals, which typically scan multiple journals for relevant research (Glasziou, 2006), or organizing interprofessional journal clubs where recent research can be discussed.

Translating research into practice requires changes not only in attitudes but also in behavior. Most models for clinical practice change, such as Promoting Action on Research in Health Services, Rosswurm and Larrabee's Model for Change to Evidence-Based Practice, or the Iowa Model of Evidence-Based Practice (Eastwood, O'Connell, & Gardner, 2008), advocate the development of collaborative interprofessional teams to promote changes in practice. The members of these teams are variable and dependent on the practice site, the expertise of the individual members, and the current problem or patient issue being examined.

For many years, APNs have been the bridge between nursing, medicine, and other health care professionals and patients. APNs should assume a major role in interprofessional collaborative teams. They can serve as mentors for nursing staff and allied health care professionals in the implementation of EBP and can function as the translators or interpreters of research in these teams.

Meso Level Solutions

Application of evidence into nursing or clinical practice is unlikely unless it is integrated into work flow (Bakken, Currie, Lee, Roberts, Collins, & Cimino, 2008). Institutional support for the integration of research into practice can come through the development of computer information systems (CIS). Information systems that provide immediate access to databases with synopses of best evidence that is relevant and has undergone critical review are necessary for practitioners to make informed or evidence-based choices. CIS with embedded guidelines can prompt the clinicians to integrate EBP into clinical decision making.

The development of CIS should be a collaborative effort between the clinicians and the institution rather than the institution purchasing a system that may or may not meet the needs of the practitioner. APNs that have been prepared at the DNP level or have expertise in informatics have the skills necessary to be members of the CIS design team. If they are not directly involved in CIS design, APNs should work with institutions when decisions are being made to purchase or design informatics systems for enhancing clinical services.

Institutional investment in human capital is important if research is to be translated into clinical services. This investment includes such activities as staff training, cultivating and supporting research implementation, mentoring, and providing resources (time and fiscal support) for developing a research agenda.

Armed with the knowledge of health care systems, APNs can function as change agents within organizations. They have the leadership skills to garner institutional support, engage the stakeholders, and institute changes that support EBP at all levels of care delivery.

Macro Level Solutions

Health care providers do not function in a vacuum. Practitioners must function within an economic and political system. Health care is governed by the "cost of doing business." When they are considering the adoption of new practices, clinicians are forced to consider the cost to the patient. Obviously, if the cost exceeds the patient's resources, often the intervention will not be followed or will be unsuccessful. Even if the evidence supports a new technology or drug, the feasibility is determined by the economic impact.

The issue of cost transcends the individual patient and permeates all health care delivery systems. On a systems level, administrators have to evaluate the fiscal impact of new interventions. Administrators must weigh the new method against the old and determine the added value of the new treatment plan. If APNs believe that a new intervention is in the best interest of patient care, these clinicians must be prepared to evaluate the cost-benefit ratio of new practice.

APNs should also become astute fiscal managers. They must appreciate that EBP does not suggest that all new evidence can or should be the standard of care. Most APNs have been trained to focus on the delivery of care to the individual patient; however, in the current health system with its limited resources, the emphasis must shift to a population perspective and cost containment.

Politicians are not health care experts and rely on multiple sources for information regarding EBP. In general, the goals of the politician are to allocate limited resources to accomplish the greatest good and to regulate health care systems and providers to protect the public from harm.

As members of the nursing profession and as part of the largest health care provider network, APNs have considerable political clout and should use this power to influence politicians. When advocating for the adoption of new evidence, the APN must be mindful of the goals of the policy makers.

SUMMARY

Becoming competent practitioners requires not only the acquisition of clinical skills but the ability to use research to guide their practice. With the proliferation of new evidence, APNs must be able to critically analyze and evaluate the evidence and appraise its utility. Applying the skills acquired during their educational experience, APNs can and should become the translators of research into practice.

APNs have the skill set to understand the research process, and they are effective change agents. Therefore, they are in the position to identify the determinants of the clinician's and patient behavior and to design models that will facilitate not only the transfer of knowledge into clinical practice but assist in the implementation process. APNs, particularly those prepared at the clinical doctorate level, can become interpretive researchers or context adaptors (Chelsa, 2008). This role consists of applying new interventions designed in academic research centers to primary care clinics.

Even when research is adapted to the primary care setting, there is no guarantee that this will facilitate implementation. As we discussed earlier, the models that currently exist to promote adoption and implementation of research into practice are inadequate. The evidence is clear that provider education, detailing, computerized clinical support, and financial incentives have minimal or modest effect on increasing the use of EBP. The answer may be in utilizing the best of all models and formulating a new paradigm to bridge the gap between research and practice.

The doctorate of nursing practice (DNP) expands the APN's skill set to include becoming a change agent, understanding and developing informatic systems, and appreciating the operations of health care systems. Therefore, APNs prepared at the doctoral level are in the position to expand and put into operation the previously discussed systems engineering and social innovation models for the dissemination and application of research. In this way, they can further elaborate the translation of research into practice.

As APNs assume leadership roles in health care, they should become proactive in removing the barriers to translating research into practice. Now and in the future, APNs can and should change health care delivery systems. This change is possible if APNs become consumers of research.

REFERENCES

Bakken, S., Currie, L. M., Lee, N., Roberts, W. D., Collins, S. A., & Cimino, J. J. (2008). Integrating evidence into clinical information systems for nursing decision support. *International Journal of Medical Informatics, 77*(6), 413–420.

Bostrom, A., Kajermo, K. N., Nordstrom, G., & Wallin, L. (2008). Barriers to research utilization and research use among registered nurses working in the care of older people: Does BARRIER Scale discriminate between research users and non-research users on perceptions of barriers? *Implementation Science, 3*, 24–32.

Bradley, E. H., Schlesinger, M., Webster, T. R., Baker, D., & Inouye, S. K. (2004). Translating research into clinical practice: Making change happen. *Journal of American Geriatric Society, 52* (11), 1875–1882.

Chelsa, C. A. (2008). Translational research: Essential contributions from interpretive nursing science. *Research in Nursing and Health, 31*, 381–390.

Claxton, K., Cohen, J., & Neumann, P. J. (2005). When is evidence sufficient? *Health Affairs, 24*(1), 93–101.

Cleary-Holdforth, J., & Leufer, T. (2008). Essential elements in developing evidence-based practice. *Nursing Standard, 23*(2), 42–43.

Col, N. F. (2005). Challenges in translating research into practice. *Journal of Women's Health, 14*(1), 87–95.

Coopey, M., Nix, M., & Clancy, C. M. (2006). Translating research into evidence-based nursing practice and evaluating effectiveness. *Journal of Nursing Care Quality, 21*(3), 195–202.

Eastwood, G. M., O'Connell, B., & Gardner, A. (2008). Selecting the right integration of research into practice strategy. *Journal of Nursing Quality Care, 23*(3), 258–265.

Genius, S. K., & Genius, S. J. (2006). Exploring the continuum: Medical information of effective clinical practice. Paper I: The translation of knowledge into clinical practice. *Journal of Evaluation of Clinical Practice, 12*(1), 49–62.

Glasgow, R. E., Magid, D. J., Beck, A., Ritzwoller, D., & Estabrooks, P. A. (2005). Practical clinical trials for translating research to practice: Design and measurement recommendations. *Medical Care, 43*(6), 551–557.

Glasziou, P. (2006). Managing the evidence flood. *Surgical Clinics of North America, 86*, 193–199.

Helfand, M. (2005). Using evidence reports: Progress and challenges in evidence-based decision making. *Health Affairs 24*(1), 123–127.

Jeffers, B., Robinson, S., Luxner, K., & Redding, D. (2008). Nursing faculty mentors as facilitators for evidence-based nursing practice. *Journal of Staff Development 24*(5), E8–E12.

Kottke, T. E., Solberg, L. I., Nelson, A. F., Belcher, D. W., Caplan, W., Green, L. W., et al. (2008). Optimizing practice through research: A new perspective to solve an old problem. *Annals of Family Medicine, 6*(5), 459–462.

Lang, E. S., Wyer, P. S., & Haynes, R. B. (2007). Knowledge translation: Closing the evidence-to-practice gap. *Annals of Emergency Medicine, 49*(3), 355–363.

McCloskey, D. J. (2008). Nurses' perceptions of research utilization in a corporate health care system. *Journal of Nursing Scholarship, 40*(1), 39–45.

Meats, E., Brassey, J., Heneghan, C., & Glasziou, P. (2007). Using the Turning Research into Practice (TRIP) database: How do clinicians really search? *Journal of the Medical Library Association, 95*(2), 156–163.

Mendelson, D., & Carino, T. (2005) Evidence-based medicine in the United States— De rigueur or dream deferred? *Health Affairs, 24*(1), 133–136.

Miser, W. F. (2006a). An introduction to evidence-based medicine. *Primary Clinical Office Practice, 33,* 811–829.

Miser, W. F. (2006b). Finding the truth from medical literature: How to critically evaluate an article. *Primary Care Clinical Office Practice, 33,* 839–862.

Munroe, D., Duffy, P., & Fisher, C. (2008). Nurse knowledge, skills and attitudes related to evidence based practice: Before and after organizational supports. *Medical Surgical Nursing, 17*(1), 55–60.

Newhouse, R. (2008). Evidence based behavioral practice: An exemplar of interprofessional collaboration. *Journal of Nursing Administration, 38* (10), 414–416.

Newhouse, R., Dearholf, S., Poe, S., Pugh, L., & White, K.M. (2005). Evidence-based practice: A practical approach to implementation. *Journal of Nursing Administration, 35*(1), 35–40.

Richardson, A., Turnock, C., & Gibson, V. (2007). Development of a critical care nursing research strategy: A tripartite approach. *British Journal of Nursing, 16*(19), 1201–1207.

Sackett, D. L., Rosenberg, M., Gray, J. A., Haynes, R. B., & Richardson, W. S. (1996). Evidence-based medicine: What it is and what it isn't. *British Medical Journal, 312,* 71–72.

Scott, I. A. (2007). The evolving science of translating research evidence into clinical practice. *ACP Journal Club, 146* (3), Suppl. 8, 9–11.

Singleton, J. (2008). Strategies for learning evidence-based practice: Critically appraising clinical practice guidelines. *Journal of Nursing Education, 47*(8), 380–383.

Singleton, J., & Levin, R. (2008). Strategies for learning evidence-based practice: Critically appraising clinical practice guidelines. *Journal of Nursing Education, 47*(8), 380–383.

Smith-Strom, H., & Norvetvedt, M. (2007). Evaluation of evidence-based methods used to teach nursing students to critically appraise the evidence. *Journal of Nursing Education, 47*(8), 372–375

Spenceley, S. M., O'Leary, K. A., Chizawsky, L. L., Ross, A. J., & Estabrooks, C. A. (2008). Sources of information used by nurses to inform practice: An integrative review. *International Journal of Nursing Science 45,* 954–970.

Tierney, W. M., Oppenheimer, C. C., Hudson, B. L., Benz, J., Finn, A., Hickner, J. M., Lanier, D., & Gaylin, D. S. (2007). A national survey of primary care practice-based research networks . *Annals of Family Medicine, 5*(3), 242–249.

Werch, C., Grenard, J. L., Burnett, J., Watkins, J. A., Ames, S., & Jobli, E. (2006) Translation as a function of modality: Potential of brief interventions. *Evaluation and the Health Professions, 29*(1), 89–125.

Wilson, K. M., & Fridinger, F. (2008). Focusing on public health: A different look at translating research into practice. *Journal of Women's Health 17*(2), 173–179.

Weingarten, S. (2000). Translating practice guidelines into patient care. *Chest, 118,* 4S–7S.

Zwarestein, M., .& Reeves, S. (2006). Knowledge translation and interprofessional collaboration: Where the rubber of evidence-based care hits the road of teamwork. *The Journal of Continuing Education in the Health Professions, 26*(1), 46–54.

Informatics for Advanced Practice Nurses

13

JANE PEACE
PAMELA SCHEIBEL

The Information Age presents new tools, opportunities, and challenges to advanced practice nurses (APNs). With the increase in published research reports, practice guidelines, and professional Web-based resources, the kind and type of information available and necessary for APN practice is growing at an unprecedented rate. Fortunately, technology and the tools available for locating, organizing, and managing information are also maturing, enabling levels of evidence-based practice and patient safety that were impossible without computerization. Most noticeable here are advanced search tools that assist APNs in locating pertinent research findings among thousands of reports, and medication references on handheld computing devices that are automatically updated for convenient access to drug dosing information. Indeed, in their groundbreaking report on health care quality, the Institute of Medicine (IOM) identified the use of information technology as one of four primary target areas to improve the quality of health care in the United States (Institute of Medicine [U.S.] Committee on Quality of Health Care in America, 2001). Therefore, familiarity and competency with technology, particularly computers, is an important skill for APNs.

Nursing informatics refers to the management and use of data and information to support nursing practice and delivery of nursing care (Graves & Corcoran, 1989). Nurses in practice need basic competency in informatics, much as they need competency in communication or physical assessment. Although nursing organizations have not yet issued a comprehensive and conclusive statement about specific informatics competencies for nurses, the National League for Nursing (NLN) (NLN, 2008) has identified the need to do so.

Working toward developing consensus about nursing informatics competencies, expert panels and nurse informaticists have suggested basic informatics competencies for nurses. For example, a group of nursing informatics experts derived a list of informatics competencies for nurses based on literature review and expert consensus, which has since been widely cited (Staggers, Gassert, & Curran, 2001, 2002a, 2002b). The competencies they identified for beginning nurses focus on basic computer skills, familiarity with common applications, use of electronic communications such as e-mail, and recognition of privacy and security concerns (Staggers et al., 2002b). Competencies at the expert level are then related to the nurse's area of expertise, such as the use of staff scheduling applications for those in administration, testing software for nurse educators, or public health databases for nurses in public health practice (Staggers et al., 2002b).

Although the competencies developed by Staggers and colleagues (2002a) are widely cited and applied, one limitation of their work involves competencies that are not necessary for all nurses, but that may or may not be attained depending on the type of practice a particular nurse is engaged in. Curran (2003) reported on work at several universities to develop a list of informatics competencies for nurse practitioners informed by the work of Staggers and colleagues (2002a) but specific to the role of nurse practitioner. These competencies are relatively applicable to all APNs because they focus on broad informatics competencies for advanced practice. The list of competencies for nurse practitioners appears in Exhibit 13.1.

Many of the informatics competencies identified for APNs in Exhibit 13.1 and by other authors as well are related to recognizing information needs and then making efficient use of the resources available for locating, managing, and applying information for practice. Bakken (2001), in identifying informatics competencies necessary for evidence-based nursing practice, wrote that nurses must be able to retrieve relevant sources of information and critically analyze evidence for applicability to practice. Information and evidence may be drawn from a variety of sources, from electronic patient records to databases of research publications to proprietary

Exhibit 13.1

APN INFORMATICS COMPETENCIES

Computer skills
- Accesses shared data sets°
- Extracts data from clinical data sets°
- Extracts selected literature resources and integrates them to a personally usable file°
- Uses applications to aggregate and analyze data for forecasting, accreditation, clinical value, nurse-sensitive outcomes, evidence-based practice, and quality improvement
- Uses applications to format and present data and information
- Uses decision support systems, expert systems, and aids for differential diagnosis
- Uses interactive communication devices with patients and other health care providers

Informatics Knowledge
- Supports efforts toward development and use of structured languages°
- Promotes the integrity of nursing information and access necessary for patient care within an integrated computer-based patient record°
- Evaluates computer-assisted instruction (CAI) as a teaching tool°
- Provides for efficient data collection°
- Discusses the impact of computerized information management on the role of the nurse°
- Describes ways to protect data°
- Describes general applications systems to support clinical care°
- Describes general applications available for research°
- Understands the principles of data display to facilitate analysis
- Is knowledgeable regarding optimal search strategies to locate clinically sound and useful studies from information resources
- Critically analyzes data, information, and knowledge for use in site-specific evidence-based practice
- Identifies, evaluates, and applies the most relevant information
- Synthesizes best evidence

(Continued)

Exhibit 13.1 (Continued)

Informatics Skills

- Converts information needs into answerable questions
- Uses data and statistical analyses to describe and evaluate practice
- Evaluates health information on the Internet using a structured critique format
- Assists patients to use databases to make informed decisions°
- Acts as an advocate of system users including patients and colleagues°
- Performs basic troubleshooting in applications°
- Incorporates structured languages into practice
- Applies the principles of data integrity, professional ethics, and legal requirements for patient confidentiality and data security
- Designs and uses database reports
- Demonstrates knowledge and clinical decision-making processes within site-specific practice
- Evaluates the appropriateness of the monitoring system for the type of data needed
- Converts data into information and then knowledge

Source: Curran (2003). Reprinted with permission.
°Competency from the research-based work of Staggers et al. (2002a).

consumer health websites. This chapter will review some important informatics resources and tools that may help APNs access and manage these often valuable but potentially overwhelming treasure troves of information.

Informatics advances rapidly. Therefore, the resources described in this chapter should be viewed only as a representative sample of the informatics tools available to APNs, not as an exhaustive list. Because new resources are constantly being developed, the reader is encouraged to use this chapter as a starting point for considering informatics resources for practice. Many mechanisms for staying abreast of current technology, such as professional development and APN journals, provide opportunities to learn about and evaluate new informatics innovations as they become available.

INFORMATIC RESOURCES FOR APNS AND PATIENTS

Hopefully, we are working toward a future in which informatics innovations will interface seamlessly with one another and with APN practice. Evidence and relevant information will be presented whenever and wherever it is needed. Electronic health record systems will receive input from the devices that monitor patients; access databases to collect relevant evidence, literature, and guidelines; and output appropriate support for clinical decision making for both provider and patient. The technology ideally becomes so well integrated and ubiquitous that it is not even noticed but is incorporated into the everyday practice of the APN. When and if that goal is attained, discussing specific informatics resources and tools as discrete and separate entities will be difficult.

Currently, some informatics innovations do interface and overlap, but many are not seamlessly incorporated into practice, relying instead on the APN to actively engage them to support practice. For example, a patient's record from one practice setting may not interface with the same patient's record in another setting; information maintained by the patient in a personal electronic health record may not be available within the health record maintained by a health care organization; and some information resources must be opened and manually searched by the APN rather than providing information in an anticipatory fashion. However, progress is being made, as is evidenced by certain decision support systems.

Electronic Health Record Systems

The ideal electronic health record (EHR) system is a system in which the computer-based health records of diverse organizations and the health records maintained by laypersons all interface to share information in an optimal manner to support health and health care. The IOM has identified the key functionalities of an electronic health record system as

(1) longitudinal collection of electronic health information for and about persons, where health information is defined as information pertaining to the health of an individual or health care provided to an individual; (2) immediate electronic access to person- and population-level information by authorized, and only authorized, users; (3) provision of knowledge and decision support that enhance the quality, safety, and efficiency of patient care; and (4) support of efficient processes for health care delivery. Critical building blocks of an EHR system are the electronic health records (EHR)

maintained by providers (e.g., hospitals, nursing homes, ambulatory settings) and by individuals (also called personal health records). (Institute of Medicine, 2003, p. 1)

National initiatives are pushing for the adoption of electronic records in all health care settings by 2014 (National League for Nursing, 2008). Although some experts predict adoption will require as much as a decade longer (Ford, Menachemi, & Phillips, 2006), electronic health records are becoming more common. Under the umbrella term *electronic health record (EHR)* are included both the electronic medical record (EMR) maintained by health care organizations and the personal health record (PHR) primarily owned and intended for use by consumers (Stead, Kelly, & Kolodner, 2005).

Electronic Medical Records (EMRs)

Electronic medical record (EMR) is currently the preferred term to describe the electronic records used by clinicians in a health care organization. These computerized records partially or fully replace paper-based charts as the repository of information about a client's care within the organization. EMRs range from records that are essentially computer-based versions of the old paper patient chart to interactive electronic record systems incorporating powerful applications to facilitate evidence-based practice and support clinical decision making. Consensus is emerging that basic components of an EMR are electronic documentation of clinicians' notes, the ability to review laboratory and radiology reports, and ordering and prescribing medications and treatments (Jha et al., 2006).

The IOM has identified EMRs and information technology as important tools to adopt in order to improve quality of care and patient safety (IOM, 2003; IOM Committee on Quality of Health Care in America, 2001). By enabling clinicians at different physical locations to access the complete medical record and incorporate resources such as access to literature databases and support for clinical decision making, EMRs have the potential to improve care, enhance safety, and promote evidence-based practice. EMRs may be especially helpful in the care of patients with chronic diseases because these electronic records have the ability to provide all clinicians involved in the patient's care with access to all relevant clinical information, regardless of where or by whom services were provided.

Patient Portals

EMR systems maintained by health care organizations sometimes provide patient portals. These Web-based applications enable the consumer to view certain parts of his EMR and carry out simple tasks, including ordering prescription refills, requesting an appointment, and sending a question to a nurse. Patient portals enable consumers to view parts of their records under certain circumstances. For example, some lab values may be shown to the consumer immediately, primarily those that require little interpretation and are familiar to consumers, such as cholesterol level. Other lab results might be revealed to the patient after review and interpretation by the provider, including thyroid stimulating hormone and hematocrit. Still others might never be available through the Web-based application due to privacy concerns, such as the results of an HIV test or genetic screening result. Overall, consumer reaction to patient portals has been positive (Hassol et al., 2004; Masys, Baker, Butros, & Cowles, 2002).

PHRs

Personal health records (PHRs) are electronic health records maintained and owned by consumers. Although the exact definition of PHR continues to evolve (Halamka, Mandl, & Tang, 2008), PHRs are generally described as repositories for health data contributed by the consumer and providers, including tools that assist consumers to take an active role in their health care (Tang, Ash, Bates, Overhage, & Sands, 2006). Therefore, PHRs may range from simple files containing lists of appointments and prescriptions to powerful and interactive applications helping consumers to control and manage their own health.

Microsoft HealthVault® and Google Health® are examples of proprietary PHRs now available in Beta versions, indicating that they are available for use but are still undergoing intense development and evaluation. The primary goals of these PHR applications are to provide seamless information sharing to import and export information from providers' records and personally entered data and to provide relevant consumer health information.

Google Health® is a free consumer tool that enables consumers to enter medical diagnoses and medications. It also provides links to related information when available. This basic PHR application enables consumers to import medical records from participating providers, including clinics, hospitals, and pharmacies, and allows them to export a Google Health® profile to online services that serve as a link to providers who in turn may access that information. Details about Google Health® are available online at www.google.com/health, as are instructions on how to sign up for a free Google Health® account.

Microsoft HealthVault® similarly aims to provide an information link between consumers, providers, insurers, and personal health services, with a goal of enabling consumers to store all of their health information in one place so that it is always organized and available online. HealthVault® includes support for uploading information from personal health monitoring devices such as heart rate monitors. Microsoft provides a home page for consumers and a separate home page for providers about HealthVault®, available at www.healthvault.com.

PHRs are currently the subject of much research and development. Many more PHR products and exciting advances may be expected in the next few years.

Clinical Decision Support Systems

A clinical decision support system (CDSS) is a software system typically embedded in an EHR system. The CDSS integrates information about a particular patient with a knowledge base to generate patient-specific evaluations and recommendations to aid the provider or patient in making health-related decisions (Hunt, Haynes, Hanna, & Smith, 1998; IOM Committee on Quality of Health Care in America, 2001). The term *patient* in this context may refer to an individual or to a specific population.

The IOM report *Crossing the Quality Chasm* (IOM Committee on Quality of Health Care in America, 2001) summarized the literature on the effectiveness of CDSSs and concluded that CDSS systems have been demonstrated to improve prevention and monitoring practices. In addition, some evidence exists that CDSS use for drug dosing is also effective. At the time of the report, data about the effectiveness of CDSS use for drug selection, avoidance of drug interactions, and screening for adverse effects was limited; the development of such systems was limited by the amount and complexity of knowledge involved.

CDSS use for diagnosis and management is more complex still, and little data about its effectiveness was available at the time of the IOM report. However, the committee noted that advances in science and technology indicated that CDSSs had the potential to grow and to improve the quality of health care.

A number of research reports about CDSSs have been published since the IOM report became available, indicating that the IOM committee's prediction was correct. A review of CDSSs in ambulatory primary care settings demonstrated that types and implementations of CDSSs in primary care varied greatly, but overall CDSSs appeared to have potential to improve outcomes (Bryan & Boren, 2008). Another review found that a CDSS to improve prescribing practices for the elderly showed benefits (Yourman, Concato, & Agostini, 2008).

Although less has been published about CDSSs specifically for nursing, Lyerla (2008) reported the successful implementation of a nursing CDSS to prevent ventilator-associated pneumonia by using alerts to maintain semirecumbant patient positioning. Bakken (2006) described the potential for nursing CDSSs to improve patient safety in such areas as fall prevention, prevention of pressure ulcers, and medication administration, but noted that although process-oriented research about nursing decision support exists, there is a need for more outcomes-based research.

PUBLIC HEALTH DATABASES

Rich databases of public health data and statistics are available online. APNs may use these sources of national, state, county, and regional data for a variety of purposes, including the detection of problems specific to their population, identification of important targets for health promotion campaigns, and evaluation of disease outbreaks such as influenza or arsenic poisoning.

To access these databases, the APN must simply know where to begin. For example, national data related to Healthy People 2010 goals are available at www.healthypeople.gov.

The U.S. Centers for Disease Control (CDC) National Center for Health Statistics (available at www.cdc.gov/nchs) provides links to a wealth of national data, such as the annual number of deaths attributed to the leading causes of death and the results of the National Health Care Surveys; as well as related reports and publications that in some cases compile and distill the data into a format that may be easier to use.

State-level data are available from the CDC website for some data sets. Additional state databases are made available by state agencies themselves. For example, health statistics related to Healthy People 2010 goals are available from the Wisconsin Department of Health

Services on the Wisconsin State Health Plan website (http://dhs. wisconsin.gov/statehealthplan). The availability and location of state, county, and regional data varies from one location to another; the state government's website is a reasonable location from which to begin a search. Local public health practitioners and libraries are also valuable resources for locating this data.

LITERATURE DATABASES

The literature available to APNs for practice is growing at an impressive rate. Because nurses cannot possibly be aware of all that is being published, bibliographic databases become more important as the amount of literature grows. PubMed and the Cumulative Index to Nursing and Allied Health Literature (CINAHL) are two important bibliographic databases for APNs, and each has a unique purpose and contribution to APN practice.

PubMed (available to everyone at www.ncbi.nlm.nih.gov/pubmed/) is the database of biomedical journal citations and abstracts created by the U.S. National Library of Medicine (NLM). The largest component of PubMed is MEDLINE (an acronym for Medical Literature Analysis and Retrieval System Online), which indexes the biomedical literature from 1949 to the present. Resources indexed in PubMed in addition to those included in MEDLINE include citations for articles that have been published very recently and are not yet included in MEDLINE, and citations for some life sciences journals that are beyond the scope of MEDLINE or not yet included in it. PubMed indexing uses medical subject headings (MeSH) terms, and the PubMed website includes a MeSH browser that enables users to locate search terms related to their concept of interest.

Literature search features enable the user to place limits on searches, including year of publication (useful if, for example, the APN is only interested in articles published in the past 5 years), type of research subjects (many users limit searches to research with humans), and type of article (RCTs, review articles, etc.). PubMed also provides links to full-text articles when they are available. Although performing a good PubMed search can be daunting at first, the PubMed website includes short tutorials and resources helpful for novice users.

CINAHL is owned and operated by EBSCO Publishing and is available through most medical and nursing libraries and many public libraries.

This bibliographic database indexes the nursing and allied health literature for the years 1982 to the present, using CINAHL subject headings that were developed to reflect nursing and allied health terminologies. Some full-text articles are available through CINAHL as well. In addition to journal articles, CINAHL includes dissertations, book chapters, nurse practice acts, and audiovisual materials. Although PubMed includes much nursing literature, it does not include much of the material indexed in CINAHL. CINAHL, on the other hand, indexes most of the nursing literature, but does not include much of the biomedical literature that might also be important for APNs. An often useful strategy is to perform both a PubMed search and a CINAHL search if one database is not clearly more relevant for a particular information need.

Other bibliographic databases may also be very useful in specific circumstances. For example, PsycINFO, a database produced and copyrighted by the American Psychological Association, may produce the most relevant results if the information need is in the domain of psychology. PsycINFO is a database of psychological literature abstracts from the 1800s to the present. Or the APN might search the Cochrane Library exclusively if a rigorous review of the existing literature about a specific topic is required. The Cochrane Library is a subscription service available through most medical and nursing libraries. In addition, access to the abstracts and summaries when they are available for all Cochrane systematic reviews are free to everyone at www.cochrane.org/reviews.

Tips for searching online bibliographic databases such as those described above focus on formulating a question, devising a sound search strategy, and leveraging the features of the bibliographic database search engine. Most include tutorials, tips for use, and instructions online. The reader is encouraged to use these online resources and also to take advantage of classes offered at medical and nursing libraries to improve literature searching skills.

Clinical Information Resources and Clearinghouses

Many applications and resources, both commercial and public, are available to help APNs find answers to clinical questions. The National Guideline Clearinghouse (NGC) is an online repository of evidence-based guidelines for clinical practice. Maintained by the Agency for Healthcare Research and Quality (AHRQ), the NGC provides access to guidelines from a variety of authoritative sources that are vetted and updated regularly. Special features of the website include side-by-side display of guidelines for comparison, annotated bibliographies associated with each guideline, and the ability to download guidelines to handheld devices (e.g., PDAs). The NGC is freely available to everyone at www .guideline.gov. Users may browse or search for guidelines by disease or condition. Like the bibliographic databases described above, the NGC website includes instructions and tips for searching the database.

In the commercial realm, UpToDate is a resource that summarizes and combines information from journals and other sources to provide evidence-based information for practice. Available online or as a download for desktop or handheld computers, UpToDate is a popular resource for evidence-based, peer-reviewed information for providers and consumers. MD Consult and Nursing Consult are additional examples of commercial resources for evidence-based practice information. The choice of resource for most APNs is based on availability; health care organizations may offer one or more of these resources to providers, or partnerships with academic institutions may facilitate APN access through library systems. Resources such as these are valuable in helping APNs deal with the often overwhelming amounts of information available for practice, and their use is likely to expand as health-related information grows and evidence-based practice is emphasized.

Genomics Resources

As genomics and genetic science progresses, genetic testing and genomic knowledge are becoming important in APN practice. Clients and clinicians alike will have more genetic questions. Excellent resources exist online to help answer these questions. Much of the literature is available through the databases mentioned above, but resources exist to help with specific genetic questions as well.

For example, the Genetic Home Reference is a resource created and maintained by the National Library of Medicine and is freely available to everyone at http://ghr.nlm.nih.gov/. This resource includes information appropriate for consumers that may also be useful to APNs whose specialty is not genetics. Included are basic science content about genes, chromosomes, and DNA; information about specific genetic conditions; a glossary of terms associated with genetics; and links to other genetics resources, including resources for the public and resources for providers. APNs may find that beginning a search for genetic information with the Genetic Home Reference and then extending the search to other professional resources as they are needed is a useful strategy.

The U.S. Centers for Disease Control and Prevention (CDC) National Office of Public Health Genomics (www.cdc.gov/genomics) maintains a Web resource of general information about public health genomics, updates, and links to CDC public health genomics publications. This resource is another useful source of genetic and genomic information for APNs, and the site also links to other resources.

The National Center for Biotechnology Information (NCBI) is the U.S. national resource for molecular biology information. The NCBI makes Web resources available at www.ncbi.nlm.nih.gov. The NCBI website provides access to sophisticated genetic resources that some APNs may find useful, although the level may be most appropriate to genetics researchers and practitioners who specialize in genetics. Available resources include software tools for analyzing genomic data, genetic and molecular databases, and education resources. The NCBI is free to everyone and serves a vital role in helping genomic researchers to share data and tools and to disseminate findings.

PDAs and Applications

Efficient time management is the hallmark of a good practitioner. One aspect of efficient time management is having the right information, at the right time, to make the right decision. This concept has been true since the use of the abacus. As people became more mobile, the need for a portable machine that could give them the right information, at the right time, became important. Not surprisingly, the first company to address this need was Apple; in 1993 they developed a personal digital assistant (PDA) called the Newton. The product had minimal success but did start a revolution of mobile handheld devices. Other companies also developed PDAs, but the market remained weak until 1996, when a relatively unknown company called Palm, Inc., released its first Palm Pilot PDA. If timing is everything, then the timing was right for this product, and an explosion in the use of handhelds PDAs was established.

Practitioners have found the clinical benefits of the PDA to be multiple, often referring to PDAs as their "peripheral brain." The device is easy to use and provides timely access to up-to-date nursing and medical information. The result is improved patient safety, satisfaction, and quality care. In addition, the portability of the device saves time while reducing medical errors.

A vast library of third-party applications (more than 20,000) have been written for the PDA. Generally, the most common applications in use by practitioners fall into the following categories:

- Medication reference tools
- Electronic textbooks
- Clinical computational programs
- Clinical decision support software
- Practice guidelines

We will explore each of these categories beginning with medication reference tools.

Medication reference tools are the most popular application used on the PDA by practitioners. In a study by Rothschild et al. (2002) of electronic drug reference users, 83% of respondents reported being better able to inform patients about medication use. The study further revealed that half of the respondents estimated that use of medication reference software had prevented at least one adverse drug event per week. Micromedex is a pharmacy database that includes drug–drug and drug–food interactions. Micromedex is considered one of the most authoritative resources available, is supported by over 150 advanced degree specialists, and is used in over 3,200 facilities in the United States and Canada. The material is accessible both on the personal computer and is downloadable to the PalmOS and Pocket PC. An important feature of the product is that it is extremely reliable and accurate.

A second popular medication reference is ePocrates Rx. Similar to Micromedex, ePocrates Rx provides drug information easily and quickly with many of the same features of Micromedex. It is used extensively in private practice. The interface on ePocrates Rx is easy to read, loads faster than Micromedex, and has a pediatric dosage calculator built in. ePocrates Rx is free and has a feature called Doc Alert that alerts physicians to new information; however, it does contain advertisements and promotions when displayed. A useful comparison of various drug databases was published by Clausan and colleagues (2004).

Electronic textbooks such as 5-Minute Clinical Consult are used in the clinical setting for a variety of purposes. The most commonly used content of 5-Minute Clinical Consult is the sign and symptom index, which supports practitioners in the diagnosis, treatment, and follow-up of a patient's complaint. Over 704 medical conditions are outlined. The screen is easy to read with brief, bulleted points organized by disease topics. Quarterly content updates are available online. The software has the ICS-9-CM code index, facilitating classifying and coding diseases. Other medical references exist, such as MD Consult and Ferri's Clinical Advisor, to name two other examples.

Calculations of any kind are hard to remember and time consuming to do on paper. The PDA can store and do calculations in moments. MedCalc, which provides over 80 unique calculation formulas, is the most common software used for this purpose on the PDA. Included are calculators for IV flow rate, BMI, Glasgow coma scale, fluid replacement after burns, pregnancy calculation, and red blood indices. MedCalc is free, another advantage to this software.

Clinical decision support systems (CDSSs) as described above related to EHRs are also making their way into PDA applications. Because of previous limitation on memory size in PDAs, it was difficult to place many of the computer-based support systems into a handheld device. However, with new technology and increases in storage capacity, more of these expert systems are available. An example is BiliTool (http://bilitool.evidencebasedcare.org/). In the past, clinicians needed to manually plot an infant's age on a Bhutani nomogram, introducing the possibility for human error. The BiliTool facilitates hyperbilirubinemia risk stratification in newborns by doing this calculation automatically, using expert information and decreasing human error.

Many of the programs mentioned above have incorporated practice guidelines. However, some specific practice guideline resources that can be loaded onto a handheld device are important to highlight. One site is "Shots" at www.immunizationed.org. This site is a necessity for any practitioner who is involved in giving immunizations. The reference guide is a collaboration of the Academy of Pediatrics, the Advisory Committee on Immunization Practices, and the American Academy of Family Practice. The site gives schedule information for not only first-time immunizations but for difficult-to-remember timelines for patients who are off schedule. The American Heart Association has collaborated with the American College of Cardiology in making numerous practice guidelines available. For example, pocket guidelines are available for the management of chronic heart failure in the adult and for the management of patients with atrial fibrillation (www.apprisor.com). The CDC also has practice guidelines for a variety of diseases such as tuberculosis and HIV (www.openclinical.org/appPDA_CDC_TB.html). The National Heart, Lung and Blood institute provides a download from their website on asthma treatment guidelines (http://hp2010.nhlbihin.net/as_palm.htm).

A helpful cholesterol management implantation tool is also downloadable from their website (http://hp2010.nhlbihin.net/atpiii/atp3palm.htm).

The acceptance of the PDA as an important part of medicine is widespread. With rapidly changing information, patient safety issues, and time pressures, these devices are another tool in a practitioner's toolbox. However, the future of the PDA is unclear in light of the newer smart phones. Many of the applications mentioned above are now available on the iPhone and Blackberry. The lines between specific types of technology may blur and overlap, but the advantages of handheld information for APN practice are obvious regardless of the device that is used.

TELEHEALTH

Connecting with people at a distance is not a new phenomenon. Ancient populations used smoke signals. Two-way radios were used in remote villages. Alexander Graham Bell's famous invention increased the population's ability to communicate at a distance. In health care, providers have been using the telephone since its invention as a way to connect with patients. In the 1960s, a new facet was added to the use of communication in health care when NASA monitored the physiologic parameters of astronauts in space and made clinical decisions based on the information received. The space program demonstrated the first real application of telemedicine. After a slight decline in the early 1980s, the use of telemedicine tools has risen steadily. Increases in broadband access and transmission quality, declines in costs of transmission and tools, and improvements in reimbursement have led to this increase in use.

Telemedicine may be divided into three types: real time, store and forward (asynchronous), and home health monitoring. Real-time telemedicine uses live video between providers and a patient, most often for specialty consultations. The technology brings the expert to the patient and provider, eliminating distance as a factor and enabling specialist care for the patient. Psychiatry and cardiology are examples of specialty consultations routinely done by telemedicine. In addition, many hospitals are using telemedicine in emergency departments (EDs) and intensive care units (ICUs) for direct access to specialist care. In California, some rural ERs are connected to medical center pediatric specialists for assistance in providing care for emergencies and injured children (Marcin et al., 2004). Another example is the recent adoption of e-ICU's. Here a critical care specialist, critical care nurses, and data managers monitor

ICU patients at different hospitals from one central location. The advantage is another set of eyes on critically ill patients helping to make decisions with real-time data and improving patient outcomes (Breslow, Rosenfeld, Doerler, Burke, & Yates, et al, 2004).

Store and forward telemedicine is used for consultations in which simultaneous participation of both health care providers is not needed. Radiology is a good example of this use and is currently the most common telemedicine specialty practice. Radiographs are digitized, transmitted, and read at a distance. The practice is often used at night when a radiologist is not on site or in large departments that use outside specialty radiologists (Thrall, 2007). Other store and forward telemedicine specialties include ophthalmology and dermatology.

The third common type of telemedicine is home health monitoring, which allows remote observation of patient status using technology. The Veterans Administration (VA) has been using telemedicine successfully for home health monitoring for many years. The VA has demonstrated the value of telemonitoring using a Health Hero System (https://www .healthhero.com) in the home. In this system, patients are instructed in a variety of devices that connect to the Hero System to monitor their health conditions.

For example, the system has a scale that the patient stands on that automatically transmits their weight through a phone line to a central server, which is then accessible by a nurse who monitors a caseload of patients. The advantage of the system is that the nurse monitors the patient daily, allowing recognition of subtle changes in the patient's condition from the data that is uploaded. The nurse can then contact the patient and other health care providers as needed. The VA has found the monitoring process to be very effective in decreasing hospital days and clinic visits (Chumbler et al., 2005). Telemonitoring equipment available for use in the home includes scales, blood pressure monitors, pulse oximeters, glucose monitoring equipment, EKG monitoring equipment, and peak flow meters, all used to monitor patients from a distance.

Telehealth is a broader concept than telemedicine. The Health Resources Services Administration (HRSA) has defined telehealth as "the use of electronic information and telecommunications technologies to support long-distance clinical health care, patient and professional health-related education, public health and health administration" (www .hrsa.gov/telehealth). Generally, telehealth tools include online medical knowledge sources for health professionals, decision support tools, and online and video-based education. For example, practitioners may

log on to the Internet and obtain medical information as needed (www
.ebmny.org/cpg.html). Webcasts, online continuing medical education
or CEs, grand rounds, and distance education are available through portals such as Medscape (www.medscape.com/home).

Medline Plus

A favorite of beginning nursing students, Medline Plus is the consumer
health site of the National Library of Medicine (NLM). Freely available
to everyone at http://medlineplus.gov/, this website is the first choice
for patient education about a wide variety of health topics. Vetted and
maintained by the NLM, Medline Plus is also useful as a firstline reference for APNs about topics outside their area of expertise. Included is
information about specific diseases and conditions, wellness topics, and
medications and supplements, as well as a dictionary of medical terms
and a medical encyclopedia. Directories for finding providers and other
resources such as libraries, health organizations, and services are also
included.

Consumer Health Applications and Websites

Health-related websites for consumers vary in scope, accuracy, and purpose. Some websites have a primary goal of selling products that may or
may not have been properly evaluated for safety and efficacy, whereas
others offer predominantly unbiased health information, generally
financed by space devoted to advertisement on the website. Consumer
websites may enable users to connect with a community of people who
share a common concern or struggle. For example, eDiets and Weight
Watchers offer an online community and support as well as weight management and activity tools, information, and resources that some consumers may find valuable.

In addition to Medline Plus, other not-for-profit consumer websites exist. For example, the U.S. Department of Agriculture (USDA)
created and maintains MyPyramid.gov (available at www.mypyramid
.gov), a website that not only offers information on nutrition but enables
the consumer to track food and caloric intake and activity. My Family
Health Portrait (https://familyhistory.hhs.gov/) is an online tool created
by the Office of the U.S. Surgeon General that enables consumers to
enter their family health history information and obtain a printout and a

pedigree to review with their health care providers. T tool does not offer any interpretation or decision support.

Some consumer websites are proprietary but are reasonably well regulated. Pharmaceutical websites for consumers fall into this category; they are a type of direct-to-consumer marketing for medications. Other commercial websites offer testing services, like 23andMe (https://www.23andme.com), which enables the consumer to obtain genomic testing. The impact and value of such consumer-driven testing have not been established.

Consumers have varying degrees of discrimination in using Web-based health resources. Some consumers believe nearly everything they find online, some believe none of it, and most fall somewhere in between. APNs can serve a valuable role in helping their patients navigate Internet health resources. By recommending reputable websites, APNs can steer patients to trustworthy resources such as Medline Plus, either as a primary source of information or as an alternative to a less trustworthy site.

In evaluating health information online, an important step is to determine who runs the website. Sites run by trusted entities such as universities, government agencies (e.g., the USDA), health care systems, or established health organizations (e.g., the American Cancer Society) can likely be trusted. APNs and consumers should be wary of websites run by commercial enterprises, bearing in mind that the primary objective may be to make a profit rather than to support consumer health.

Consumers often bring information that they have discovered online to their providers. A useful strategy for APNs in this situation is to discuss the information while avoiding defensiveness. APNs can educate their patients about evaluating Web resources. The National Library of Medicine offers several resources that evaluate the quality of health information on the Internet. Through MedlinePlus, APNs and consumers can access a short tutorial on evaluating health websites (www.nlm.nih.gov/medlineplus/webeval) and a "Guide to Healthy Web Surfing" with easy-to-understand tips for evaluating health information on the Web (www.nlm.nih.gov/medlineplus/healthywebsurfing.html or by search from the homepage). The Health on the Net Foundation (HON) is a nongovernmental organization committed to ensuring quality health information online. This foundation certifies trusted health-related websites and provides a certification to those that meet its criteria for quality. Certified websites post the HONcode certification symbol, and the foundation uses sophisticated Web surveillance to ensure that all sites using their certification have actually been certified. It is important to stress that the absence of HONcode certification does not mean that a website is of poor quality because certification is by request.

PRIVACY ISSUES RELATED TO INFORMATICS

Privacy of electronic information, including health information as well as financial, scholastic, and other private information maintained on computer systems, is a ubiquitous concern. Security of EHRs has been the subject of much investigation and discussion. Several common measures to protect privacy, such as authentication of users, access controls, audit trails, and encryption of electronic communication, are generally agreed upon and adhered to in the U.S. health care industry (Halamka, Szolovits, Rind, & Safran, 1997). It is worth noting that the biggest threats to security tend to be low tech, such as failure to log off or to use a screensaver to secure a work station, incorrectly addressing e-mail messages, and sharing user accounts (Sands, 2004). Avoiding these low-tech threats to security may be the most important step an APN can take toward safeguarding patients' privacy when using an EHR system.

The security issues involved with electronic communication with patients deserve special mention. The two major types of electronic communication available to providers and their patients are e-mail and Web messaging. APNs may choose to communicate electronically with patients for several reasons. Electronic communication offers certain advantages over telephone communication. For example, a permanent record of the interaction is maintained. Telephone tag and interruptions for pages may be minimized. The ability to embed links to related online information is another benefit of electronic communication, as well as the ability to provide information that the patient would otherwise have to write down (Kane & Sands, 1998; Sands, 2004).

If an APN chooses to communicate with patients via e-mail or Web messaging, it is vital to have guidelines in place about the use of electronic communications. The American Medical Informatics Association (AMIA) has provided straightforward guidelines for providers and administrators regarding the use of e-mail with patients (Kane & Sands, 1998). Examples of these guidelines are establishing a turnaround time for answering e-mail messages; establishing what types of transactions will be handled via e-mail (e.g., prescription refills); informing patients about who will see their e-mail messages; including copies of all messages in the patient's record; not sharing professional email accounts with family members or others; and using encryption. APNs considering using e-mail or Web messaging with patients should explore their health care organization's policies and guidelines regarding electronic communications.

CONCLUSION

Informatics resources and tools are available to help nurses and consumers locate and manage information, support decision making, and improve safety. Recognizing the need for information and knowing about resources that can help to provide relevant information are vital skills for APNs. By keeping abreast of technology, APNs will be able to benefit from the latest and greatest informatics tools, resources, and innovations.

REFERENCES

Bakken, S. (2001). An informatics infrastructure is essential for evidence-based practice. *Journal of American Medical Informatics Association, 8*(3), 199–201.

Bakken, S. (2006). Informatics for patient safety: A nursing research perspective. *Annual Review of Nursing Research, 24,* 219–254.

Breslow, M. J., Rosenfeld, B. A., Doerfler, M., Burke, G., Yates, G., Stone, D. J., Tomaszewicz, P., Hochman, R., & Plocher, D. W. (2004). Effect of a multiple-site intensive care unit telemedicine program on clinical and economic outcomes: An alternative paradigm for intensivist staffing. *Critical Care Medicine, 32*(1), 31–38.

Bryan, C., & Boren, S. A. (2008). The use and effectiveness of electronic clinical decision support tools in the ambulatory/primary care setting: A systematic review of the literature. *Informatics in Primary Care, 16*(2), 79–91.

Chumbler, N. R., Neugaard, B., Kobb, R., Ryan, P., Qin, H., & Joo, Y. (2005). Evaluation of a care coordination/home-telehealth program for veterans with diabetes: Health services utilization and health-related quality of life. *Evaluation and the Health Professions, 28*(4), 464–478.

Clauson, K. A., Seamon, M. J., Clauson, A. S., & Van, T. B. (2004). Evaluation of drug information databases for personal digital assistants. *American Journal of Health Systems Pharmacy, 61*(10), 1015–1024.

Curran, C. R. (2003). Informatics competencies for nurse practitioners. *AACN Clinical Issues, 14*(3), 320–330.

Ford, E. W., Menachemi, N., & Phillips, M. T. (2006). Predicting the adoption of electronic health records by physicians: When will health care be paperless? *Journal of American Medical Informatics Association, 13*(1), 106–112.

Graves, J. R., & Corcoran, S. (1989). The study of nursing informatics. *Image—the Journal of Nursing Scholarship*, 21(4), 227–231.

Halamka, J. D., Mandl, K. D., & Tang, P. C. (2008). Early experiences with personal health records. *Journal of American Medical Informatics Association*, 15(1), 1–7.

Halamka, J. D., Szolovits, P., Rind, D., & Safran, C. (1997). A WWW implementation of national recommendations for protecting electronic health information. *Journal of American Medical Informatics Association*, 4(6), 458–464.

Hassol, A., Walker, J. M., Kidder, D., Rokita, K., Young, D., Pierdon, S., et al. (2004). Patient experiences and attitudes about access to a patient electronic health care record and linked web messaging. *Journal of American Medical Informatics Association*, 11(6), 505–513.

Hunt, D. L., Haynes, R. B., Hanna, S. E., & Smith, K. (1998). Effects of computer-based clinical decision support systems on physician performance and patient outcomes: A systematic review. *Journal of American Medical Association*, 280(15), 1339–1346.

Institute of Medicine. (2003). Key capabilities of an electronic health record system: Letter report. Retrieved October 30, 2008, from www.nap.edu/catalog/10781.html

Institute of Medicine (U.S.). Committee on Quality of Health Care in America. (2001). Crossing the quality chasm: A new health system for the 21st century. Washington DC: National Academy Press.

Jha, A. K., Ferris, T. G., Donelan, K., DesRoches, C., Shields, A., Rosenbaum, S., et al. (2006). How common are electronic health records in the United States? A summary of the evidence. *Health Affairs (Millwood)*, 25(6), w496–507.

Kane, B., & Sands, D. Z. (1998). Guidelines for the clinical use of electronic mail with patients. The AMIA Internet Working Group, Task Force on Guidelines for the Use of Clinic–Patient Electronic Mail. *Journal of American Medical Informatics Association*, 5(1), 104–111.

Lyerla, F. (2008). Design and implementation of a nursing clinical decision support system to promote guideline adherence. *Computers, Informatics, Nursing*, 26(4), 227–233.

Marcin, J. P., Nesbitt, T. S., Kallas, H. J., Struve, S. N., Traugott, C. A., & Dimand, R. J. (2004). Use of telemedicine to provide pediatric critical care inpatient consultations to underserved rural northern California. *Journal of Pediatrics*, 144(3), 375–380.

Masys, D., Baker, D., Butros, A., & Cowles, K. E. (2002). Giving patients access to their medical records via the internet: The PCASSO experience. *Journal of American Medical Informatics Association*, 9(2), 181–191.

National League for Nursing. (2008). Position statement: Preparing the next generation of nurses to practice in a technology-rich environment: An informatics agenda. New York: Author.

Rothschild, J. M., Lee, T. H., Bae, T., & Bates, D. W. (2002). Clinician use of a palmtop drug reference guide. *Journal of American Medical Informatics Association*, 9(3), 223–229.

Sands, D. Z. (2004). Help for physicians contemplating use of e-mail with patients. *Journal of American Medical Informatics Association*, 11(4), 268–269.

Staggers, N., Gassert, C. A., & Curran, C. (2001). Informatics competencies for nurses at four levels of practice. *Journal of Nursing Education*, 40(7), 303–316.

Staggers, N., Gassert, C. A., & Curran, C. (2002a). A Delphi study to determine informatics competencies for nurses at four levels of practice. *Nursing Research, 51*(6), 383–390.

Staggers, N., Gassert, C. A., & Curran, C. (2002b). Results of a Delphi Study to Determine Informatics Competencies for Nurses at Four Levels of Practice. Retrieved October 20, 2008, from www.nurs.utah.edu/informatics/competencies.pdf

Stead, W. W., Kelly, B. J., & Kolodner, R. M. (2005). Achievable steps toward building a National Health Information infrastructure in the United States. *Journal of American Medical Informatics Association, 12*(2), 113–120.

Tang, P. C., Ash, J. S., Bates, D. W., Overhage, J. M., & Sands, D. Z. (2006). Personal health records: Definitions, benefits, and strategies for overcoming barriers to adoption. *Journal of American Medical Informatics Association, 13*(2), 121–126.

Thrall, J. H. (2007). Teleradiology. Part I. History and clinical applications. *Radiology, 243*(3), 613–617.

Yourman, L., Concato, J., & Agostini, J. V. (2008). Use of computer decision support interventions to improve medication prescribing in older adults: A systematic review. *American Journal of Geriatric Pharmacotherapeutics, 6*(2), 119–129.

Transitions to the Advanced Practice Role

PART III

14 Scholarship of Practice

CECELIA R. ZORN

You receive an invitation to view vacation pictures at your neighbor Leslie's home. To be friendly, you grudgingly agree. Hugging a bowl of fruit salad, you and your partner walk over to Leslie's house Friday evening to watch a digital picture show from his winter break in Hawaii. Anticipating the delicious buffet to follow, you patiently sit through the show, which includes 62 pictures of the sunset on Waikiki. Shifting around on the couch with each passing minute, you find yourself forcing excitement into your muttered "ooohs" and "aaahs."

Reflecting on the long and tedious evening, you realize that what was missing in the pictures was Leslie. How was Leslie affected by the sunset? What meaning did the sunset have for him? You also realize that *you* were not "in the picture." Instead, you were passively squirming on the couch, doing your best to act engaged from the margins.

So it is with writing and presenting. You, as the photographer–author, and the sunset, which is the content or the substance of your message, *must both be visible* in your professional writing and presenting. The content cannot stand alone; it needs to be you and the content. What meaning does the content have for you? How were you changed through learning the content? It follows naturally, of course, that you should also focus on how the readers might be changed. What meaning does the sunset have for the reader or the audience? Publishing and presenting then must include you, the reader, and the sunset; otherwise, the result is a dull Friday evening.

The invitation in this chapter is to examine the publishing and presenting process with an emphasis on linking yourself with the reader and the sunset. In an advanced practice nursing role with a doctorate in nursing practice (DNP), you will be expected to disseminate your scholarship through presentation and publishing. As you transition to that role, these guidelines will enhance your success as a writer and presenter.

MAKING THE TRANSITION

The transition begins where you are now. Your life is bubbling over with graduate course work, research requirements, employment, family, friends, and personal activities. In all of this bubbling, you are developing new expertise and feeling the growing wings of confidence (at least on most days). As part of the graduate school experience, your "voice" changes and intensifies.

Olshansky summarized the role that writing plays in developing a person's voice: writing demands introspection, which leads to self-reflection, and then growth occurs. Being self-reflective is essential as you accept the new challenges of the advanced practice role. "Writing is a way of living the examined life" (Olshansky, 2003, p. 177), and the examined life is necessary for a healthy transition.

This transition into the advanced practice role does not begin after graduate degree completion. It really began when you first started thinking about graduate school: Is graduate school for me? Can I be successful? Do I have the skills? How will it help me, and how might my professional work be different? Similarly, writing for publication and polishing your professional presentation skills must begin while you are in the graduate program. Waiting until "after I'm finished" means it may never happen.

I recently served on a committee searching for potential faculty for a university undergraduate and graduate nursing program. I recall several specific conversations from interested applicants. One individual admitted, "I'm very interested in your faculty position. I completed my DNP a year ago, and I was planning to write an article once I began working as an NP, but that never happened. What do I do about this now in my application portfolio?" Another individual was also concerned, "I'm worried about my publishing history. I wrote one article in a CNS journal four years ago when I was a student. . . . how will this be viewed?"

I believe that both applicants possessed the thinking skills necessary for an educator position. The problem, however, was that their identities as advanced practice nurses did not include professional writing and presentation, regardless of their future interest or career goals. Because of this gap, their expertise and contributions to the nursing body of knowledge were missing. They were disengaged from this medium of professional discourse, which "allows us to grapple with controversies and sift out the various arguments in the hopes of making decisions and advancing the discipline" (Olshansky, 2003, p. 177).

An advanced practice role must include professional writing and presenting. These are both opportunities and responsibilities and are an integral part of your identity in this new role. By not valuing, practicing, and developing these skills while you are in graduate school, it is easy to slide down the slippery slope into a technical conceptualization of the role.

Transition models often include some notion of "connectedness." For example, Bridges (1991) described the reorientation phase as a final step in transition. In this phase, connectedness is associated with a redefinition, new meanings, and a new identity. According to his three-step model, transition commences in an ending phase, in which familiar ways are "let go." A neutral phase follows as a bridge to reorientation. Confusion, disequilibrium, and a loss of harmony and familiarity often fill the neutral phase, in which the person recognizes that previous expectations or actions no longer work.

In reorientation then nurses in advanced practice redefine themselves as leaders. In this new identity, publishing and presenting are critical leadership actions. It is through dissemination that others' thinking and acting are influenced—and that is leadership.

ONE GRADUATE STUDENT'S STORY

So how is this transition experienced? What insights can be learned from connecting with publishing and presenting? I recently enjoyed a luncheon discussion with a current master's degree student nurse about her experience with the publishing process. Rose (not her real name) is a coauthor of one article in press and a second submitted manuscript, both reports of nursing education research.

Rose related several key things that she learned. First, she realized that "normal people write," not only the established, nationally known nurse scholars who are authors. "It could be a new father writing at the kitchen table with a child in the high chair next to him, or a young mom in the dining room with a toddler throwing food across the table," she laughed. For Rose, it also changed the way she examined articles, focusing on author biographies, thinking about positions they held, and placing herself more intimately in the "hall of authors."

Second, Rose gained a deeper insight into the writing process. Not only did she develop skill in condensing and identifying major points (e.g., editing a six-page literature review to five paragraphs), but she also appreciated writing as hard work (sometimes even bordering on drudgery). "I may not always feel inspired . . . it may not always flow naturally," she was quick to point out, but "it was always fulfilling . . . and I improved with practice." A helpful strategy, particularly during the more difficult, less inspired writing, was to break the entire piece down into smaller, more manageable components.

This and other approaches are described creatively in *Bird by Bird,* in which Lamott (1994) presented various lessons about writing. Beginning with lessons learned on the floor of her father's study as a child, she described such topics as getting started, short assignments, perfectionism, help along the way, and publication. Lamott warned, however, "Publication is not all that it is cracked up to be. But writing is. Writing has so much to give, so much to teach, so many surprises" (p. xxvi).

Finally, Rose appreciated the power of professional discourse. In this process, she developed a keener ability to review others' writing and also to open herself more to peer critique of her own writing. This fostered a richer relationship with the co-authors. Also, the manuscript submission procedure was demystified: "I could do this myself now." Through this professional discourse, Rose felt a greater sense of responsibility in her authorship than in papers she had written merely as course requirements: "This was something *real* people will use, I knew it had to be true and it had to make sense. . . . Our articles really may influence how other people teach. . . . I found this experience was good for me and good for others."

THINKING ABOUT THE READER OR THE AUDIENCE

Health care professionals read the professional literature for a reason, and you need to figure out the reason. This underpins the move from writer-based presentation, in which the description was focused primarily on what you learned or what happened to you, to reader-based presentation. Hooking the reader or the conference attendee is the goal.

Begin with an issue or question from the reader and one for which you have some response. What have you solved, developed, or examined that will be useful to others? This may be a method, a population-specific intervention, a program, or an insight. The unique idea may relate to direct patient care, to a resource issue, or to collaboration within the unit or larger system of health care. You may already have done a substantial examination and some writing about the readers' issue or question. Furthermore, in a persuasive piece, you may convince the readers that they have an issue or a question that begs exploration and that you have a valuable perspective.

In his classic handbook for writers, John Trimble (1975) stressed this reader focus when he distinguished between novice writer and veteran writer thinking. In writing for the reader, veteran writer thinking is indispensable.

The veteran writer persuades the reader by writing simply, with deep conviction and straightforwardness. Veteran writers want readers to buy both their ideas and their source (which is you, the writer). In other words, as a veteran writer you are selling your idea and yourself. To accomplish this, veteran writers serve the reader by developing empathy with the reader and presenting ideas clearly and logically. Additionally, veteran writers imagine that the reader is just waiting for a reason to "tune out." As a veteran writer, your goal is to have readers forget everything else and stay with you because they cannot put your piece down.

Veteran writing is in contrast to novice writing. Novice writers write for themselves, not the reader. According to Trimble (1975), novice writers are egocentric and focus on being clear for themselves and do not emphasize communicating with the reader. Novice writers do not consider, persuade, or charm the reader.

To become a veteran writer, then, demands that you know the reader. In your daily advanced nursing practice, you will meet the readers as your nurse colleagues. Reviewing the target audience of a particular journal or the attendees at a conference where you will be presenting is also essential. Are the nurse practitioners involved directly with clients and families? Are they clinical nurse specialists working largely with staff development? Are they nurses as well as non-nurses? Are they educators or researchers? Several months ago, a colleague asked me to review a manuscript she was close to submitting. "What journal are you planning to submit this to? And who are the readers?" were the first questions I asked. Believing her manuscript was nearly "polished," she quickly realized it was not "shaped" for the intended readers, because the journal—and, hence, the audience—had not been considered.

Your own graduate student experiences in selecting a journal for manuscript submission will be helpful. What journals have you found to be comprehensive and pertinent to the content area? What is the research base in their articles? For whom are the articles intended? How organized, clear, practical, and accurate is the writing? If you have found numerous errors in the references, for example, or heavy use of secondary sources framed as primary sources, you may suspect other credibility gaps as well.

In addition to your practice and reading experiences, journals also publish a brief section guiding authors. Identified as "information for authors" or "manuscript guidelines," this information is available in the printed journal and online. Reviewing these guidelines carefully is a must because the manuscript types and content areas that are accepted by the journal are delineated (e.g., practice focus, research, literature reviews, policy, opinion pieces). Also, skimming articles in a recent issue to examine style, tone, research base, and intended audience will help you decide if your manuscript "seems to fit." Finally, the journal's information for authors will identify the specific writing format to be used in preparing the manuscript, for example, the guidelines of the American Psychological Association (APA) (APA, 2001) or Modern Language Association (MLA) (Gibaldi, 2003).

Several references guiding journal selection and examining readership are available. Northam, Trubenbach, and Bentov (2000) published results of a nursing journal survey, including numerous characteristics of over 70 journals such as areas of focus, acceptance rate, reasons for rejection, and acceptance-to-publication details (i.e., time for acceptance, time for publication, editorial style, etc.). Daly (2000) also summarized descriptions of nursing periodicals in a useful handbook format.

Selecting a journal that is peer reviewed is a basic criterion. In the peer-review process, two or three content and/or method experts provide a double-blind review to assist the journal editor in making publication recommendations to the authors. The peer-review process ensures that a minimum standard of quality exists in the published literature. For beginning writers, however, it may be advantageous to select state, regional, or national newsletters or other non-peer-reviewed publications as initial writing outlets. Not only is there a faster turnaround time to dissemination, but the submission process is less complex and the writer's confidence is boosted along the way. Moving toward a peer-reviewed publication then can often follow more easily.

A quick e-mail inquiry to the editor is beneficial in selecting a journal. In your inquiry it will be helpful to review your topic and manuscript thesis, describe your target audience, and summarize the format, tone, and structure of your manuscript. Doing your homework about journal selection is a must—don't neglect this.

GUIDELINES AND STRATEGIES

And now let's look at the sunset. Thinking about the reader or audience frequently occurs simultaneously with the process and structure of writing. Several key writing tips are provided in Exhibit 14.1, such as overcoming writer's block, focusing on detail and structure, writing with others, and seeking a mentor.

Exhibit 14.1

GUIDELINES AND STRATEGIES FOR WRITING AND PRESENTING

Overcoming writer's block
- Use free-writes, lists, thinking out loud
- Write small pieces

Focusing on detail and structure
- Organization
- Specific and dense content
- Readability

Writing and presenting with others
- Peer review and dialogue
- Consensus building and order of authors

Seeking a mentor
- Be deliberate
- Stay connected with academia
- Develop a network with other scholars
- Provide mentorship to others

Often, the most challenging barrier is to work through an idea or even to select one of many swirling ideas. Using a free-writing exercise, put your pen to paper (or fingers to keyboard) and simply write anything that comes to your mind, without stopping, for a limited period of time (e.g., 10 to 15 minutes). To get started, begin with the phrase, "I don't know what to write, but . . ." Free-writing exercises can be done on several different occasions, a few days apart. After some time away, go back and circle "hot spots" (a new or key idea, an insight) that may provide an impetus for a manuscript or even a thesis statement. Compiling a list of anything that comes to mind without deleting an idea because it "doesn't seem very good" also can generate or shape ideas. Thinking out loud with a skilled listener who can probe with questions that unravel your web of ideas serves a similar purpose.

In advising emerging scholarly writers, an English professor friend maintained that a top priority is specific and dense content: "Provide an example with a few words . . . it needs to be tight and sparkling . . . you want the reader to quickly say, 'I got it!'" To achieve this writing density, she suggested brevity: "Write a piece, and then cut it in half. . . . use one- or two-syllable words, not four- or five-syllable words."

In my own writing, being specific and detailed with examples has not come easily. It seems that my writing naturally stops at the abstract and vague level. To illustrate, I often end after a sentence such as, "*Students are learning-wedged in the detailed swirl and gritty memorization of nursing.*" But the reader probably is left puzzled and confused about the exact meaning of this sentence. So I am learning to add more detail: "*Students are learning-wedged in the detailed swirl and gritty memorization of nursing. They lug textbooks exceeding 10 pounds each, and their backs screech as their backpacks overflow. And each passing year stretches the length of textbook reading assignments.*"

In addition to detail and density, the writing structure must be organized so that the reader can move quickly and easily through the writing. If the reader is struggling to stay with you in format, language, or organization, your message may be lost no matter how notable the content; cognitive leaps and disorganization prevent the reader from "getting it." Award-winning ideas can be lost in murky, musty writing swamps.

To help the reader "get it" and follow the content of your message, use transitions between sentences generously. Initially, using transitions may seem forced, even artificial, especially if this has not been part of your writing style. Also, design the first sentence of each paragraph as a bridge sentence that links the previous paragraph to the next one. In the following example, the first paragraph contains few transitions and the second paragraph has been revised using both a bridge sentence and transitions to strengthen the flow and connections.

Two Examples to Demonstrate the Use of Transitions

Transitions Missing

The teacher must help students hear and internalize the significant contribution novel reading can make to their learning about nursing. Spending planned time in class describing the "why" of a learning activity is central. It is important to highlight specific novels and how they can help us understand relationships among and between individuals and groups; learn to ask questions; examine sociological, economic, and family systems; and study topics such as prevention, leadership, and autonomy. Devoting class time affirms the assignment's importance. Neglecting a discussion altogether, or "yelping" brief comments as students pack their bags, turn on their cell phones, and walk out the door signals "busywork"—a curricular "snub," if you will.

If course requirements . . .

Transitions Added

In addition to selecting the novel, the teacher must *also* help students hear and internalize the significant contribution novel reading can make to their learning about nursing. *First,* spending planned time in class describing the "why" of *this* learning activity is central. *For example, the "why" may be illustrated by* highlighting specific novels and how they can help us understand relationships among and between individuals and groups; learn to ask questions; examine sociological, economic, and family systems; and study topics such as prevention, leadership, and autonomy. Devoting class time affirms the assignment's importance. Neglecting *this* discussion altogether or "yelping" brief comments as students pack their bags, turn on their cell phones, and walk out the door signals "busywork"—a curricular "snub," if you will.

Second, if course requirements . . .

Other Strategies

Besides the use of transitions within and between paragraphs, there are other strategies that help the reader stay engaged with your writing. First, lively quotes bring the page to life. A word of caution, though:

use quotes sparingly, select them purposefully, and keep them brief. Remember, the reader wants to hear your voice, not line after line lifted from another source.

Second, regard the verb in the sentence as the powerhouse. Rather than overusing the passive "be" verbs, consider using more action verbs. For example, because the following sentence contains several "be" verbs, dull and flaccid writing results:

> The young Algonquin mother *was* panicked when her infant's cry *became* a gasping moan as hunger *was* increasing during the Arctic winter.

Revising the sentence with action verbs absorbs the reader more intimately:

> Hearing her infant's cry *muffle* to a gasping moan as hunger *slithered* into the Arctic winter, the young Algonquin mother *shivered* in terror.

There are many handbooks for writers beginning the scholarly publication process. Dexter (2000) described writing tips, including strategies to enhance clarity, precision, accuracy, logic, and depth. For beginning writers, the following may be helpful: (1) use an outline to plan and organize the paper; (2) after setting aside a manuscript, read it out loud (grammar problems, incomplete sentences, extra long sentences or paragraphs will be more easily heard than seen); and (3) paraphrase and use references precisely. Additionally, Silvia (2007) has a bright and practical little book that stresses the need for a weekly writing schedule, how to address common writing barriers, and specific motivational tools. If a structured week-by-week approach appeals to you, Belcher's (2009) book helps academic authors overcome anxieties, learn a particular feature of a strong manuscript every week, and send their own work to a journal at the end of 12 weeks.

Writing or presenting with others is also a strategy that may be beneficial. By providing feedback and receiving critique from co-authors, your writing abilities will further develop. In addition, meetings and scheduled timelines with others provide structure; after all, you may be tempted to set aside writing opportunities. Of course, sharing the brainstorming and dialogue enriches and enlivens the process. However, especially with multiple authors who have not written together, consensus building and blending different writing styles can take more time. Another word of caution: clearly determine author order (primary, secondary, etc.) at the outset, based on agreed-upon contributions and responsibilities.

Mentorship in publication and presentation is essential. Mentoring relationships are more long-term, collegial, and transformational for both parties than a preceptor. As a beginning writer, be deliberate in choosing one or several individuals who agree to be your writing coaches. More recently it has been recognized that mentoring relationships rely not only on the mentor seeking and supporting the mentee, but also on the mentee explicitly asking for mentorship.

The connectedness, as well as the new identity and meanings of the reorientation phase in transition, continue as lifelong endeavors. Publication and presentation do not end with graduate education or the years that immediately follow. Staying connected with mentors from your academic setting will provide continuing support of your scholarship. This can be done individually, or through alumni associations, honor societies, or school-sponsored activities, as well as through an adjunct faculty position. Establishing links with other scholars who are involved in publishing and presenting in your work setting or in professional organizations will also expand your network. Professional journal meetings, co-authorships, or unit-based presentations are examples.

Finally, in your transition to publishing and presenting, take nurse colleagues with you. All too often, nurses in advanced practice roles move away from the staff nurses, literally and figuratively.

MOVING AN IDEA FORWARD

Here we will provide a brief overview of the publication and presentation process. Nemcek (2000) and Oermann (2002) have described this process in detail, and their discussion will be helpful to both beginning and more seasoned writers.

As can be seen in Exhibit 14.2, selecting publication or presentation is an early decision. Presentations may be appealing for those who are less attracted to writing as a medium, and dissemination via presentation usually occurs more quickly. Often, early presentations may involve a description of what is being done in your work setting. With this type of content, being a national expert is not expected. You are presenting a practice change, for example, "what is being done in my setting . . . and what we have learned." Recognizing that others value your message and want to learn from your experiences is empowering and confidence

Exhibit 14.2

THE PUBLICATION AND PRESENTATION PROCESS

- Publication or presentation?
- Peer review from colleagues
- Submission, following manuscript guidelines
- Awaiting the journal or organization response
- Preparing the presentation
- Celebrate the dissemination

building. On the other hand, presentations often demand more spontaneity, including dialogue with conference attendees, whereas writing tends to be less public and at a pace that may better suit your personality. Finally, a mentor early in my career suggested that I first present a topic at a conference, learn from the dialogue, and then revise and shape the piece for publication. She assured me that this sequence would result in a greater chance of publication and a stronger article.

In addition to choosing presentation or publication as a method of dissemination, presenting with a poster format is also a possibility and is sometimes seen as less intimidating. In poster presentations, content is summarized visually using text, pictures, graphs, models, and the like. Posters are then exhibited in an open area with an opportunity for dialogue with interested individuals. Frequently, networks are established and maintained around an area of interest in this format. Also, poster abstracts are often included in conference proceedings for later reference.

Securing peer review from colleagues is a second component of both publishing and presenting. It is helpful to form a circle of writers with a variety of skills: a conceptual, abstract thinker; an organized, structured, logical thinker and writer; and an "editor-type" detailed reviewer. Everyone in the writing circle must be committed to honest and thorough feedback. Skimpy or superficial responses, such as "this is a good piece" or "suitable for presentation" are rather useless.

Precise adherence to the manuscript guidelines or the organization's call for abstracts, particularly page limits or word counts, format, and content focus, is essential. A response from the journal editor after manuscript submission can vary from 6 weeks to nearly a year. Following the ethics of publishing, a manuscript can only be submitted to one journal at a time. The editor's response also may vary; he or she compiles the peer reviewers' appraisal and then typically decides to (1) publish as is, (2) reconsider after suggested revisions, or (3) not publish.

Interestingly, I have received peer reviews on the same manuscript from the same journal from both ends of the continuum: "publish as is" from one reviewer and "do not publish" from the second reviewer. After receiving the review from the two peer reviewers, the editor took the middle ground, recommended revisions (which I did), and published the article. I learned about the "humanness" of the process and the value of perseverance.

Thoughtfully preparing a professional presentation for a conference meeting is a must. There is nothing duller than listening to a paper read word for word for 20 or 30 minutes. Times and formats for presentations vary significantly; they can be grouped into five to six 10-minute summaries in 1 hour, or they can be 60 to 90 minutes long for one detailed presentation and dialogue. There is usually a format choice to be made when submitting the abstract. Because most conferences provide abstracts online or as CDs, simplicity, directness, and clarity are even more essential with this information abundance. Further, English may be a second or third language for many readers and conference attendees, so using short, expressive, and familiar terms is crucial. Finally, as with publications, the same principle applies to professional presentations: they must contain you, the audience, and the sunset.

With both manuscript and abstract submission, rejection is a possibility. Recognizing that everyone has a "pink slip" in their file, mentors are invaluable in helping you stand back up, dust yourself off, and revise, reshape, and resubmit. It may also be worthwhile to invite another co-author to the manuscript for a fresh look at additions and revisions.

Regardless of the outcome of your article or presentation, you must celebrate your achievement. Not only is basking in the warmth of the accomplishment important, but it also reenergizes a forward movement. As the publishing and presenting process unfolds, there is value in having several different pieces in various phases, rather than a single linear progression (i.e., write, publish, write again, publish, etc.). If one article is rejected, another may be accepted, and you can sustain a livelier momentum by keeping several "irons in the fire."

Delineating an individual development plan is part of professional evolution—it demonstrates your reorientation to a new and different place. Career goals around employment, position, setting, and client population are highlighted in your plan; however, constructing an area of expertise is also necessary. This area of expertise is sustained through presenting and publishing that must begin now.

CONCLUSION

Throughout this chapter you have been examining yourself in transition to professional writing and presentation, considering the reader, and exploring guidelines and "how-to's" with regard to content (the sunset). This transition is never complete. These lines from *The Journey* by Mary Oliver (1986) reflect the patience and calling, as well as the pleasure and personal nature of moving forward: "But little by little, as you left their voices behind, the stars began to burn through the sheets of clouds, and there was a new voice, which you slowly recognized as your own, that kept you company as you strode deeper and deeper into the world." May your journey into the world of publishing and presenting be filled with the joyful challenges of intellectual inquiry and the glow of living the examined life.

ACKNOWLEDGMENT

My deepest gratitude to Wilma Clark, Mary Thelen, and John Hildebrand for teaching and learning with me about the writing journey, the bumps along the road, and the sunset.

REFERENCES

American Psychological Association. (2001). *Publication manual of the American Psychological Association* (5th ed.). Washington DC: Author.

Belcher, W. L. (2009). *Writing your journal article in twelve weeks: A guide to academic publishing success.* Thousand Oaks, CA: Sage Publications.

Bridges, W. (1991). *Managing transitions: Making the most of change.* Reading, MA: Addison-Wesley.

Daly, J. M. (2000). *Writer's guide to nursing periodicals.* Thousand Oaks, CA: Sage Publications.

Dexter, P. (2000). Tips for scholarly writing in nursing. *Journal of Professional Nursing, 16*(1), 6–12.

Gibaldi, J. (2003). *MLA handbook for writers of research papers.* New York: The Modern Language Association of America.

Lamott, A. (1994). *Bird by bird: Some instructions on writing and life.* New York: Anchor Books Doubleday.

Nemcek, M. A. (2000). Getting published online and in print: Understanding the publication process. *American Association of Occupational Health Nurses Journal, 48*(7), 344–347.

Northam, S., Trubenbach, M., & Bentov, L. (2000). Nursing journal survey: Information to help you publish. *Nurse Educator, 25*(5), 227–236.

Oermann, M. H. (2002). *Writing for publication in nursing.* Philadelphia: Lippincott, Williams & Wilkins.

Oliver, M. (1986). *Dream work.* Boston: Atlantic Monthly Press.

Olshansky, E. (2003). Why write? *Journal of Professional Nursing, 19*(4), 177–178.

Silvia, P. J. (2007). *How to write a lot: A practical guide to productive academic writing.* Washington DC: American Psychological Association.

Trimble, J. R. (1975). *Writing with style: Conversations on the art of writing.* Englewood Cliffs, NJ: Prentice Hall.

Employment Strategies for Advanced Practice Nurses

JENNIFER PETERS

Most advanced practice nurses (APNs) are on the hunt for their dream job—not just a paycheck but an opportunity to build a professional career. Looking for advanced practice employment is an exciting, challenging, and ultimately rewarding process. It is also time-consuming, mentally demanding, and occasionally frustrating. This chapter addresses strategies that APNs can use to find employment and to position themselves for successful and dynamic careers.

IMPACT OF THE HEALTH CARE SYSTEM ON APN EMPLOYMENT

Understanding the realities of the health care delivery system enables APNs to anticipate career opportunities and find their job niche. Demonstrating awareness of these factors during the employment process is attractive to potential employers. Over the next decade, the following characteristics of the U.S. health care system will likely affect the careers of APNs (Bodenheimer & Grumbach, 2005; Institute of Medicine, 2003; Porter-O'Grady, 2003).

- Expanded efforts to control health care costs
- Consumer and payer demands for care that is safe, of high quality, accessible, equitable, effective, and individualized
- Increased competition between providers for market share
- Use of evidence-based systems to guide clinical interventions and analyze outcomes
- Reduction in institutional care, particularly acute care services
- Increasing focus on primary care, including alternative and nontraditional therapies
- Greater demand for chronic care services, particularly for an aging population
- Development of service models to address increasing ethnic diversity
- Expansion of capitated, subscriber-based systems
- Development of interdependent, rather than independent, practice models
- Rapid growth of medical and pharmaceutical technology
- Expansion of computer information systems for service delivery, outcomes analysis, and cost control
- Persistence of the registered nurse shortage
- Contraction of the overall job market, with increasing competition for desirable positions

UNDERSTANDING AND USING MARKETING APPROACHES

Success in a competitive marketplace is dependent on the ability of APNs to deliver valuable services and to effectively market these services (Lachman, 1996). Marketing is determining what the client wants or needs, designing a product or service to meet that need, and then communicating information about the product or service to potential clients (Dayhoff & Moore, 2004; Lachman, 1996). The marketing process is guided by four concepts, the four Ps: product, price, place, and promotion. In addition, the potential client, market segment, or target population of the marketing effort must be identified.

For some APNs, marketing may seem uncomfortable or even unprofessional. Negative images of salespeople, the "hard sell," and aggressive advertising may come to mind. Actually, marketing is not like any of these portrayals. In essence, marketing is about establishing a relationship between the APN and potential clients that demonstrates the competence, necessity, and value of APN services in meeting a need of the client (Dayhoff & Moore, 2004).

Depending on their career stage, APNs target their marketing efforts to diverse prospective clients. During a job search, APNs market themselves and the APN role to potential employers. Current employers may be the focus of marketing to diversify services or achieve a job promotion. Consumers, the community, and other health care providers may be customers for entrepreneurial or independent practice ventures. Whatever the target market, the characteristics of potential clients should be examined. Geographic, demographic, economic, and psychosocial variables should be explored (Pakis, 1997). Sources of information on potential clients include census data, newspaper and media reports, human resource departments of potential employers, needs surveys, focal groups, websites, and personal contact with potential customers. The objective is to focus on potential clients and work with them to identify the services they need and want (Dayhoff & Moore, 2004).

The first P of marketing, product, refers to APNs themselves. Components of the APN "product" include education, certification, experience, and achievement. Unique and special characteristics should be highlighted to distinguish the individual APN from competitors. The individual APN should seek to define a personal niche.

The second P of marketing, price, involves exploration of the worth of the APN product in the market. Salaries and fringe benefits should be carefully analyzed for specific geographic regions and work environments. Once again, analyzing the competition and the current market through personal, informal contact is helpful. Much salary information is also available on the websites of APN associations.

The third P, place, refers to the geographic places and health care institutions in which APN services are to be delivered. Questions to explore include: Are APNs currently practicing in this environment? How many? What kind? What are the characteristics of the environment that are conducive to APN practice? What barriers to APN practice exist?

The fourth P of the marketing process, promotion, or selling a service, should only occur after the product, price, and place of the service have been identified.

Specific APN Marketing Strategies

Knowledge Building

Demonstration of clinical knowledge and competency is the cornerstone of the APN marketing process. In addition to clinical knowledge, APNs must also possess knowledge about professional issues, the health care needs of the community, and the marketing process. To successfully market yourself and the APN role, APNs must develop a working knowledge of:

- Standards for clinical practice in the specialty area, including current research
- Regulations affecting advanced practice, including licensure, certification, prescriptive privileges, institutional credentialing, and collaborative practice
- Reimbursement patterns and regulations
- Health care services and unmet needs in the target market
- The role and services of competitors in the target market
- Communication skills, including professional networking and negotiation skills
- The target market's perception and utilization of APNs

Sources of information include professional APN associations, APN publications, and government websites. It is critical for the APN to visit state Board of Nursing websites early in the employment process because regulations affecting the scope and parameters of APN practice vary widely from state to state. The *American Journal for Nurse Practitioners* annually publishes state-by-state reviews of legislative issues and regulations affecting APNs (Pearson, 2008) (www. webnp.net). Excellent information on issues, job opportunities, clinical guidelines, and regulation affecting the different APN specialties is available online from the following organizations:

- *National Association of Clinical Nurse Specialists* (www.nacns.org)
- *American College of Nurse Midwives* (www.midwife.org)
- *American Association of Nurse Anesthetists* (www.aana.com)
- *American Academy of Nurse Practitioners* (www.aanp.org)
- *American College of Nurse Practitioners* (www.acnpweb.org)

Self-Inventory

Self-inventory and reflection are elemental components of APN career development and must occur as precursors to the market plan. They are part of an ongoing process that is initiated many months in advance of a job search. Critical, reflective questions to ask include:

- Who am I?
- What do I believe and value?

- Where and what do I come from?
- Where am I now?
- Where am I going and why that direction?
- How will I get there?
- How will I know when I have attained my goals? (Neubauer, 1998, p. 3)

During self-reflection, Price (1998) suggests the exploration of five points: abilities, interests, values, needs, and characteristics. Abilities can be analyzed through identification of skills, achievements, and failures. In addition to clinical and caregiving skills, APNs should consider abilities such as communication, teaching, consultation, research, leadership, organization, computer proficiency, mentoring, writing, political action, and others. Interests may be identified by listing desirable professional activities. Values are those principles or qualities that guide life and work. Listing and prioritizing values can clarify the relative importance of competing interests such as career, family, friends, and other demands.

Needs are identified by listing satisfiers and dissatisfiers in prior work situations. Desired levels of control, power, salary, independence, security, recognition, creativity, and achievement often appear on a list of needs. Finally, individual physical, emotional, and intellectual characteristics relevant to career and job performance should be listed. Factors such as physical limitations, endurance, stress tolerance, enthusiasm, creativity, sensitivity, knowledge level, and learning ability are but a few individual characteristics to inventory (Price, 1998). For APNs unfamiliar with self-inventory, detailed and helpful formats are available in the popular press (Bolles, 2008).

For APNs seeking employment or promotion, developing an ideal job description can be a helpful step in self-inventory. It is important to be specific about desired job functions and job benefits. Specific dollar amounts should be attached to salary and monetary benefits. Specific amounts of time should be identified for vacation and leave time. Specific percentages of time spent in various job functions should be considered.

Once completed, the self-inventory provides a guide for the job search and interview process. It is important to ascertain how well each prospective job fits the "ideal." Exhibit 15.1 provides a self-inventory guide that can be used during the job search and interview process (Bolles, 2008; Shapiro & Rosenberg, 2002).

Exhibit 15.1

APN SELF-INVENTORY

- What are my strengths as an APN? What is special about me?
- What are my weaknesses, and how am I working to improve them?
- What type of APN job am I looking for?
- What do I enjoy most about working as an APN? Least?
- Where do I want to live? What things are important about the place I live? How much am I willing to travel for work?
- What kinds of people do I like to work with? What kinds of people are difficult for me to work with?
- What things are stressful to me in my work? What do I need to manage stress?
- Am I comfortable working with a lot of autonomy? Would I prefer working closely with others? How much supervision is best for me?
- How many hours a day am I willing to work? How much call? How much weekend, evening, and night service? How many holidays?
- What is my ideal salary? What is an acceptable salary? Would I be willing to work for an hourly wage? Am I looking for productivity incentives in my pay?
- How important are the following benefits? How much of each do I prefer?
  - Paid vacation days
  - Paid sick days
  - Paid holidays
  - Retirement benefits (type, employer contribution, vesting)
  - Medical and dental insurance (individual and family coverage, portability, pre-existing condition coverage, pregnancy coverage, prescription coverage, long-term care options)
  - Life insurance
  - Short- and long-term disability insurance
  - Malpractice insurance (occurrence or claims made, gap or tail coverage requirements)
  - Licensing and certification fee reimbursement
  - Orientation period (duration and content)

(Continued)

Exhibit 15.1 (Continued)

- ◆ Continuing education (travel, fees, meals, lodging)
- ◆ Tuition reimbursement or waivers
- ◆ Professional membership dues
- ◆ Subscriptions to texts/journals
- ◆ Office and supplies: private office, computer, e-mail/Internet access, medical supplies/equipment, personal digital assistant (PDA), cellphone, pager, parking
- ◆ Mileage reimbursement
- ◆ Interview and relocation expense reimbursement
- ◆ Profit sharing

Market Inventory

An inventory of the APN target market is the next step. At this point, APNs seek to determine what opportunities are available that may fit their "ideal" position. Analysis and inventory of the APN market is ideally begun 6 to 12 months in advance of actual employment. It continues throughout the interview process as the APN evaluates the pros and cons of each potential employment setting. Many seasoned APNs will continually inventory the employment market to identify career opportunities and trends. Exhibit 15.2 provides a sample APN market inventory.

Developing a Career Portfolio

Career portfolios are personal files containing evidence of professional knowledge, development, and achievement (McMullan et al., 2003). Development of the portfolio continues throughout an individual's career. The career portfolio is the resource from which documentation can be selected to use in marketing. Most persons maintain two types of portfolios, closed and open. The closed portfolio is personal, only viewed by the individual, and serves as the master file documenting career achievement. The open portfolio is used as a marketing tool and shared with potential employers and target markets. The open portfolio contains selected elements of the closed portfolio that are relevant to the current market. Open portfolios can be very powerful tools in the marketing or job search process because they demonstrate achievement and an organized approach to marketing (Weinstein, 2002). All professionals

Exhibit 15.2

APN MARKET INVENTORY

- What national standards will affect my practice?
  - ◆ Specialty certification requirements
  - ◆ Specialty certification process and time frame
- How will regulations from the state Board of Nursing affect me?
  - ◆ Registered nurse licensure
  - ◆ APN recognition/licensure
  - ◆ APN scope of practice
  - ◆ Prescriptive authority regulations
  - ◆ Collaborative practice regulations
- What characteristics of this region are important to me?
  - ◆ Urban, small town, or rural nature
  - ◆ Population size, age distribution, ethnicity, and socioeconomic status
  - ◆ Educational system for me, my family, others
  - ◆ Cost of living
  - ◆ Health care organizations: type, size, focus
  - ◆ Transportation availability and accessibility
  - ◆ APN practice in the area: roles/numbers of APNs, practice settings, networks, typical salaries/benefits
- What characteristics of this organization will affect my practice?
  - ◆ Type of practice: acute/long-term/clinic, rural/urban, size, location, referral networks, satellite facilities, reimbursement mix
  - ◆ Organizational philosophy: Medicaid services, indigent care, community outreach, educational partnerships, health promotion, research
  - ◆ Stability of the organization: age, financial stability, reputation
  - ◆ Types of patients: age, gender, education, socioeconomic status, ethnicity, chronic/acute illness mix, diagnoses/conditions
  - ◆ Medical providers (numbers/types/roles): physicians, registered and licensed practice nurses, physician assistants, therapists, medical assistants
  - ◆ Support staff (numbers/types/roles): assistants, administrators, billing, medical records

(Continued)

Exhibit 15.2 (Continued)

- Organizational policies/procedures: documentation, billing, quality improvement, performance appraisal
- Other APNs in the organization (numbers/types/roles)
- My role & responsibilities in the organization
  - ◆ Scope of clinical practice: typical patients, procedures, skill requirements
  - ◆ Level of autonomy, access to supervision, position in organizational structure
  - ◆ Collaborative practice policies, agreements, protocols
  - ◆ Employment contracts and stipulations
  - ◆ Credentialing requirements and procedures
  - ◆ Clinical productivity expectations: patient visits, call, weekend coverage, evening/night coverage, holiday coverage
  - ◆ Nonclinical responsibilities: administrative duties, committee work, education/precepting, research
  - ◆ Access to support services: billing, medical records, secretarial
  - ◆ Salary/benefit structure (see Exhibit 15.1 for detailed considerations)
  - ◆ Resource availability: office, computer, Internet/e-mail access, pager, cellphone, personal digital assistant (PDA), medical equipment, journals/texts, parking
  - ◆ Performance appraisal frequency, criteria, evaluators
  - ◆ Opportunities for growth: orientation, in-service training, continuing education

should maintain a hard-copy portfolio to bring to job interviews, usually in the format of a neatly organized plastic binder. However, electronic portfolios are also available through academic websites. Exhibit 15.3 lists items that APNs may want to include in a closed or open personal career portfolio.

One important element of the portfolio is the list of references. References should be individuals who can attest to the APN's professional abilities, competence, and achievements. Ideally, the APN will have a list of three to five professionals who are willing to serve as references. The APN must contact each person to determine his or her willingness

Exhibit 15.3

APN PROFESSIONAL PORTFOLIO

- Current resumé and curriculum vitae
- Official transcripts of all academic programs after high school
- Copies of nursing licenses and certifications
- Current list of references with addresses, phone numbers, and e-mail addresses
- Malpractice insurance policies
- Records of continuing education attendance
- Reprints of publications
- Abstracts or brochures documenting conference presentations
- Newspaper or media recognition
- Evidence of honors or awards
- Prior references, recommendations, and performance evaluations
- A sample job description listing desirable job functions and benefits
- Examples of clinical and leadership achievements such as patient education programs/tools; history and physical examinations; quality improvement projects; and research utilization projects
- Professional organization memberships
- Health records pertinent to APN employment
- Volunteer and community activities

to provide a positive recommendation. The portfolio must include the reference's name, professional title, and complete contact information (address, phone, and e-mail).

The APN role is relatively new and often poorly understood in some potential markets; thus, it is helpful to maintain a master portfolio of documents describing and validating the APN role. Sharing this information with potential employers or markets can be very helpful. This portfolio includes research articles demonstrating the effectiveness of APNs, copies of APN practice regulations, and brochures from practice organizations that document the role of APNs.

Resumés and Curricula Vitae

Resumés and curricula vitae (CVs) are powerful tools for individual marketing. A current resumé and CV are essential components of the APN portfolio. They are used to communicate professional credentials to prospective employers, current employers, and colleagues. Although both describe professional and educational accomplishments, they differ in format and application.

Resumés are one- or two-page overviews of an individual's professional career. They are used to quickly communicate your credentials and abilities to potential employers. Brevity is important. There is no single correct format for a resumé; it should be tailored to the prospective position. Functional resumés highlight areas of skill and expertise. Chronological resumés present the job history in chronological order. Critical information for any resumé includes name, address, phone numbers, e-mail addresses, FAX numbers, education and degrees earned, professional employment, and licensure and certification (no license numbers). If space allows, selected information about publications, honors and awards, research and grants, presentations, teaching experience, consulting experience, membership in professional organizations, specific clinical or professional objectives, languages spoken, community service, or military service may be included. Information is often presented in reverse chronological order, with the most recent events listed first in each category of the resumé. Exhibit 15.4 shows a typical chronological resumé for an APN.

Curricula vitae are more lengthy descriptions of professional career and qualifications. They are often called academic resumés because of their use in academic settings. There is no maximum length for a CV; they will typically address all of the essential and additional information categories listed in the preceding discussion of resumés.

Resumés and CVs are usually designed by APNs on a personal computer. Use of the personal computer enables updating and individualizing for prospective employers. Books, journal articles, and software are readily available to guide those less familiar with the process. Inexpensive, helpful resources include *What Color Is Your Parachute 2009* (Bolles, 2008) and *Resumés for Nursing Careers* (McGraw Hill, 2007). Most academic institutions have free-access websites available to assist with resumé and CV composition. Online resumé-building services are also available at the websites of the American Nurses Association (http://nursingworld.org) and most of the APN organizations listed earlier. The APN should design the resumé for paper and electronic use because some organizations require electronic submission of resumés.

The physical appearance of these documents is extremely important. They are often the first impression a potential employer has of an APN.

Exhibit 15.4

SAMPLE APN RESUMÉ

Maria R. Lewis, MSN, RN
2231 Echo Lane
St. Paul, MN 55105
(615) 222-2222

Objective	Gerontological Nurse Practitioner in a Community Setting
Education	2008 Master of Science in Nursing, University of Minnesota, Minneapolis, MN
	1992 Bachelor of Science in Nursing, University of Michigan, Ann Arbor, MI
Experience	1995–present Clinical Coordinator, Eastbrook Long-Term Care Center, Roseville, MN
	1993–1995 Nurse Manager—Coronary Care Unit Midwest Regional Medical Center, Ann Arbor, MI
	1990–1993 Staff Nurse—Coronary Care Unit Midwest Regional Medical Center, Ann Arbor, MI
Licensure certification	RN, Minnesota Gerontological Nurse Practitioner, ANCC
Honors/Awards	1997 Gerontology Scholarship, University of Minnesota, Minneapolis, MN
	1990 Sigma Theta Tau
Publications	Lewis, M. (2008). Assessing cardiac function in older adults. *Long-term Care Nursing, 12,* 221–223.
Professional organizations	American Nurses Association, Minnesota Gerontology Association
Languages	Fluent in Spanish and French
References	Available on request

A poorly designed resumé or CV may close the door to interviews with prospective employers. Resumés should be neat, concise, well organized, and visually appealing, and should contain no errors in spelling or punctuation. High-quality paper should be used in printing. White or off-white paper with black print is most commonly used to give a traditional, professional appearance to the resumé or CV. It is helpful to have colleagues review and proofread these documents.

Information on resumés and CVs must be accurate and truthful. Many prospective employers define the information or format that should be used. Some things should not appear on the resumé or CV, including professional license numbers; social security numbers; names of references; salary expectations; and personal information such as age, gender, ethnic background, height, weight, marital status, or health status and disabilities.

When a resumé or CV is sent to a prospective employer, a cover letter should always accompany it. The cover letter introduces the APN to the prospective employer. It should be individualized to a position and express enthusiasm for future employment. The cover letter is direct, brief (no more than one page), and written in standard business format. Whenever possible, address the cover letter to a specific person. The letter should include the reason for writing and briefly highlight your accomplishments. The previously suggested resources for resumé writing also have many helpful examples of cover letters. Exhibit 15.5 is a sample cover letter to accompany an APN resumé or CV. It is important to follow up by telephone or mail on all resumés and CVs that have been sent to prospective employers. Follow-up indicates enthusiasm and persistence, two attractive qualities in potential employees. This communication should be initiated within two weeks of sending these documents.

Locating Opportunities

For most APNs, career opportunities do not just materialize; finding a great position is not just a matter of luck. Preparation, persistence, and personal contacts are fundamental requirements. Most positions are located through personal contacts or networks. Developing a network is not difficult, but it does require the willingness to meet and communicate with new people. Every person the APN knows or knows of should be considered a potential contact. Helpful networks for APNs to explore include local professional organizations, other APNs already working in the same role, nurse managers in local health care organizations, faculty,

Exhibit 15.5

SAMPLE APN COVER LETTER

Maria R. Lewis, MSN, RN
2231 Echo Lane
St. Paul, MN 55105

September 1, 2008

Jane S. Parsons, PhD, RN
Director, Clinical Services
Gerontology Nurse Associates
3640 Simpson Street
Minneapolis, MN 55455

Dear Dr. Parsons:

We spoke briefly at the Minnesota Long-Term Care Conference about a position for a nurse practitioner at Gerontology Nurse Associates. I am writing to express my interest in that position.

I have recently completed my graduate nursing studies and have received my certification as a gerontological nurse practitioner. I would like to pursue a career as a GNP in community and long-term care settings. My prior clinical and leadership experience in long-term care and cardiovascular nursing provides me with an excellent background for this field. In addition, my fluency in several languages is an asset in today's health care environment.

I have enclosed a copy of my resumé for your review. I am interested in interviewing for the position, and I can be reached at (615) 222-2222 or at lewis1234@online.com. Thank you for your consideration. I look forward to speaking with you.

Sincerely,
Maria R. Lewis, MSN, RN

Enclosure

and anyone else who may have knowledge of APN opportunities. Blogs of APN networks can often be located on professional websites. Telephone contacts and personal meetings are both effective means of making contact. Meeting people over breakfast or lunch is a tried and true networking technique.

Traditional job search strategies should not be ignored. Weekly review of newspaper and website employment listings is important. In addition, professional journals often advertise for APNs. Mass mailings of resumés are generally not advisable unless they are preceded by personal contact (Bolles, 2008). For APNs planning to use a professional job search firm, it is advisable to thoroughly research the track record of the firm and their experience and success in placing APNs.

Interviewing

Many books have been written about job interviewing; however, successful interviewing is not difficult. Essentially, the interview is an opportunity for the applicant and the prospective employer to meet, exchange information, and evaluate whether there is a "fit" between the organization and the candidate. Both parties are trying to determine if they have something to offer each other by exchanging very subjective information and cues.

In a competitive environment, APNs should expect to complete several interviews before locating an acceptable position. Typically, employers will utilize a series of interviews when hiring for APN positions. Applicants are screened in initial interviews. Follow-up interviews are scheduled for applicants who progress beyond the screening. The interview process may take many weeks to complete. Usually APNs will meet with several individuals from the organization during the interview process. Patience is important. Hiring organizations may take several months to fill their vacant positions.

Interviewing requires homework. As previously discussed, APNs should be informed about the characteristics of organizations they are interested in. Exhibits 15.1 and 15.2 provide topics to examine before and during the interview. Physical preparation for the interview is also important; first impressions count enormously. Dress neatly and conservatively. Arrive for the interview on time. Bring the organized open portfolio in a folder that can be left with the interviewers. Psychological preparation is essential. Although nervousness during an interview is typical, the ability to project self-confidence is important. For APNs unfamiliar with interviewing, Bolles (2008) offers detailed strategies for coping with interview anxiety. Anticipating questions that interviewers are likely to ask and developing a list of questions to ask are two means of reducing the anxiety of interviewing. Questions for APNs to ask during an interview are easily generated from the ideal job description. The following are questions typically asked of APNs in the interview process:

- What type of position are you interested in?
- Could you tell me about yourself?
- What are your strengths? Your weaknesses?
- What do you know about our company?
- What would you do in this situation (typical situation described)?
- Why are you leaving your present job?
- What are your professional or career goals?
- What do you enjoy most about work? Least? Why?
- Why should we hire you for this position?
- What salary do you expect?
- What questions do you have about this position? This company?

Federal law prohibits asking certain questions during the interview. It is unlawful for an interviewer to ask about age, date of birth, children, age of children, race or ethnicity, religious affiliation, marital status, military discharge status, arrest records, home ownership, spousal employment, and organization and club memberships (Bolles, 2008). When such questions are asked, it is usually not out of malicious intent. However, it is best to prepare a gracious way of not answering these questions.

During the interview project, maintain a positive attitude, interest, and enthusiasm. Be friendly, smile, and make eye contact. Listen as well as speak. Be professional in all interactions. Focus on the position, qualifications, and experience. Ask for the job. Thank the interviewer for the opportunity and ask when the hiring decision will be made. Finally, follow up with a written letter expressing thanks and continued interest in the position.

Negotiation and Employment Contracts

At some point in the interviewing process, the parties are likely to have different perspectives about the position, responsibilities, salary, or benefits. Negotiation is the process of resolving these differences. Negotiation should not be considered a win–lose, adversarial interaction. Rather, it is a win–win, or a gain–gain situation for all parties (Laubach,

1997). Successful negotiation requires preparation, innovative thinking, integrity, respect for the other party, and superior listening skills. Both parties must recognize their priorities and areas where flexibility is possible. Negotiations should be focused on outcomes and results rather than emotions (Shapiro & Rosenberg, 2002). The time to begin negotiation is after the prospective employer has expressed interest in hiring, but before the APN has agreed to take the job.

In the managed care marketplace, one of the most critical factors for APNs to understand and negotiate is the employment relationship. It is imperative to be absolutely clear on whether the position is classified as independent contractor or employee. In addition, critical questions about billing, primary provider listing, and productivity expectations should be clarified. Finally, the level of collaboration or independent control APNs have over practice issues such as ordering tests, diagnostic procedures, and specialty care requires attention (Cady, 2001; Shapiro & Rosenberg, 2002; Stuart 2001).

As part of the negotiations, the issue of whether an employment contract will be used should be discussed. In the past, APNs were often hired based on an informal verbal contract and handshake. Today it is much more likely that APNs will be asked to sign formal employment contracts or agreements. Employment agreements are legally binding contracts between employers and employees stating the terms of a working relationship. The employment contract provides for job security in that it limits and specifies the reasons for termination. In addition, the contract provides a vehicle to describe salary, benefits, liability insurance coverage, productivity expectations, job functions, and hours of work. Before signing an employment contract, the APN should carefully review the contract, negotiate areas of confusion, and seek legal advice (Shapiro & Rosenberg, 2002; Stuart, 2001).

Employees hired without a contract are termed "at will." Technically, "at-will" employees may be terminated at any time without cause. Most state laws provide some protection for employees who face termination without contract protection, but accessing this protection may be a lengthy process requiring legal advice (Cady, 2001).

When negotiating an employment contract, APNs should note covenants not to compete and termination clauses in the contract. A covenant not to compete is a contract clause that restricts an employee from practicing within a certain number of miles from an employer's business for a certain period of time after the employee leaves the employer's business. Covenants not to compete are legal and enforceable if the

Exhibit 15.6

CONTRACT AGREEMENTS AND CLAUSES

Covenants Not to Compete

Restrictive: "Upon termination of employment for any reason, the CRNA agrees not to practice within 50 miles of any present or future office of this practice for a period of 5 years."

Less Restrictive: "Upon termination of employment for any reason, the CRNA agrees not to practice within 25 miles of the current office of this practice for a period of 1 year."

Termination Clauses

Termination for Cause: "The employer may terminate this agreement at any time by written notice to the CRNA for any of the following reasons:

a. The CRNA dies or becomes permanently disabled.

b. The CRNA loses his or her professional license.

c. The CRNA is restricted by any governmental authority from rendering the required professional services.

d. The CRNA loses his or her staff privileges.

e. The CRNA conducts him- or herself in a grossly negligent way."

Termination without Cause: "The employer may terminate this agreement at any time, for any reason, after giving the CRNA 30 days written notice."

courts deem them reasonable. They protect the employer from APN competition in the event the APN leaves the employer. However, they restrict the ability of the APN to continue to practice in a geographic area. Exhibit 15.6 contains an example of covenants not to compete. If possible, APNs should seek a contract that does not contain a covenant not to compete. If the employer insists on including the clause, the APN should seek a clause that is less restrictive in terms of duration or geographic area (Blumenreich, 1996; Buppert, 1997; Stuart, 2001).

A typical employment contract contains a termination section that lists events that are bases for termination of the employee "with cause." These events may include loss of license or certification, gross negligence, death, or conviction of a felony. Some contracts include a termination "without cause" clause that states that the employee may be terminated at any time, for any reason, with 30 days notice. Rarely should APNs sign a contract containing a termination "without cause" statement. It effectively removes the employee job security that the contract provides. The only circumstance in which "without cause" termination would be acceptable is when the APN is unable to commit to the full duration of the contract (Buppert, 1997). Exhibit 15.6 contains examples of "with cause" and "without cause" termination clauses.

Contracts are likely to specify the amount and type of liability insurance coverage. The APN is likely to encounter two different types of liability insurance coverage: occurrence or claims made. Occurrence insurance covers an incident that occurred during the year of coverage regardless of when the claim is made. Claims-made insurance covers claims made during the year of coverage. Gap or tail insurance may be needed when the APN leaves an organization that provided claims-made coverage. Coverage limits (amounts) are usually specified by amount per claim and annual aggregate amount. Typical contract language would be "$1,000,000 occurrence/$3,000,000 aggregate." This means the insurance would cover $1,000,000 per claim and up to three claims a year of $1,000,000. Coverage amounts vary, but per claim coverage should be at least $1,000,000. A helpful guide to the language and issues surrounding liability insurance is available online at www.npjobs.com/malpractice.

Liability insurance coverage is a critical contract issue for all APNs; but particularly so for nurse-midwives and nurse anesthetists. In some practice settings, APNs will want to purchase their own coverage in addition to that provided by an employer. Once again, questions arising about the complexities of contract provisions in this area may be best addressed by seeking legal advice.

Collaborative Practice Agreements

Many states and organizations require the APN to maintain a written practice agreement with a medical doctor. Terms for this agreement include collaborative practice agreements, patient care guides, protocols, and standing orders. The purpose of the agreement is to specify guidelines for provision of APN care, including prescriptive authority. The scope and nature of APN practice is identified and agreed to by the nurse and physician(s). The agreement should be viewed as a positive mechanism to enhance interdisciplinary collaboration and integrate the delivery of health care.

Before establishing any practice agreement, APNs must first review any state Board of Nursing requirements for the agreement. These can be accessed online. Some states allow APNs to practice independently without physician collaboration. Others require on-site physician supervision for APN practice. Most states require some degree of collaboration and/or supervision with a written agreement specifying the terms. In addition, health care organizations may require a practice agreement for APNs. State boards of nursing and organizations often have examples or samples of practice agreements available. During the interview process, it is important to ask about the nature of such agreements and view any available examples.

Practice agreements can be controversial. Too much specificity in the agreement will limit the APN's ability to individualize care and will also leave the APN open to legal claims if the specifics are violated. It is not desirable to craft extensive protocols to address the details of every clinical situation. Minimal and flexible guidelines that recognize APN competence are preferred to those with extreme detail. The practice agreement should not prevent APNs from delivering care that is within their scope of practice, education, and competence. In addition, the practice agreement should not require a level of supervision that limits effective clinical practice or reimbursement.

The agreement is signed by the APN and collaborating MDs. Any change to the agreement should include the date of the revision, the change, and the signatures of the APN and physician. Exhibit 15.7 provides an example of a collaborative practice agreement that would be considered minimalist or flexible in terms of guidelines or protocols. More restrictive agreements can run to many pages.

SUMMARY

Changes in the health care marketplace will continue to generate opportunities for APNs who demonstrate competence, enthusiasm, and commitment to the role. Marketing strategies enable APNs to take full and timely advantage of these opportunities. Knowledge building, self-inventory, market inventory, and positive negotiation can be used to build a successful and rewarding APN career.

Exhibit 15.7

SAMPLE APN PRACTICE AGREEMENT

1. Purpose: This agreement describes the professional collaborative relationship between Mary N. Adams RN, MSN, CANP, a certified and registered adult nurse practitioner and physicians at XYZ Healthcare Clinics.

2. Setting for Practice: The nurse practitioner will practice at the facilities of XYZ Healthcare Clinics in Anytown, Address, USA, and within a 50-mile radius of this location.

3. Scope of Practice: Mary N. Adams is a nurse with current licensure as a registered nurse in XX state and current registration with this state's Board of Nursing as an advanced practice nurse practitioner. She is prepared for her advanced practice role by virtue of post-baccalaureate education and national specialty certification as an adult nurse practitioner. The collaborating nurse practitioner and physicians agree that the nurse practitioner performs the functions outlined below for adult patients. These functions include, but are not limited to:

    a. History taking and physical examination, including ordering and interpreting diagnostic tests
    b. Differential diagnosis
    c. Health promotion and disease prevention
    d. Management of acute and chronic health care programs
    e. Emergency treatment and stabilization
    f. Referral to other health care providers
    g. Prescription of therapeutic regimens and medical devices
    h. Prescription of medications, pharmaceutical substances, and controlled substances as consistent with federal and state laws
    i. Documentation of all care, procedures, and contacts in the clinical record of the patient

4. Delegated Medical Functions: The nurse practitioner has received specialized training in the following medical functions and may perform them as necessary for adult patients:

    a. Suturing of simple lacerations
    b. Incision and drainage of abscesses

(Continued)

Exhibit 15.7 (Continued)

5. Practice Guidelines: The nurse practitioner is authorized to diagnose and treat conditions using the following current guidelines:
   a. *Physician's Desk Reference*
   b. OSHA guidelines
   c. CDC guidelines for immunization and management of infectious diseases
   d. *JNC VII* Guidelines for Management of Hypertension
   e. American Diabetes Association Guidelines for Management of Diabetes
   f. Barker, L., Fiebach, N., Kern, D., et al. (2006). *Principles of ambulatory medicine* (7th ed.). Philadelphia: Lippincott, Williams, & Wilkins
   g. Edmunds, M., & Mayhew, M. (2002). *Procedures for primary care practitioners.* St. Louis: Mosby
   h. Fauci, A., Braunwald, E., Kasper, D., et al. (2008). *Harrison's principles of internal medicine* (17th ed.). New York: McGraw Hill
   i. Wolff, K., Johnson, R., & Suurmond, R. (2005). *Fitzpatrick's color atlas and synopsis of clinical dermatology* (5th ed.). New York: McGraw-Hill
6. Consultation: The nurse practitioner will consult with a collaborating physician for the following situations. A physician collaborator will be available to the nurse practitioner on site, by telephone, or by e-mail for all such situations.
   a. Situations that go beyond the competence, scope of practice, or experience of the nurse practitioner
   b. Whenever the patient's condition fails to respond to the management plan within an acceptable time frame
   c. Upon patient's request
   d. For all emergency situations after initial stabilizing care has been initiated
7. Signatures of Collaborating Parties: We, the undersigned, agree to the terms of this practice agreement and will review the terms no less than annually.

(Continued)

Exhibit 15.7 (Continued)

_____Mary N. Adams, RN, MSN, CANP
_____XYZ Healthcare Clinics Physician
_____XYZ Healthcare Clinics Physician
_____XYZ Healthcare Clinics Physician
_____XYZ Healthcare Clinics Physician
Agreement date_____

REFERENCES

Blumenreich, G. A. (1996). Covenants not to compete. *Journal of the American Association of Nurse Anesthetists, 64*, 317–319.

Bodenheimer, T. S., & Grumbach, K. (2005). *Understanding health policy: A clinical approach* (4th ed.). New York: McGraw-Hill.

Bolles, R. N. (2008). *What color is your parachute? 2009: A practical guide for job hunters and career changes.* Berkeley, CA: Ten Speed Press.

Buppert, C. (1997). Employment agreements: Clauses that can change an NP's life. *The Nurse Practitioner, 22*, 108–109, 112, 117–119.

Cady, R. J. (2001). The legal forum. *JONA's Healthcare, Law, Ethics, and Regulation, 3*, 35–39.

Dayhoff, N. E., & Moore, P. S. (2004). CNS entrepreneurship: Marketing 101. *Clinical Nurse Specialist: The Journal for Advanced Nursing Practice, 18*, 123–125.

Institute of Medicine, National Academy of Sciences. (2003). *Crossing the quality chasm: A new health system for the 21st century.* Washington DC: National Academies Press.

Lachman, V. D. (1996). Positioning your business in the marketplace. *Advanced Practice Nursing Quarterly, 2*, 27–32.

Laubach, C. (1997). Negotiating a gain–gain agreement. *Healthcare Executive, 12*, 12–17.

McGraw Hill Editors. *Resumés for Nursing Careers.* (2007) New York: McGraw Hill Companies.

McMullan, M., Endacott, R., Gray, M., Jasper, M., Miller, C., Scholed, J., et al. (2003). Portfolios and assessment of competence: A review of the literature. *Journal of Advanced Nursing, 41*, 283–294.

Neubauer, J. (1998). Personal development: A lifelong journey. *Advanced Practice Nursing Quarterly, 3*, 1–9.

Pakis, S. (1997). Managing the marketing function for advanced nurse practitioners in a managed care environment. *Seminars for Nurse Managers, 5*, 149–153.

Pearson, L. (2008). The Pearson report. *The American Journal for Nurse Practitioners, 12*, 9–80. (available online at webnp.net)

Porter-O'Grady, T. (2003). Of hubris and hope: Transforming nursing for a new age. *Nursing Economics, 21*, 59–64.

Price, J. L. (1998). A reflective approach to career trajectory in advanced practice nursing. *Advanced Practice Nursing Quarterly, 3,* 35–39.

Shapiro, D., & Rosenberg, N. (2002). Acute care nurse practitioner Collaborative practice negotiation. *AACN Clinical Issues. Advanced Practice in Acute Critical Care, 13,* 470–478.

Stuart, J. G. (2001). Steps toward forging a successful initial employment arrangement. *The Journal of Bone and Joint Surgery, 83,* 1915–1919.

Weinstein, S. (2002). A nursing portfolio: Documenting your professional journey. *Journal of Infusion Nursing, 25,* 357–364.

Launching Your Career as an Advanced Practice Nurse

MARY ZWYGART-STAUFFACHER
MICHAELENE P. JANSEN

Oh, the places you'll go. Today is your day. You're off to Great Places! You're off and away!

—*Dr. Seuss*

Dr. Seuss (Geisel & Geisel, 1990) encourages graduates to risk, enjoy, and see what is ahead of them without apprehension and with excitement. This is excellent advice, and yet for advanced practice nurses completing scholarly projects, graduating, and beginning their first positions, that time can be quite overwhelming. Transitions of any kind hold an opportunity for great growth and reward for participants, but transitions can also be very challenging and even very frightening at times. This array of emotions is all occurring during a very important time in the APN's professional life.

Certainly, you have heard horror stories of new APNs overwhelmed with their new positions, yet there are thousands of APNs every year who complete their first week with feelings of great satisfaction and excitement about the weeks ahead. What can you expect during that first year? Are additional responsibilities expected from me as a DNP? What are some of the strategies that have been identified to assist me as a new APN in assimilating this new role? How do I not only survive, but also thrive, during those first few months in the new role? These are only a few of the many questions you may face as an APN who is anticipating

307

and entering the transition from graduate student to graduate prepared advanced practice nurse.

ROLE SOCIALIZATION

Role socialization and professional role development literature is replete with theories and strategies on role transition. Brykczynski (2009) identifies the component process including (1) aspects of adult development, (2) development of clinical expertise, (3) modification of self-identity through initial socializing in school, (4) development and integration of professional subrole components, and (5) subsequent resocialization in the work setting. The APN begins the role transition while in graduate school with the acquisition of new knowledge and role performance expectations and implements this role socialization during the work experience. Role stress can occur at any time along this continuum. Great stress can occur for the new graduate nursing student, moving from the role of very capable experienced BSN-prepared nurse to that of graduate student (Cusson & Viggaino, 2002). This role transition also occurs for newly graduated APNs as they launch into their first position.

The classic work of Kramer (1974) has been identified as having relevance for role socialization for APNs (Andrews, 2001). Kramer contends that reality shock could be diminished for novices if they were provided with real-world situations during their formal education. This work served as impetus for many schools of nursing to consider utilizing preceptorships for graduate nursing programs.

Kelly and Matthews (2001) in their qualitative study on the transition to the first position as a nurse practitioner found that participants, when asked to give a word or thought that would describe how they felt during the transition, included responses such as, "exciting, nervous anxiety, overwhelmed, scared, uncertain, panicky, novice, inadequate, halting, stressful, and frustration" (p. 3). Clearly, this time can be a very emotional one for the new APN.

ROLE TRANSITION

Five essential factors have been found to influence role transitions (Schumacher & Meleis, 1994). They are: (1) the personal meanings of the transition while related to the degree of identity crisis experienced; (2) the degree of planning, which involves the time and energy devoted to anticipating the change; (3) environmental barriers and supports, which refer to peer, school, family, and others; (4) level of knowledge and skill, which relate to prior experience and school experiences, and (5) expectations, which are related to role models, literature, media, etc. Therefore, the role transition one experiences following graduate studies is a process that begins as the student enters graduate school. During graduate school, students experience role acquisition as they rehearse new roles, develop clinical knowledge, and create support networks (Brykczynski, 2009).

A research-based model developed by Brown and Olshansky (1997; 1998) provides the new APN with helpful and practical guidance during the first year of practice. Initially based on the nurse practitioner's role transition, it has been referenced as a model with probable utility for all advanced practice nurses. The process they describe is "limbo to legitimacy" with four categories or stages and several subcategories. Stage 1, laying the foundation, is the time period immediately after finishing graduate studies when the student is not yet a certified advanced practice nurse. Time is spent recuperating from school, negotiating the bureaucracy related to licensure and certification, and job searching. All the worry associated with these activities consumes the new APN. The time requires the APN to be busy doing both the external work of becoming a legitimate APN and the internal work of establishing a new personal role identity. It is important to keep in mind that there is no "perfect APN" position, only the more ideal beginning position for each individual. Therefore, new APNs must be clear on what their needs and desires are, not what the expectations of others may be. Taking the needed time to prepare for the initial position is important, and the APN should not rush to start the new position.

Stage 2, launching, occurs at the beginning of the first position and continues for at least 3 months. An underlying aspect of this stage is a transition from the self-confident, competent RN to the uncertain APN. The APN works hard at "getting through the day" and is concerned about feeling real anxiety. It is also a stage in which APNs battles time, being slow with the tasks and functions of the new role, and also impatient with themselves. Enormous effort is required to get through the day and perform the tasks required of the position. Basic daily work activities are strenuous; therefore, the APN has few reserves. There also never seems to be enough time, and the new APN needs to schedule additional time for new tasks and be willing to accept help and guidance from others.

Stage 3 is meeting the challenge. During this stage, APNs become more realistic about the expectations of the role as they become more competent and more comfortable in the system. They begin to build internal support systems to help meet professional challenges, and they have increased competence as defined by external manifestation measurements or the behavior that reflects skillful professionals.

Stage 4, broadening the perspective, occurs when the APN has a feeling of enhanced self-esteem and a solid feeling of legitimacy and competence. The APN is affirming progress based on feedback from others and is now able to seek opportunities to develop even more complex skills. Comfort in the role and a strong sense of accomplishment are achieved, and the APN is seen as a fully contributing member of the agency.

As the APN moves through the transition to managing the changes and challenges ahead, Draye and Brown (2000) provide helpful suggestions in their work, *Surviving the Proving Ground: Lessons in Change from NP Pioneers*. These include suggestions such as working to ensure their competence, maintaining a clear nursing identity, and preserving their autonomy. Additionally, APNs should recognize that control over their own practice is essential when making decisions regarding clinical care and management, investing in the APN collective, advocating for quality care, and strengthening networks.

No role transition is ever without challenge, and for some APNs, the first position may not hold all that was anticipated. So what do advanced practice nurses do if their first position is not what they expected? Sometimes, even after a careful and thorough job search, an APN can find himself or herself in an agency that simply is not a good or healthy fit. Thankfully, this does not happen very often, and if it does occur, the APN should carefully explore other options and be sure that a change in position versus a change in approach or attitude is what is truly needed. Hopefully, with an understanding of the transition process, new APNs will be able to discern if the conflicts and anxieties experienced are consistent with the role development or if there is clearly a misfit.

Transitioning to the role of the APN can be a very rewarding and exciting career phase. Dr. Loretta Ford's shared words may be most fitting, "My final word for current NPs . . . is to take risks, chart new directions, study the results, learn from your mistakes, and enjoy the change" (Ford, 1997, p. 6). "For today is your day! Your mountain is waiting. . . . So, get on your way!" (Geisel & Geisel, 1990).

REFERENCES

Andrews, J. (2001). Roles of the advanced practice nurse. In D. Robinson & C. Kish, *Core concepts in advanced practice in nursing* (pp. 261–268). St. Louis, MO: C. V. Mosby.

Brown, M., & Olshansky, E. (1997). From limbo to legitimacy: A theoretical model of the transition to the primary care nurse practitioner role. *Nursing Research, 48*(1), 46–51.

Brown, M., & Olshansky, E. (1998). Becoming a primary care nurse practitioner: Challenges of the initial year of practice. *Nurse Practitioner, 23*(7), 46.

Brykczynski, K. (2009). Role development of the advanced practice nurse. In A. Hamric, J. Spross, & C. Hanson (Eds.), *Advanced practice nursing* (p 95–120). St. Louis, MO: Saunders.

Cusson, R., & Viggaino, N. (2002). Transition to the neonatal nurse practitioner role: Making the change from side to the head of the bed. *Neonatal Network, 21*(2), 21–28.

Draye, M., & Brown, M. (2000). Surviving the proving ground: Lessons in change from NP pioneers. *Nurse Practitioner, 25*(10), 60–68.

Ford, L. (1997). A voice from the past: 30 fascinating years as a nurse practitioner. *Clinical Excellence for Nurse Practitioners: The International Journal NPACE, 1*(1), 3–6.

Geisel, T. S., & Geisel, A. (Dr. Seuss). (1990). *Oh, the places you'll go*. New York: Random House.

Kelly, N., & Matthews, M. (2001). The transition to first positions as nurse practitioner. *Journal of Nursing Education, 40*(4), 156–157.

Kramer, M. (1974). *Reality shock*. St Louis, MO: C. V. Mosby.

Schumacher, K., & Meleis, A. (1994). Transitions: A central concept in nursing. *Image: The Journal of Nursing scholarship, 26*, 119–127.

Appendix

APN WEBSITES

www.aana.com	American Association of Nurse Anesthetists
www.aanp.org	American Academy of Nurse Practitioners
www.aacn.org	American Association of Critical Care Nurses
www.acnm	American College of Nurse Midwives
www.nacns.org	National Association of Clinical Nurse Specialists
www.awhonn.org	Association of Women's Health, Obstetrics and Neonatal Nursing
www.aacn.nche.edu	American Association of Colleges of Nursing
www.nursingworld.org	American Nurses Association
www.aone.org	American Organization of Nurse Executives
www.napnap.org	National Organization of Pediatric Nurse Practitioners
www.nursingworld.org/ojin	Online *Journal of Issues in Nursing*
www.cms.hhs.gov	Center for Medicare and Medicaid Services
www.medicare.gov	Medicare (consumer)

www.dea.gov	Drug Enforcement Agency
www.icn-apnetwork.org	International Nurse Practitioner/ Advanced Practice Nursing Network
www.thomas.loc.gov	Legislative Information on the Internet—Library of Congress
www.georgetown.edu/research/kie	The Kennedy Institute of Ethics
www.thehastingscenter.org	Hastings Center
www.nursingethicsnetwork.org	Nursing Ethics network
www.hartfordign.org	Hartford Institute for Geriatric Nursing
www.ispub.com/journals/ija.htm	Internet *Journal of Advanced Nursing Practice*
www.nih.gov	National Institutes of Health
www.ahcpr.gov	Agency for Healthcare Research and Quality
www.guideline.gov	National Guideline Clearinghouse
www.nurse.org.acnp	American College of Nurse Practitioners
www.npwh.org	National Association of Nurse Practitioners in Women's Health
www.nursecredentialing.org	American Nurses Credentialing Center
www.nonpf.org	National Organization of Nurse Practitioner Faculties

Index

Note: Page numbers followed by "*t*," "*f*," or an "*e*" indicate the reference is to a table, figure, or exhibit respectively on the indicated page.